THE NEUROBIOLOGY OF AUTISM

The Neurobiology of Autism

EDITED BY

MARGARET L. BAUMAN, M.D.

Department of Neurology
Harvard Medical School, Boston, Massachusetts

AND

THOMAS L. KEMPER, M.D.

Departments of Neurology, Anatomy, and Pathology
Boston University School of Medicine, Boston, Massachusetts

THE JOHNS HOPKINS UNIVERSITY PRESS

Baltimore and London

Johns Hopkins Paperbacks edition, 1997
06 05 04 03 02 01 00 99 98   5 4 3 2

The Johns Hopkins University Press
2715 North Charles Street
Baltimore, Maryland 21218

Library of Congress Cataloging-in-Publication Data

The Neurobiology of autism / edited by Margaret L. Bauman and Thomas L. Kemper
p.   cm. — (The Johns Hopkins series in psychiatry and neuroscience)
    Includes index.
ISBN 0-8018-4764-8 (hc : alk. paper)
    1. Autism—Pathophysiology.   2. Neurobiology.   3. Autism-Etiology.
    4. Autism—Imaging.   I. Bauman, Margaret L.   II. Kemper, Thomas L.   III. Series
    [DNLM: 1. Autism—physiopathology.   2. Diagnostic Imaging.   3. Brain—
physiopathology   WM 203.5 N4945   1994]
RC553.A88N5   1994
616.89'8207—dc20   DNLM/DLC
for Library of Congress   93-5358

A catalog record for this book is available from the British Library.

ISBN 0-8018-5680-9 (pbk.)

CONTENTS

CONTRIBUTORS

George M. Anderson, Ph.D., Research Scientist, Department of Laboratory Medicine, Yale University School of Medicine, New Haven, Connecticut

Jocelyne Bachevalier, Ph.D., Associate Professor, Department of Neurobiology and Anatomy, University of Texas Medical School, Houston, Texas

Stephen M. Dombrowski, B.S., Research Associate, Western Psychiatric Institute and Clinic, University of Pittsburgh School of Medicine, Pittsburgh, Pennsylvania

Michelle Dunn, Ph.D., Instructor, Department of Neurology, Albert Einstein College of Medicine, Bronx, New York

Susan Folstein, M.D., Professor, Department of Child and Adolescent Psychiatry, Tufts University School of Medicine, Boston, Massachusetts

Barry Horwitz, Ph.D., Chief, Unit on Brain Imaging and Computers, Laboratory of Neurosciences, National Institute on Aging, Bethesda, Maryland

Ronald J. Killiany, Ph.D., Research Associate, Department of Anatomy and Neurobiology, Boston University School of Medicine, Boston, Massachusetts

Nancy J. Minshew, M.D., Associate Professor, Western Psychiatric Institute and Clinic, University of Pittsburgh School of Medicine, Pittsburgh, Pennsylvania

Mark B. Moss, Ph.D., Associate Professor, Department of Anatomy and Neurobiology and Department of Neurology, Boston University School of Medicine, Boston, Massachusetts

Joseph Piven, M.D., Assistant Professor, Department of Psychiatry, University of Iowa College of Medicine, Iowa City, Iowa

Isabelle Rapin, M.D., Professor, Department of Neurology, Department of Pediatrics, and Rose F. Kennedy Center for Research in Mental Retardation and Human Development, Albert Einstein College of Medicine, Bronx, New York

Judith M. Rumsey, Ph.D., Chief, Autism Program, Child Psychiatry Branch, National Institute of Mental Health, Bethesda, Maryland

Jeremy D. Schmahmann, M.D., Assistant Professor, Department of Neurology, Harvard Medical School, Boston, Massachusetts

PREFACE

Significant advances have been made over the past decade in the clinical and biologic research in autism. It has become apparent that autism is a developmental disorder of the central nervous system that is associated with a characteristic set of behaviors, including impairment of social interaction, disordered verbal and nonverbal communication, limited ability to participate in imaginative play, a preference for routine and an insistence on sameness, and, in some cases, repetitive and stereotypic mannerisms. The clinical evaluation of these and other distinguishing features of the disorder has become more refined. We have come to appreciate the fact that there may be many subtypes of autism and that a spectrum of symptoms, in terms of both appearance and severity, characterize children and adults with this disorder.

The etiology of autism in most cases remains unknown. There is as yet no metabolic, radiographic, or genetic marker to aid in the diagnosis or in predicting the clinical severity. There is still no form of treatment to improve predictably the social, cognitive, and behavioral impairments that limit the daily functioning of most autistic children and adults. Thus, although we have achieved much in the past decade, we still have much to learn and to accomplish.

The purpose of this book is to bring together some of the research currently under way that is directly or indirectly related to the many puzzling clinical and biomedical questions that surround the spectrum of autistic disorders. We hope that, by having this information in a single source, clinical investigators and basic scientists will be able to begin to speculate about the seemingly disparate pieces of information already available, consider how they might fit together, and develop new ideas and avenues for future research.

We dedicate this book to our autistic patients, and to their families, teachers, therapists, and physicians, who are working toward helping these children and young adults achieve an improved quality of life.

THE NEUROBIOLOGY OF AUTISM

1

INTRODUCTION AND OVERVIEW

Isabelle Rapin, M.D.

THE HISTORY OF AUTISM

We owe the term *early infantile autism* to Kanner (1943), from Balti-more. He borrowed the term *autism* from Bleuler, who used it to de-scribe schizophrenic patients' deficient ability to relate to other people and their withdrawal from social interaction. Almost simultaneously, Asperger (1944) used the term *autistic psychopathy* to describe similar children in Vienna. Kanner and Asperger each described individual children without obvious signs of focal cerebral disease and with the now classic symptoms of severely impaired social interaction, a bizarre and narrow range of interests, language and communication abnormal-ities, and, in at least some cases, preserved intellect.

Kanner and Asperger were not the first to observe children with this behavioral constellation. Heller (1908), a Viennese educator, had vividly described six children with an insidious loss of language and mental abilities between three and four years of age which left them se-verely impaired with symptomatology essentially identical to that of autistic children (Rapin, 1965). Both Kanner and Asperger speculated that early infantile autism was the sign of abnormal brain function, al-though they mentioned that the parents of the children they were de-scribing tended to be highly intelligent and educated. In retrospect, that observation reflects the often unrepresentative characteristics of small samples. Asperger, impressed with behavioral similarities between some of the parents and their children, speculated about possible ge-netic factors in autistic psychopathy.

The work of Spitz (1945) on the dire physical and behavioral conse-quences of a lack of consistent mothering in institutionally raised in-fants and the strong influence of Freud, who stressed the deleterious effects of early childhood experiences on later behavior, no doubt in-fluenced the psychiatrists, educators, and other professionals caring for autistic children in the direction of a psychogenic theory of autism. This theory seemed supported by Kanner's description of autistic children's parents as distant from their children (Kanner, 1943, 1971; Kanner and Eisenberg, 1956). The unevenness of some of the children's cognitive skills, with islands of normal or even hypertrophied abilities, such as calendar calculation, rote memory, and musical talent also supported this. The theory was bolstered by the inconsistencies in children's behaviors, speaking a few sentences one day and saying nothing for days thereafter. Heller (1908) had stressed the bright-eyed and alert look of these children, contrasted with the dull facies of many severely mentally deficient children. The psychogenic theory was a hopeful one because it implied that if only one could reach the children in their isolated world, break the "glass ball" in which they lived (Junker, 1964), and provide them with the opportunity to relive their early infantile experiences in a more normal way, then the person hidden within the shell would recover and emerge as a normal child. Heroic psychoanalytically based efforts, targeted at the parents as often as at the children, were anecdotally reported as salvaging a few cases. Unfortunately, these efforts were ineffective in the overwhelming majority of autistic children.

The autistic children of today continue to pay a price for the parenting hypothesis: autism has been criminalized. Many professionals still hesitate to offer this diagnosis, especially to the parents of less severely affected children, since the label is viewed as stigmatizing and as tantamount to accusing the parents of ineptitude or neglect.

Refutation of the psychogenic hypothesis came about in the 1960s and 1970s through several lines of evidence: observation that a highly significant proportion of autistic children developed epilepsy (e.g., Schain and Yannet, 1960; Deykin and MacMahon, 1979); the realization that children born of the 1964 rubella epidemic were at a disproportionately high risk for autism (Chess et al., 1971); and the demonstration that the parenting skills of parents of autistic children were equal to those of parents of normal children and of children with other handicaps (DeMyer et al., 1972; Cantwell et al., 1979).

The realization, in the 1970s, that the majority of autistic children are truly mentally deficient (Rutter, 1979) and that autism is a life-long deficit has perpetuated the reluctance of clinicians to voice an unvarnished diagnosis of autism, especially in mildly affected children (Frith, 1991; Wing, 1991). Autism is incurable in the present state of knowledge and, of all the developmental disorders of brain function, it is most often associated with behaviors that are extremely difficult to manage and socially unacceptable. The diagnosis of autism is the schizophrenia or cancer of the developmental disorders. It is a diagnosis to whisper, avoid altogether, or couch in less-damaging terms such as "not autistic but with autistic traits," Asperger syndrome, pervasive developmental disorder, atypical child, communication disorder with impaired pragmatics, and others.

Epidemiologic studies (reviewed in Nelson, 1991), genetic studies (reviewed in Folstein and Piven, 1991), longitudinal studies (e.g., Lockyer and Rutter, 1970; DeMyer et al., 1973; Gillberg and Steffenburg, 1987), and neurologic studies (e.g., Piven et al., 1990; Steffenburg, 1991; Tuchman et al., 1991) provide evidence that autism is but one of the developmental disorders of brain function. Autism is a behaviorally defined syndrome with a variety of different etiologies (Gillberg, 1992). There is no longer any rational reason to eschew this diagnosis, although it will take a major effort to convince professionals, the public, school systems, and insurance companies of this fact.

DIAGNOSTIC CRITERIA

Because of the lack of biologic behavior markers for most psychiatric conditions, American psychiatrists have attempted to develop criteria that would enable them to provide a firm basis upon which to diagnose psychiatric disorders. The *Diagnostic and Statistical Manual of Mental Disorders,* third edition (DSM-III) (American Psychiatric Association, 1980), separated autism from childhood schizophrenia for the first time and introduced the term *pervasive developmental disorder* (PDD) for children with early onset of distortions of multiple psychological functions involving social behavior and language. PDD included three disorders: "infantile autism, full syndrome present"; "childhood onset PDD" (COPDD), for children who met all the criteria for "infantile autism" but with onset after thirty months; and "atypical PDD," for children who did not meet these criteria. In addition, there were "infantile autism, residual state" and "COPDD, residual state" for children who previously fulfilled all the criteria for these diagnoses, but no longer did. DSM-III criteria for infantile autism are provided in Table 1.1.

The DSM-III definition of *infantile autism* was viewed as too rigid in several respects, notably the requirements for onset before thirty months and for pervasive lack of social responsiveness rather than atypical social responsiveness. DSM-III-R (American Psychiatric Association, 1987) removed the arbitrary age of onset and defined autism with a somewhat different list of descriptors (Table 1.2) divided into three behavioral categories: impaired reciprocal social skills, impaired verbal and nonverbal communication, and impaired development of imaginative activity. To be called *autistic,* a child must exhibit a given number of qualitatively impaired behaviors in each of the three categories. DSM-III-R placed children with autistic symptomatology who fulfill fewer criteria in the category "PDD not otherwise specified" (PDDNOS), the

Table 1.1. Diagnostic Criteria for Autism and Pervasive Developmental Disorders, DSM-III (1980)

299.0x   Infantile Autism: Diagnostic Criteria
A. Onset before thirty months of age.
B. Pervasive lack of responsiveness to other people (autism).
C. Gross deficits in language development.
D. If speech is present, peculiar speech patterns such as immediate and delayed echolalia, metaphorical language, pronominal reversal.
E. Bizarre responses to various aspects of the environment (e.g., resistance to change, peculiar interest in or attachments to animate or inanimate objects).
F. Absence of delusions, hallucinations, loosening of associations, and incoherence as in Schizophrenia

299.00   Infantile Autism, Full Syndrome Present
Currently meets the criteria of Infantile Autism.

299.01   Infantile Autism, Residual State: Diagnostic Criteria
A. Once had an illness that met the criteria for Infantile Autism.
B. The current clinical picture no longer meets the full criteria for Infantile Autism, but signs of the illness have persisted to the present, such as oddities of communication and social awkwardness.

299.9x   Childhood Onset Pervasive Developmental Disorder:
Diagnostic Criteria
A. Gross and sustained impairment in social relationships (e.g., lack of appropriate affective responsivity, inappropriate clinging, asociality, lack of empathy).
B. At least three of the following:
   (1) Sudden excessive anxiety manifested by such symptoms as free-floating anxiety, catastrophic reactions to everyday occurrences, inability to be consoled when upset, unexplained panic attacks.
   (2) Constricted or inappropriate affect, including lack of appropriate fear reactions, unexplained rage reactions, and extreme mood lability.
   (3) Resistance to change in the environment (e.g., upset if dinner time is changed), or insistence on doing things in the same manner every time (e.g., putting on clothes always in the same order).
   (4) Oddities of motor movement, such as peculiar posturing, peculiar hand or finger movements, or walking on tiptoe.
   (5) Abnormalities of speech, such as questionlike melody, monotonous voice.
   (6) Hyper- or hyposensitivity to sensory stimuli (e.g., hyperacusis).
   (7) Self-mutilation (e.g., biting or hitting self, head banging).
C. Onset of the full syndrome after thirty months of age and before twelve years of age.
D. Absence of delusions, hallucinations, incoherence, or marked loosening of associations.

299.90   Childhood Onset Pervasive Developmental Disorder, Full Syndrome Present
Currently meets the criteria for Childhood Onset Pervasive Developmental Disorder.

299.91   Childhood Onset Pervasive Developmental Disorder, Residual State:
Diagnostic Criteria
A. Once had an illness that met the criteria for Childhood Onset Pervasive Developmental Disorder.

B. The current clinical picture no longer meets the full criteria for the disorder, but signs of the illness have persisted to the present, such as oddities of communication and social awkwardness.

299.8x   Atypical Pervasive Developmental Disorder
This category should be used for children with distortions in the development of multiple basic psychological functions that are involved in the development of social skills and language and that cannot be classified as either Infantile Autism or Childhood Onset Pervasive Developmental Disorder.

Source: American Psychiatric Association, 1980.

only other pervasive developmental disorder. Children with disintegrative psychosis (Kurita, 1988; Burd et al., 1989) or so-called Heller syndrome are classified as having either infantile autism or PDDNOS. This classification is praised by those who view autism as encompassing a broad spectrum of children sharing common behavioral deficits and is criticized by those who feel that the current definition is too broad.

DSM-III-R introduced a problematic qualification: It specified that autistic symptoms must be "out of proportion to the person's developmental level." This statement implies that if these qualitatively aberrant symptoms appear in the face of mental deficiency, which may be severe or even profound in autism, one should not diagnose infantile autism. DSM-III-R stated that stereotypies and self-injurious behaviors are common in severe-to-profound mental deficiency; however, they did not indicate that, when present, they should suggest autism. Yet DSM-III-R stressed that there is an associated diagnosis of mental deficiency in most autistic persons even though intelligence is not a defining feature of the disorder.

It seems logical that, inasmuch as autism is a behaviorally defined syndrome, any person with a behavioral constellation that fulfills the criteria for a diagnosis of autism (or PDDNOS) should be considered as being on the autistic spectrum, regardless of IQ. A recent population-based study of autism in Goteborg, Sweden (Steffenburg, 1991), that included a mentally deficient comparison group supported this view. On purely statistical grounds, the more severe the brain damage, the more likely it is to affect whatever brain systems are responsible for the occurrence of autistic symptomatology. From this vantage point, self-injurious behaviors, stereotypies, and lack of social responsiveness are considered autistic behaviors in whomever they occur (DSM-III-R stated that there are no exclusionary criteria for a diagnosis of autism), including in severely mentally deficient persons. Specifying the autistic nature of these behaviors in any person who exhibits them has explanatory value for the

Table 1.2. Diagnostic Criteria for Autism and Pervasive Developmental Disorders, DSM-III-R (1987)

299.00   Autistic Disorder
The essential features constitute a severe form of Pervasive Developmental Disorder, with onset in infancy or childhood.

Diagnostic criteria for 299.00 Autistic Disorder
At least eight of the following sixteen items are present, these to include at least two items from A, one from B, and one from C.
Note: Consider a criterion to be met only if the behavior is abnormal for the person's developmental level.
A. Qualitative impairment in reciprocal social interaction as manifested by the following: (The examples within parentheses are arranged so that those first mentioned are more likely to apply to younger or more handicapped, and the later ones to older or less-handicapped persons with this disorder.)
   (1) Marked lack of awareness of the existence or feelings of others (e.g., treats a person as if he or she were a piece of furniture; does not notice another person's distress; apparently has no concept of the need of others for privacy).
   (2) No or abnormal seeking of comfort at times of distress (e.g., does not come for comfort even when ill, hurt, or tired; seeks comfort in a stereotyped way, that is, says "cheese, cheese, cheese" whenever hurt).
   (3) No or impaired imitation (e.g., does not wave bye-bye; does not copy mother's domestic activities; mechanical imitation of others' actions out of context).
   (4) No or abnormal social play (e.g., does not actively participate in simple games; prefers solitary play activities; involves other children in play only as "mechanical aids").
   (5) Gross impairment in ability to make peer friendships (e.g., no interest in making peer friendships; despite interest in making friends, demonstrates lack of understanding of conventions of social interaction; for example, reads phone book to uninterested peer).
B. Qualitative impairment in verbal and nonverbal communication, and in imaginative activity, as manifested by the following:
   (The numbered items are arranged so that those first listed are more likely to apply to younger or more handicapped, and the later ones to older or less-handicapped persons with this disorder.)
   (1) No mode of communication, such as communicative babbling, facial expression, gesture, mime, or spoken language.
   (2) Markedly abnormal nonverbal communication, as in the use or eye-to-eye gaze, facial expression, body posture, or gestures to initiate or modulate social interaction (e.g., does not anticipate being held, stiffens when held, does not look at the person or smile when making a social approach, does not greet parents or visitors, has afixed stare in social situations).
   (3) Absence of imaginative activity, such as playacting of adult roles, fantasy characters, or animals; lack of interest in stories about imaginary events.
   (4) Marked abnormalities in the production of speech, including volume, pitch, stress, rate, rhythm, and intonation (e.g., monotonous tone, questionlike melody, or high pitch).
   (5) Marked abnormalities in the form or content of speech, including stereotyped and repetitive use of speech (e.g., immediate echolalia or mechanical repetition of television commercial); use of "you" when "I" is meant (e.g., using "You want cookie?" to mean "I want a cookie"); idiosyncratic use of words or phrases (e.g.,

"Go on green riding: to mean "I want to go on the swing"); or frequent irrelevant remarks (e.g., starts talking about train schedules during a conversation about sports).

(6) Marked impairment in the ability to initiate or sustain a conversation with others, despite adequate speech (e.g., indulging in lengthy monologues on one subject regardless of interjections from others).

C. Markedly restricted repertoire of activities and interests, as manifested by the following:

(1) Stereotyped body movements (e.g., hand-flicking or -twisting, spinning, head-banging, complex whole-body movements).

(2) Persistent preoccupation with parts of objects (e.g., sniffing or smelling objects, repetitive feeling of texture of materials, spinning wheels of toy cars) or attachment of unusual objects (e.g., when a vase is moved from usual position.

(4) Unreasonable insistence on following routines in precise detail, e.g., insisting that exactly the same route always be followed when shopping.

(5) Markedly restricted range of interests and a preoccupation with one narrow interest, e.g., interested only in lining up objects, in amassing facts about meteorology, or in pretending to be a fantasy character.

D. Onset during infancy or childhood.
Specify if childhood onset (after thirty-six months of age).

299.80 Pervasive Developmental Disorder Not Otherwise Specified
This category should be used when there is a qualitative impairment in the development of reciprocal social interaction and of verbal and nonverbal communication skills, but the criteria are not met for Autistic Disorder, Schizophrenia, or Schizotypal or Schizoid Personality Disorder. Some people with this diagnosis will exhibit a markedly restricted repertoire of activities and interests, but others will not.

Source: American Psychiatric Association, 1987.

caretakers of autistic persons, who are often baffled by these aberrant behaviors and the difficulty controlling them. It may have clinical implications once the pathophysiology of autism is unraveled and efficacious pharmacologic agents to control some of these symptoms become available. As DeMyer et al. (1981) pointed out, it is a strength of DSM to have introduced the concept of multiaxial diagnoses and comorbidity.

There are clinicians who feel that broadening the criteria for a diagnosis of autism has resulted in such a lack of specificity that they prefer not to use the term at all. All would agree that there is an urgent need to develop a validated typology that is widely accepted and that is based on sharply defined specific criteria.

NOSOLOGY

An unresolved issue is whether autism should be considered a single syndrome with highly variable severity (the autistic spectrum) or an aggregate of specific disorders that share some common features (Wing and Gould, 1979; Dahl et al., 1986; Allen, 1988; Minshew and Payton, 1988). The answer is clear as far as etiology is concerned: Autism has many etiologies. There is no reason to expect, however, that distinct etiologies will be manifest as distinct behavioral syndromes if autism results from the dysfunction of one or more, probably widely distributed, brain systems and from a variable array of signs and symptoms that reflect co-occurring dysfunction in other brain systems.

An etiologic typology of autism divides autistic children into etiologically defined subtypes (e.g., cases due to congenital rubella, fragile X, tuberous sclerosis, etc.). (Note that none of these etiologies is invariably associated with autistic behaviors.) The advantage of an etiological typology is that it elucidates the cause of the syndrome in an individual child and thus provides a basis for genetic counseling. In the present state of knowledge, the most serious drawback of an etiologic typology is that it does not encompass the great majority of children in whom etiology remains unknown.

Gaining an understanding of the pathophysiology of autism, that is, identifying the brain system(s) that is (are) dysfunctional in autistic children, requires the development of a validated typology based on behavioral criteria. The hypothesis underlying such an effort is that the dysfunction of particular brain systems produces reasonably predictable behavioral deficits. This hypothesis justifies the assumption that children grouped on the basis of similar behavioral symptoms may share a detectable dysfunction in the same or related brain systems. A behaviorally defined typology has the advantage of encompassing all children with autistic symptomatology and the practical advantage of grouping those whose similar behavioral deficits may be amenable to similar interventions.

Investigators are far from having achieved consensus on a behaviorally defined typology of autism. Is there a fundamental difference between children in whom behavioral abnormalities were already evident in infancy and those whose parents report a regression or prolonged plateau in the development of language, sociability, and play? Is there a fundamental difference between children whose autistic regression occurred between one and three years, which is the rule, and the less-common cases with later regression? Cases with late regression are often referred to as *disintegrative psychosis* (Kurita, 1988; Burd et al., 1989) and probably correspond to those described as Heller syndrome. What is the relationship of cases with regression and cases of acquired epileptic aphasia or Landau–Kleffner syndrome (Landau and Kleffner, 1957), which is often associated with frankly autistic symptomatology (Kurita, 1988; Burd et al., 1989)? Equally unclear is the boundary, if any, between autism and Asperger syndrome (Wing, 1981, 1991; Gillberg, 1989; Frith, 1991), a subtype of children with autistic symptomatology who speak well and who may have higher verbal than performance IQs.

Until the 1970s, autism was often considered a precocious form of schizophrenia (e.g., Bender, 1955; Goldfarb, 1964) or a childhood psychosis (Reiser, 1963), even though Asperger (1944) had pointed out that the children were not psychotic. This confusion makes some early large follow-up studies less useful than they might have been inasmuch as congenital cases and cases with onset before five years were lumped with those with onset between five and ten years, some of whom may in fact have been schizophrenic (e.g., Annell, 1963). The relationship, if any, between verbal autistic children and children with childhood-onset schizophrenia remains unresolved. A validated behavioral typology of children with autistic symptomatology is clearly needed to reduce the present nosologic confusion.

There is every reason to anticipate that even an empirically validated typology of autistic persons into behaviorally well-defined subtypes will not map onto a classification based on specific etiologic (biologic) criteria. Hybrid typologies based on a combination of biologic and behavioral criteria are guaranteed to lead to confusion. It is illogical to speak of the differential diagnosis between autism and a particular biologic condition associated with autistic symptoms. Yet a preliminary version of ICD 10 (World Health Organization, 1990) listed autism and Rett syndrome as separate conditions. Rett syndrome is believed to be a biologically specific condition that affects girls, has well-defined neurologic signs and symptoms, and, at least in infancy and early childhood, is associated with blatant autistic symptoms (Hagberg et al., 1983). Similarly, some boys with fragile X syndrome have autistic symptoms (Cohen et al., 1988). A minority of children with Down syndrome, a favorite comparison group for studies of autistic children, are also autistic. In such cases one should not speak of the differential diagnosis between autism and Rett syndrome, fragile X, or Down syndrome, but should refer to them as representing etiologically (that is, biologically) distinct subtypes among autistic children.

RESEARCH ON THE NEUROBIOLOGY OF AUTISM

The realization that autism is not a psychogenically determined syndrome has accelerated research attempting to define its cause. A large number of investigations have assessed various sensory, cognitive, social, and behavioral aspects of autism (often referred to as "childhood schizophrenia" until the 1970s), while others have addressed its etiology and underlying brain dysfunction. A major output from these many research efforts (comprehensively reviewed by DeMyer et al., 1981) is a proliferation of conflicting theories about the fundamental cause of autism.

RESPONSIVITY TO SENSORY STIMULI

Many parents of autistic children report that the children respond atypically to a variety of sensory stimuli. Impressed with the fascination of some autistic children with wheels or turning fans and with their pleasure in antigravity play and running around in circles, Ornitz (1970) studied the vestibular function of autistic children and hypothesized that impaired response to vestibular input played an important role in the genesis of autistic symptomatology.

Many studies have demonstrated that many autistic children respond atypically to auditory signals, being oblivious to some and hypersensitive to others. There is evidence that the syndrome of verbal auditory agnosia, which is more common in children with autistic symptomatology than in nonautistic children (Allen and Rapin, 1992), may be due to a deficit in auditory (Stefanatos et al., 1989) rather than phonologic perception, as earlier suggested (Rapin et al., 1977). Following a report that auditory desensitization resulted in the "cure" of one autistic girl (Stehle, 1991), parents of autistic children are currently flocking to try this "miraculous" treatment.

Autistic children regularly have better visual/spatial than auditory/verbal skills, and many have remarkable visual memories. They may be excellent at jigsaw puzzles and some draw remarkably well (Hermelin and O'Connor, 1990). Some autistic infants arch their backs and resist being cuddled and, later, touched, while others take an inordinate pleasure in tickling and rough play. Strong taste and texture aversions for certain foods and an unusual sensitivity to smell are reported by some parents.

All in all, this conflicting variety of responses indicates that the perception of and not sensitivity to sensory inputs in all modalities is atypical in these children (Frith and Baron-Cohen, 1987). This statement does not contradict the fact that there are children who are hearing impaired and autistic (Jure et al., 1991) or blind and autistic (Chase, 1968). A sensory or perceptual theory of autism is not tenable, but the reason for autistic children's aberrant reaction to many sensory stimuli remains speculative.

ATTENTIONAL DEFICITS

Unusually sustained attention to favorite activities, lack of boredom for repetitive activities, marked distractibility, disorganization, and sleep disturbances are frequent complaints by the parents of autistic children (Rapin, 1991). These observations have spawned several attentional theories of autism. Ornitz (1988) was impressed with a deficit in directed attention, Courchesne (Akshoomoff and Courchesne, 1992) with an inability to shift attention rapidly, and Kinsbourne (1991) with hyperfocused attention to compensate for overarousal. These theories raise a number of different speculations about subcortical and cortical brain dysfunctions that may underlie autism.

LANGUAGE DEFICITS

Delayed or inadequate development of language is the most frequent complaint that brings autistic children to professional attention (Tuchman et al., 1991). Although the majority of children with deafness, developmental dysphasia, and acquired aphasia are not autistic, some investigators have speculated that autism is the consequence of inadequate communicative ability or a more severe variant of developmental language disorder (see Paul, 1987, for a review). Allen and Rapin (1992) argued that preschool autistic children are both autistic and dysphasic. They were able to classify autistic children into the same dysphasic syndromes as nonautistic children with developmental language disabilities, with two exceptions: in the preschool years, autistic children invariably have comprehension deficits; and two subtypes of the language deficit—verbal auditory agnosia and the semantic–pragmatic syndrome—are considerably more prevalent in the autistic than in the nonautistic population.

Others have proposed that the language deficit of autistic children is the consequence of a primary cognitive deficit (Rutter, 1983) or of their social deficit (Fein et al., 1986). While there is a correlation between the severity of autistic children's cognitive and language deficits, longitudinal studies of the evolution of language in autistic children are needed to determine the specificity and predictive value of various preschool subtypes of language deficit.

COGNITIVE DEFICITS

Population studies indicate that the majority (some two-thirds or more) of children with autistic symptomatology are mentally deficient, many of them severely so. This leaves a sizeable number of children on the autistic spectrum who are of normal or near-normal intelligence, characteristically with quite uneven abilities across a range of different skills. All investigators of autism agree that there are even some exceptionally intelligent children on the autistic spectrum. It is to these intelligent children that terms such as Asperger syndrome, schizotypal personality, PDDNOS, and others are likely to be applied (Tuchman, 1991). The wide range of IQs among autistic children is the reason DSM places cognition on a separate axis from autism per se. Yet a number of investigators (e.g., Gillberg and Steffenburg, 1987; Wing, 1991) have pointed out that, while these intelligent children may constitute behavioral subtypes among autistic children, they do not seem to differ in a fundamental way from more classically autistic children. This makes sense if the cognitive level is not a defining feature of autistic symptomatology, even though it has a marked influence on its manifestations and outcome (e.g., Rutter, 1979).

A number of investigators, including Frith (1989, 1991) among others, have speculated that what distinguishes autistic children from other mentally deficient or learning disabled children is an inadequate ability to attribute to others emotions and viewpoints separate from their own. They attribute the children's social deficits to this inability, called the lack of a "theory of mind."

DEFICITS IN SOCIABILITY AND AFFECT

The most salient feature of autistic children is their inadequate ability to relate to others, their aloofness and flat affect often coupled with excessive anxiety and lability of mood. Impaired ability to read facial expression, body posture, and tone of voice, attributed by some investigators to dysfunction of the right hemisphere (Weintraub and Mesulam, 1984; Semrud-Clikeman and Hynd, 1990), suggests a right-hemisphere theory of autism. Other investigators invoke hypothalamic–limbic pathology to account for the lack of drive to communicate and poor response to the usual social reinforcers (Mundy and Sigman, 1989). While many studies of serotonin and catecholamines, which play an important role in the regulation of drive and affect as well as the regulation of sleep and motor activity, have been carried out in autistic persons, alterations are not reproducible in all cases.

This brief review emphasizes that there is no lack of theory about autism, but that thus far no comprehensive theory accounts for the unique syndrome represented by autistic children. To advance the field, data collected from rigorously defined groups of autistic children who are compared to well-matched controls are more likely to prove fruitful than are studies of children who encompass the entire spectrum of autism. There is a need for biologic studies as well as behavioral ones, keeping in mind their entirely different goals and levels of investigation.

UNMET NEEDS

This volume addresses current knowledge of the neurobiology of autism from both etiologic and behavioral standpoints. Data provided by clinical and neuropathologic investigations in autistic persons, together with the recent development of powerful tools for imaging cerebral metabolism during the performance of relevant behaviors, drove the selection of topics.

The application of neurobiologic tools to autism has already born fruit. While the finding of neuropathologic lesions in the cortex (Piven et al., 1990) and limbic system (Bauman and Kemper, 1985; Bauman,

1991) came as no surprise, those observed in the cerebellum (Bauman and Kemper, 1985; Bauman, 1991; Courchesne, 1991) have forced investigators to reexamine their most basic assumptions on the role of the cerebellum in functions even more complex than sensorimotor control and programing. Missing from this book, because of the dearth of prospective information, is a focus on the many potential nongenetic etiologies of the autistic spectrum and its differential diagnosis from infantile schizophrenia, schizoid and schizotypal personality disorders. DSM-III-R (American Psychiatric Association, 1987) stated that high-functioning autistic persons may show catatonic phenomena in adolescence, "an indifferentiated psychotic state with apparent delusions and hallucinations," but that these states are short-lived and appear in response to stress. It is clear that childhood schizophrenia and autism are disorders that share many features and that, until biologic markers are discovered, their borders will continue to remain fuzzy (Rumsey et al., 1985; Tantam, 1991). Is it perhaps the case that they are the manifestation of different brain disorders impinging on (some of) the same brain systems?

Another topic of interest, because of its potential therapeutic implications, that is not considered as such in this book is autistic regression. At least 40 percent of parents report that their infant or toddler, whose development may or may not have been entirely normal up to then, experienced a regression, usually insidious but occasionally abrupt, in language, sociability, and play (Tuchman et al., 1991). The regression is rarely if ever associated with a regression in motor skills or with other evidence of a neurologic illness. It is rarely associated with seizures. In some cases, regression seems to be precipitated by an environmental event, such as separation from the mother, a hospitalization, or the birth of a younger sibling. If such environmental events have any relevance to the regression, then they can be only triggers. As far as possible mechanisms for underlying regression are concerned, these tell us that the child's course is not relentlessly downhill, as would be the case in a progressive degenerative disease of the brain. Development resumes after a plateau that usually lasts for some months, but, in most cases, never returns to its previous level. Some children are left nonverbal, severely withdrawn, and mentally deficient, while others fare better, although complete recovery seems not to occur. One question, then, is whether this regression, which appears to correspond to a very early disintegrative psychosis (or Heller syndrome), might be the result of undiagnosed seizures affecting both the language areas of the left hemisphere as well as the amygdala and other limbic structures, as proposed by Deonna (1991). Many speculations have been offered, thus far without evidence, to explain autistic regression: slow viral infection, autoimmune phenomenon, lack or insufficiency of a growth factor at a particular time in development, abnormality of an excitatory neurotransmitter. Data need to be collected to investigate these speculations.

Only in the past decade have sophisticated neurobiologic tools been applied to the study of the developmental disorders of brain function, including autism. There was no known pathology of autism until the painstaking work of Bauman and Kemper (1985; Bauman, 1991) demonstrated subtle developmental cellular alterations in the cerebellum and limbic system in autistic persons. This timely volume should be an incentive to other neurobiologists to investigate this fascinating, complex, and devastating disorder of the immature brain. What will be learned will no doubt provide new insights into disorders of adults as well as those of children.

ACKNOWLEDGMENTS

The preparation of this chapter was supported in part by program project grant NS 20489 from the National Institute of Neurologic Disorders and Stroke, U.S. Public Health Service.

REFERENCES

Allen, D. A. 1988. Autistic spectrum disorders: Clinical presentation in preschool children. *Journal of Child Neurology* 3(Suppl):S48–S56.
Allen, D. A., and Rapin, I. 1992. Autistic children are also dysphasic. In H. Naruse and E.M. Ornitz, eds., *Neurobiology of Infantile Autism.* 157–68. Amsterdam: Excerpta Medica.
Akshoomoff, N. A., and Courchesne, E. 1992. A new role for the cerebellum in cognitive operations. *Behavioral Neuroscience* 106: 731–38.
American Psychiatric Association. 1980. *Diagnostic and Statistic Manual of Mental Disorders (3rd Edition).* 86–92. Washington, D.C.: American Psychiatric Association.
American Psychiatric Association. 1987. *Diagnostic and Statistic Manual of Mental Disorders (3rd Edition Revised).* 33–39. Washington, D.C.: American Psychiatric Association.
Annell, A.-L. 1963. The prognosis of psychotic syndromes in children: A follow-up study of 115 cases. *Acta Psychiatrica Scandinavica* 39:235–97.
Asperger, H. 1944. Die 'autistischen Psychopathen' im Kindesalter. *Archiv für Psychiatrie und Nervenkrankheiten* 127:76–136. Translated and annotated by U. Frith in U. Frith, ed. 1991. *Autism and Asperger Syndrome.* 37–92. Cambridge: Cambridge University Press.
Bauman, M. L., and Kemper, T. L. 1985. Histoanatomic observations of the brain in early infantile autism. *Neurology* 35:866–74.
Bauman, M. L. 1991. Microscopic neuroanatomic abnormalities in autism. *Pediatrics* 87:791–96 (supplement).
Bender, L. 1955. Twenty years of clinical research on schizophrenic children, with special reference to those under six years of age. In G. Caplan, ed., *Emotional Problems of Early Childhood.* 503–15. New York: Basic Books.

Burd, L., Fisher, W., and Kerbeshian, J. 1989. Pervasive disintegrative disorder: Are Rett syndrome and Heller dementia infantilis subtypes? *Developmental Medicine and Child Neurology* 31:609–16.

Cantwell, D. P., Baker, L., and Rutter, M. 1979. Families of autistic and dysphasic children. I: Family life and interaction patterns. *Archives of General Psychiatry* 36:682–87.

Chase, J. B. 1968. *Retrolental Fibroplasia and Autistic Symptomatology*. New York: American Foundation for the Blind.

Chess, S., Korn, S. J., and Fernandez, P. B. 1971. *Psychiatric Disorders of Children with Congenital Rubella*. New York: Brunner/Mazel.

Cohen, I. L., Fisch, G. S., Sudhalter, V., Wolf-Schein, E. G., Hanson, D., Hagerman, R., Jenkins, E. C., and Brown, W. T. 1988. Social gaze, social avoidance, and repetitive behavior in fragile X males: A controlled study. *American Journal of Mental Retardation* 92:436–46.

Courchesne, E. 1991. Neuroanatomic imaging in autism. *Pediatrics* 87:781–90 (supplement).

Dahl, E. K., Cohen, D. J., and Provence, S. 1986. Clinical and multivariate approaches to the nosology of pervasive developmental disorders. *Journal of the American Academy of Child Psychiatry* 25:170–80.

DeMyer, M. K., Barton, S., DeMyer, W. E., Norton, J. A., Allen, J., and Steele, R. 1973. Prognosis in autism: A follow-up study. *Journal of Autism and Childhood Schizophrenia* 3:199–246.

DeMyer, M. K., Hingtgen, J. N., and Jackson, R. K. 1981. Infantile autism reviewed: A decade of research. *Schizophrenia Bulletin* 7:388–451.

DeMyer, M. K., Pontius, W., Norton, J. A., Barton, S., Allen, J., and Steele, R. 1972. Parental practices and innate activity in normal, autistic, and brain-damaged infants. *Journal of Autism and Childhood Schizophrenia* 2:49–66.

Deykin, E. Y., and MacMahon, B. 1979. The incidence of seizures among children with autistic symptoms. *American Journal of Psychiatry* 136:1310–12.

Deonna, T. 1991. Acquired epileptiform aphasia in children (Landau–Kleffner syndrome). *Journal of Clinical Neurophysiology* 8:288–98.

Fein, D., Pennington, B., Markowitz, P., Braverman, M., and Waterhouse, L. 1986. Toward a neuropsychological model of infantile autism: Are the social deficits primary? *Journal of the American Academy of Child Psychiatry* 25:198–212.

Folstein, S. E., and Piven, J. 1991. The etiology of autism: Genetic influences. *Pediatrics* 87:767–73 (supplement).

Frith, U. 1989. *Autism: Explaining the Enigma*. Oxford: Blackwell.

Frith, U., ed. 1991. *Autism and Asperger Syndrome*. Cambridge: Cambridge University Press.

Frith, U., and Baron-Cohen, S. 1987. Perception in autistic children. In D. J. Cohen, A. M. Donnellan, and R. Paul, eds., *Handbook of Autism and Pervasive Developmental Disorders*. 85–102. New York: John Wiley.

Gillberg, C. 1989. Asperger syndrome in 23 Swedish children. *Developmental Medicine and Child Neurology* 31:520–31.

Gillberg, C. 1992. Subgroups in autism: Are there behavioural phenotypes typical of underlying medical conditions? *Journal of Intellectual Disability Research* 36:201–14.

Gillberg, C., and Steffenburg, S. 1987. Outcome and prognostic factors in infantile autism and similar conditions: A population study of 46 cases followed through puberty. *Journal of Autism and Developmental Disorders* 17:273–87.

Goldfarb, W. 1964. An investigation of childhood schizophrenia. *Archives of General Psychiatry* 11:620–34.

Hagberg, B., Aicardi, J., Dias, K., and Ramos, O. 1983. A progressive syndrome of autism, dementia, ataxia and loss of purposeful hand use in girls: Rett syndrome: Report of 35 cases. *Annals of Neurology* 14:471–79.

Heller, T. 1908. Über Dementia infantilis: Verblödungsprozess im Kindesalter. *Zeitschrift für die Erforschung und Behandlung jugendlichen Schwachsinns* 2:17–28.

Hermelin, B., and O'Connor, N. 1990. Art and accuracy: The drawing ability of idiot-savants. *Journal of Child Psychology and Psychiatry* 31:217–28.

Junker, K. 1964. *The Child in the Glass Ball.* Nashville: Abingdon Press.

Jure, R., Rapin, I., and Tuchman, R. F. 1991. Hearing impaired autistic children. *Developmental Medicine and Child Neurology* 33:1062–72.

Kanner, L. 1943. Autistic disturbances of affective contact. *Nervous Child* 10:217–50.

Kanner, L. 1971. Follow-up study of eleven autistic children originally reported in 1943. *Journal of Autism and Childhood Schizophrenia* 2:119–45.

Kanner, L., and Eisenberg, L. 1956. Early infantile autism 1943–1955. *American Journal of Orthopsychiatry* 26:55–65.

Kinsbourne, M. 1991. Overfocussing: An apparent subtype of attention deficit-hyperactivity disorder. In N. Amir, I. Rapin, and D. Branski, eds., *Pediatric Neurology: Behavior and Cognition of the Child with Brain Dysfunction.* 18–35. Basel: Karger.

Kurita, H. 1988. The concept and nosology of Heller's syndrome: Review of articles and report of two cases. *Japanese Journal of Psychiatry and Neurology* 42:785–93.

Landau, W. M., and Kleffner, F. R. 1957. Syndrome of acquired aphasia with convulsive disorder in children. *Neurology* 7:523–30.

Lockyer, L., and Rutter, M. 1970. A five to fifteen year follow-up study of infantile psychosis: IV. Patterns of cognitive ability. *British Journal of Social and Clinical Psychology* 31:156–63.

Minshew, N. J., and Payton, J. B. 1988. New perspectives in autism. Part I: The clinical spectrum of autism. *Current Problems in Pediatrics* 19:618–94.

Mundy, P., and Sigman, M. 1989. Specifying the nature of the social impairment in autism. In G. Dawson, ed., *Autism: Nature, Diagnosis, and Treatment.* 3–21. New York: Guilford Press.

Nelson, K. B. 1991. Prenatal and perinatal factors in the etiology of autism. *Pediatrics* 87:761–66 (supplement).

Ornitz, E. M. 1970. Vestibular dysfunction in schizophrenia and childhood autism. *Comprehensive Psychiatry* 11: 159–73.

Ornitz, E. M. 1988. Autism: A disorder of directed attention. *Brain Dysfunction* 1: 309–22.

Paul, R. 1987. Communication. In D. J. Cohen, A. M. Donnellan, and R. Paul, eds., *Handbook of Autism and Pervasive Developmental Disorders.* 61–84. New York: John Wiley.

Piven, J., Berthier, M. L., Starkstein, S. E., Nehme, E., Pearlson, G., and Folstein, S. 1990. Magnetic resonance imaging evidence for a defect of cerebral cortical development in autism. *American Journal of Psychiatry* 147:734–39.

Rapin, I. 1965. Dementia infantilis (Heller's disease). In C. H. Carter, ed., *Medical Aspects of Mental Retardation.* 760–67. Springfield, IL: Charles C. Thomas.

Rapin, I. 1991. Autistic children: Diagnosis and clinical features. *Pediatrics* 87:751–60 (supplement).

Rapin, I., Mattis, S., Rowan, A. J., and Golden, G. S. 1977. Verbal auditory agnosia in children. *Developmental Medicine and Child Neurology* 19:192–207.

Reiser, D. E. 1963. Psychosis of infancy and early childhood, as manifested by children with atypical development. *New England Journal of Medicine* 269:790–98, 844–50.

Rumsey, J., Rapoport, J., and Sceery, W. 1985. Autistic children as adults: Psychiatric, social and behavioral outcomes. *Journal of the American Academy of Child Psychiatry* 4:465–73.

Rutter, M. 1979. Language, cognition, and autism. In R. Katzman, ed., *Developmental and Acquired Disorders of Cognition*. 247–64. New York: Raven Press.

Rutter, M. 1983. Cognitive deficits in the pathogenesis of autism. *Journal of Child Psychology and Psychiatry* 24:513–31.

Schain, R., and Yannet, H. 1960. Infantile autism. *Journal of Pediatrics* 57:560–67.

Semrud-Clikeman, M., and Hynd, G. W. 1990. Right hemisphere dysfunction in nonverbal learning disabilities: Social, academic, and adaptive functioning in adults and children. *Psychological Bulletin* 107:196–209.

Spitz, R. A. 1945. Hospitalism: Inquiry into genesis of psychiatric conditions in early childhood. *Psychoanalytic Study of the Child* 1:53–74.

Stefanatos, G. A., Green, G. R. G., and Ratcliff, G. G. 1989. Neurophysiological evidence of auditory channel anomalies in developmental dysphasia. *Archives of Neurology* 46:871–75.

Steffenburg, S. 1991. Neuropsychiatric assessment of children with autism: A population-based study. *Developmental Medicine and Child Neurology* 33:495–511.

Stehle, A. 1991. *Sound of a Miracle: A Child's Triumph over Autism*. New York: Doubleday.

Tantam, D. 1991. Asperger syndrome in adulthood. In U. Frith, ed., *Autism and Asperger Syndrome*. 147–83. Cambridge: Cambridge University Press.

Tuchman, R. F. 1991. Autism: Delineating the spectrum. *International Pediatrics* 6:161–69.

Tuchman, R. F., Rapin, I., and Shinnar, S. 1991. Autistic and dysphasic children. I: Clinical characteristics. II: Epilepsy. *Pediatrics* 88:1211–18, 1219–25.

Weintraub, S., and Mesulam, M.-M. 1983. Developmental learning disabilities of the right hemisphere. *Archives of Neurology* 40:463–68.

Wing, L. 1981. Asperger's syndrome: A clinical account. *Psychologic Medicine* 11:115–29.

Wing, L. 1991. The relationship between Asperger's syndrome and Kanner's autism. In U. Frith, ed., *Autism and Asperger Syndrome*. 93–121. Cambridge: Cambridge University Press.

Wing, L., and Gould, J. 1979. Severe impairments of social interaction and associated abnormalities in children: Epidemiology and classification. *Journal of Autism and Developmental Disorders* 9:11–29.

World Health Organization. 1990, unpublished. *International Classification of Diseases: Tenth Revision*. Chapter V. Mental and behavioral disorders (including disorders of psychological development). Diagnostic criteria for research (May 1990 draft for field trials). Geneva: World Health Organization.

2

THE GENETICS OF AUTISM

Joseph Piven, M.D.
Susan Folstein, M.D.

In 1976, Hanson and Gottesman, reviewing the available literature on autism, concluded that the cause was unlikely to be genetic. However, over the last fifteen years considerable evidence has accumulated to support the importance of hereditary factors in the etiology of this disorder. In addition, the development of new technologies during this period, in both molecular genetics and cytogenetics, has substantially improved our capacity to investigate the role of genetics in neuropsychiatric disorders.

THE CHARACTERISTICS OF AUTISM

ASSESSMENT AND DIAGNOSIS

The outcome of genetic studies of psychiatric disorders is primarily determined by nosologic and epidemiologic approaches to defining the samples for study. These issues have particular relevance to autism. Fifty years ago, Kanner (1943) described eleven children who represented the core behavioral features of the condition. Kanner noted two features in these children that he felt were pathognomonic of autism: a lack of social responsiveness to others and an obsessive insistence on the preservation of sameness in the environment. Although there have been numerous revisions of Kanner's early definition, it is not clear that these changes have significantly improved on Kanner's clinical acumen.

Studies of autism have employed varying sets of criteria (e.g., Creak's criteria, Rutter's criteria, DSM III and DSM III-R criteria) and differing methods of assessment (e.g., behavioral checklists, unstandardized and standardized clinical interviews). Such approaches to diagnosis and assessment have led to variation in the definition of study samples of autistic individuals (Volkmar et al., 1988; Hertzig et al., 1990).

These discrepancies, in addition to differing methods of case ascertainment, are most likely responsible for the variability in prevalence estimates of autism (0.7 to 5.6/10,000) among epidemiologic studies (reviewed by Smalley et al., 1988) and have led to different conclusions about familial aggregation (Lotter, 1966; Piven et al., 1990). In genetic studies of autism, as with all studies concerned with elucidating the etiology of behavioral syndromes, the importance of standardized methods of assessment and diagnosis should not be underestimated. Standardized investigator-based instruments for the assessment of autism (e.g., the Autism Diagnostic Interview and the Autism Diagnostic Observation Schedule) (LeCouteur et al., 1988; Lord et al., 1988) are now available. These instruments will greatly improve our ability to establish diagnostic reliability between investigators and to describe differences between samples that may be associated with etiologic heterogeneity.

MENTAL RETARDATION

Approximately 70 percent of autistic individuals are mentally retarded (IQ less than 70) and 40 percent have IQs less than 50 (DSM-III, 1980). Although there is a strong association between autism and mental retardation, the two differ in important ways. First, while both are associated with a higher rate of perinatal complications than is found in the general population, autism is associated with more minor pre- and perinatal abnormalities (e.g., first-trimester bleeding), whereas mental retardation is associated with more severe complications (e.g., postnatal asphyxia). Second, the pattern of cognitive deficits tends to be different from that typically found in nonautistic mentally retarded individuals (reviewed by Rutter, 1988). Third, while autism and mental retardation are both associated with infantile spasms (Riikonen and Amnell, 1981), congenital rubella (Chess et al., 1971), and fragile X syndrome (Blomquist et al., 1982, 1983, 1985), there are clear differences with regard to associations with other disorders. Thus, while mental retardation is common in both cerebral palsy and Down syndrome, neither of those is associated with autism (Rutter, 1988). Finally, autism and mental retardation differ with regard to the onset of seizures. In autism, seizure disorders commonly have their onset in adolescence (Deykin and MacMahon, 1979; Volkmar and Nelson, 1989), whereas the onset is typically in infancy and early childhood in nonautistic mentally retarded individuals (Richardson et al., 1980).

Such differences between autism and mental retardation suggest that these syndromes most likely have different etiologies and that autistic probands of different IQ groups may define etiologically distinct subgroups in autism. The likelihood that IQ may indicate etiologic diversity in autism is further supported by the dramatic variation in IQ (from profound mental retardation to the superior range) in those diagnosed as autistic. An example of this is found in the mucopolysaccharidoses, previously grouped as one disorder ("gargoylism" or "Hurler syndrome") defined on the basis of similar physical features in which IQ ranges from profound retardation to normal. The current classification defines subgroups on the basis of recessive mutations at distinct genetic loci, and the IQ range in each of these subgroups is much narrower (McKusick, 1992). Similar examples exist among other genetic disorders (e.g., Marfan syndrome) that have been defined more recently on the basis of genetic loci in addition to clinical characteristics. In contrast, however, there are many examples of a unitary etiology that results in widely varying levels of intelligence (e.g., congenital rubella) as well as a wide range of qualitatively distinct characteristics. An example of the latter phenomenon, referred to as variable expressivity, is the varied manifestations in the same kindred of such genetic disorders as osteogenesis imperfecta and neurofibromatosis (Folstein and Rutter, 1988). Thus, the level of intelligence of autistic probands is an important variable to consider in interpreting genetic studies of autism.

GENETIC FACTORS

FAMILY STUDIES

The prevalence of autism in siblings of autistic probands, based on data pooled from six studies, is 2.7 percent (Smalley et al., 1988). While this number is small, it is 50–100 times greater than expected, given the rate of autism of 2–5 per 10,000 in the population (Lotter, 1966; Wing et al., 1976; Steffenburg et al., 1986; Ritvo et al., 1989a). Furthermore, this rate may be an underestimate of the actual risk of autism to siblings as a result of parents of autistic children limiting their plans for having subsequent children (Jones and Szatmari, 1988). This phenomenon occurs in the families of severely handicapped children and could decrease the likelihood of having more than one affected child in a family (Steele, 1986). The use of such "reproductive stoppage rules" was taken into account in a recent epidemiologic survey by measuring the recurrence risk of autism in siblings (i.e., considering only the siblings born *after* the proband, rather than all siblings) (Ritvo et al., 1989a). These investigators reported a recurrence risk of autism in siblings of 8.6 percent.

TWIN STUDIES

Twin studies in autism have provided substantial support for a genetic component. The first population-based twin study, carried out in Great Britain, examined twenty-one same-sexed pairs in which at least one member of the pair met the criteria for autism (Folstein and Rutter, 1977). Of the monozygotic pairs, 36 percent (4/11) were concordant for autism, versus 0 percent (0/10) of the dizygotic pairs. The 0 figure for dizygotic twins is likely to be an artifact resulting from small sample size (Rutter, 1990). The actual figure, assuming similar risk to dizygotic twins and singletons, is probably around 3 percent, the prevalence rate of autism in siblings of autistic probands. Folstein and Rutter (1977) also reported nine of eleven (82 percent) monozygotic pairs and one of ten (10 percent) dizygotic pairs to be concordant for a variety of cognitive deficits (i.e., reading, spelling, and articulation disorders; language delay and mental retardation), suggesting that a cognitive disorder, rather than autism per se, is inherited in families of autistic individuals.

These findings have been replicated by LeCouteur et al. (1989), again using an epidemiologically based twin sample in Great Britain. These investigators found a pairwise concordance rate in fourteen monozygotic pairs of 50 percent for autism and 86 percent for cognitive abnormalities, versus 0 percent concordance for autism and 9 percent concordance for cognitive abnormalities in eleven same-sexed dizygotic pairs. Significant differences between monozygotic and dizygotic twins were also reported in a population-based twin study in Scandinavia by Steffenburg et al. (1989) and a twin study by Ritvo et al. (1985a). Both of these studies reported much higher concordance rates for monozygotic twins (89 percent and 96 percent, respectively). The Steffenburg study is unusual in that there is approximately a 1:1 ratio of males to females. Furthermore, because ten of eleven monozygotic pairs were concordant for autism, hypotheses regarding the inheritance of cognitive disorder could not be examined. The study by Ritvo et al. (1989a) is the only one to report a significant concordance in dizygotic pairs (24 percent). In this latter study, a number of methodologic problems (including a bias of ascertainment, the inclusion of opposite-sexed dizygotic pairs, limited blood group testing for zygosity in many monozygotic pairs, and nonblind diagnosis) make it difficult to interpret the findings.

Folstein and Rutter (1977) examined the pre- and perinatal histories in discordant monozygotic twin pairs in their sample. They found that the nonautistic cognitively impaired co-twins had markedly fewer serious perinatal complications than did those co-twins with autism. These findings are supported by the twin study of Steffenburg et al. (1989), who reported "perinatal stress" to be much more common in the autistic co-twin of discordant pairs. These results suggested that perinatal complications increase the risk for autism in individuals with a genetic liability for this disorder. The findings on pre- and perinatal insults may not be generalizable to singletons, as these complications are more common in twins than they are in the general population (Propping and Vogel, 1976). In addition, twins are known to be at higher risk for reading and language disorder (Hay et al., 1984, 1987) and severe mental retardation (Allen and Kallman, 1955) than are singletons.

FAMILIAL AGGREGATION OF OTHER CONDITIONS

Cognitive Deficits.   The hypothesis that autism may be a severe form of cognitive disorder, based on the finding by Folstein and Rutter (1977) of a high rate of cognitive disorders in nonautistic monozygotic co-twins, prompted a number of family studies to further examine this hypothesis. August et al. (1981) directly examined the siblings of autistic and Down syndrome children and found a significantly higher rate of cognitive disorders in the siblings of autistic probands (15 versus 3 percent). However, deficits in reading and spelling were found only in siblings whose IQs were less than 90 and who were themselves siblings of mentally retarded autistic probands. Based on this finding, August et al. suggested that an aggregation of cognitive deficits may reflect an association between the inheritance of cognitive disorders and mental retardation, rather than a genetic association between cognitive deficits and autism. These results were replicated by Baird and August (1985). In addition, Minton et al. (1982) reported a higher than expected rate of mental retardation in the siblings of autistic probands, as well as a high proportion of siblings with verbal scores significantly lower than performance scores on the Wechsler intelligence tests.

The finding of cognitive deficits, however, has not been limited to the family members of low IQ probands. Bartak et al. (1975) noted a family history of language and/or speech disorder in more than one-quarter of the parents and siblings of autistic probands with a nonverbal IQ greater than 70. Piven et al. (1990), in a more recent family history study, reported 15 percent of siblings to have a history of cognitive disorder, most of which were disorders of reading and language. In this study there was no association between proband IQ and the presence of cognitive disorder in siblings. Macdonald et al. (1989) similarly reported a 15-percent rate of cognitive disorder in a larger sample of siblings of autistic probands (versus a 4.5 percent rate in the siblings of Down syndrome controls). Most of the cognitive disorders in this study involved abnormalities of speech and language rather than mental retardation. Gillberg et al. (1992), in a family history study of school-aged siblings and parents of thirty-five autistic children and forty-two children with "deficits in attention, motor control and perception," found no difference in rates of cognitive disorder. However, more than one-third of the autistic probands had associated medical conditions (e.g., trisomy 13). The possible etiologic heterogeneity of this sample limits comparison to other studies.

Two studies directly tested parents and siblings of autistic probands. Freeman et al. (1989) found that reading, spelling, and intelligence scores in parents and siblings did not differ from published norms and that there was no evidence of verbal scores being consistently lower than performance scores, as reported by Minton et al. (1982). Wzorek et al. (1991) compared 118 parents and adult siblings of 51 autistic probands to 47 parents and adult siblings of 19 Down syndrome controls and found no excess of reading and/or spelling disorders or low IQ in the autism families. Her sample contained no probands with IQ less than 30, so the absence of cognitive disorders in this sample could result from the exclusion of low IQ probands. In addition, both Freeman et al. and Wzorek et al. tested adult relatives who may have developed compensatory skills that obscured the detection of learning disabilities that may have been present at younger ages (Pennington, 1986). Studies that have shown an excess of cognitive disorders in the families of autistic individuals have all either examined young siblings or based the diagnosis of cognitive disorders on reports of functioning during childhood.

Deficits in executive function have also been noted to aggregate in the siblings of high-functioning autistic probands compared to siblings of learning-disabled controls (Ozonoff et al., 1991). Executive function is defined as the cognitive ability to maintain an appropriate problem-solving set for the attainment of a future goal; it includes behaviors such as flexibility of thought and action, and inhibition of irrelevant responses. Similar deficits have been reported in autistic subjects compared to nonautistic IQ-matched controls (Rumsey and Hamburger, 1988; Prior and Hoffman, 1990). Flexibility of action (i.e., as evidenced by extreme resistance to change) is also a defining feature of autism and was originally thought by Kanner to be one of the two pathognomonic features of this disorder (Kanner, 1943).

Personality Characteristics.   In their early descriptions of autistic children, Kanner and Eisenberg (1957) noted that a number of the parents of these children were serious-minded, perfectionistic individuals with intense interests in abstract ideas, who appeared to lack interest in developing relationships with others. These observations were incorrectly interpreted as evidence that faulty child-rearing practices caused autism. Research has confirmed that autism is not the result of child-rearing practices (Cantwell et al., 1978). Nevertheless, particular personality characteristics have been reported in the parents and siblings of autistic individuals more commonly than in controls.

In a follow-up of the original twin sample studied by Folstein and Rutter (1977), LeCouteur et al. (1989) reported a high rate of social deficits in the nonautistic co-twins of autistic probands who were reinterviewed approximately ten years after the original study. These social deficits had not been as apparent in these individuals during childhood. However, this study did not incorporate a control group. Macdonald et al. (1989), using the family history method, detected autistic-like social deficits in 12 percent of the adult first-degree relatives of autistic probands, but none in the first-degree relatives of Down syndrome controls. Two other studies (DeLong and Dwyer, 1988; Piven et al., 1990) also using the family history method reported severe social deficits in a number of the relatives of autistic probands. Individuals with social and language deficits (without significant cognitive or language delay) and circumscribed interests that are milder than but qualitatively similar to those defining autism, have been referred to as having Asperger syndrome (Tsai, 1991). DeLong and Dwyer (1988) reported that relatives with Asperger syndrome were more likely to aggregate in the families of high IQ autistic probands. Gillberg et al. (1989) compared the family histories of twenty-three children with autism and twenty-three children with Asperger syndrome and found a significantly higher number of the parents of the Asperger probands to have deficits in their social interaction and restricted range of interests. These deficits were particularly apparent in the fathers (11/23) of the children with Asperger syndrome. Gillberg et al. (1992), using the family history method, also reported the occurrence of Asperger syndrome more commonly in the parents of thirty-five autistic individuals compared to the parents of forty-two children with "deficits in attention, motor control and perception."

Wolff et al. (1988) interviewed parents of autistic and control subjects (parents of nonautistic mentally retarded children), blind to proband diagnosis, and rated their personality characteristics. Parents of autistic children were more often judged to have schizoid personality traits. Characteristics contributing to the rating of schizoid personality included a lack of emotional responsiveness and empathy, impaired rapport with the examiner, a history of and preference for solitariness, oversensitivity to experiences, special interest patterns, and oddities of social communication. Piven et al. (unpublished manuscript) carried out a similar study but used a standardized interview to assess personality. Parents ($N = 87$) of forty-eight autistic probands were more likely than the parents ($N = 38$) of twenty Down syndrome controls to describe themselves as aloof, untactful, undemonstrative, and unresponsive.

Specific Language Abnormalities.   The appearance of "social oddity" in parents and siblings has also been approached through the study of the social use of language. Wolff et al. (1988) noted that the parents of autistic children were significantly different from controls demonstrating over- and undercommunicativeness, excessive guardedness, and disinhibition. In a study that directly assessed social communication, a significantly higher rate of deficits in both social use of language (pragmatic language) (Landa et al., 1992) and story telling (narrative discourse) (Landa et al., 1991) was detected in the parents of autistic individuals compared to the parents of individuals with Down syndrome. When rated blind to family membership, approximately 30 percent of autism parents were judged to provide too much detail and to give vague accounts; these parents were also unable to give up their conversational turn and frequently misinterpreted their conversational partner's statements. Autism parents also had significantly greater difficulty than did controls in generating a complete and properly constructed story after first being told how the story begins. These findings could not be attributed to IQ or education, which were matched in the parents of autistic probands and controls.

Psychiatric Disorders.   Several studies have reported the aggregation of particular psychiatric disorders in the family members of autistic individuals (reviewed by Piven et al., 1991a). Early studies of autism suggested that schizophrenia aggregated in the families of autistic probands. These early studies could not be replicated (reviewed by Rutter, 1988) and were most likely the result of the overly inclusive diagnostic criteria used to define both autism and schizophrenia. More recently, two studies using the family history method and DSM III criteria for autism reported rates of major affective disorder in the family members of autistic individuals that were significantly higher than were those from published epidemiologic studies (DeLong and Dwyer, 1988; Piven et al., 1990). However, neither study incorporated a control group for direct comparison. When parents were directly assessed using a structured psychiatric interview (Piven et al., 1991a), they were found to have significantly higher rates of anxiety disorders than did controls. Recurrent major affective disorder (four weeks duration) was also more common in the parents of autistic probands (16 percent), although the difference compared to controls (6 percent) did not reach statistical significance. Neither anxiety disorders nor affective disorders could be explained as a result of the stress of having an autistic child because the onset of these disorders, in most cases, had occurred before the birth of the proband.

The finding of high rates of anxiety and affective disorders in families of autistic individuals has received further support in two subsequent reports employing the direct assessment of relatives. In an ongoing family study of autism, Smalley et al. (1992) detected elevated rates of affective disorder in the parents of sixteen autistic probands compared to the parents of fifteen probands with tuberous sclerosis. Rates of anxiety disorder in these relatives were not reported. Abramson et al. (1992) also noted elevated rates of anxiety and affective disorders in twenty-six first-degree and thirty-five second-degree relatives of thirteen autistic probands.

Summary. In their report of cognitive deficits in the monozygotic co-twins of autistic individuals, Folstein and Rutter (1977) hypothesized that cognitive deficits may be a milder expression of a common underlying genetic abnormality in autism. The results of these more recent studies examining personality characteristics, language deficits, executive function, and psychiatric disorder in relatives of autistic individuals suggest that a variety of different abnormalities aggregate in families of autistic individuals, and that these abnormalities may be manifestations of an underlying genetic liability to autism. While deficits in language, executive function, and personality are reliably detectable, they are often mild and not associated with significant functional impairment. Although milder, a number of these deficits are qualitatively similar to the characteristic features of autism (e.g., aloofness and pragmatic language deficits). Clarification of these abnormalities in relatives (i.e., defining the behavioral phenotype appropriate for genetic study of autism) is an important preliminary step in the genetic analysis of this disorder.

GENETIC DISORDERS ASSOCIATED WITH AUTISM

Most of the studies discussed previously that have demonstrated the familial aggregation of autism and other disorders in family members have excluded cases of autism in which the proband has a concurrent medical condition of known genetic etiology. Of interest in the quest for the etiology of autism are the occasional cases seen in association with particular genetic conditions. Only a few such conditions are reported in association with autism, so the associations do not appear to be random. Understanding the genetic and neural mechanism underlying these disorders may contribute to our understanding of the etiologies and mechanisms in autism.

Fragile X. Fragile X syndrome (or Martin–Bell syndrome) is an X-linked mental retardation disorder defined by a cytogenetic marker (or fragile site, FraX) located at Xq27.3. The fragile X syndrome is the second most common known genetic cause of mental retardation (Turner et al., 1986). In addition to mental retardation, the syndrome occasionally includes particular dysmorphic features, such as macro-orchidism, a prominent jaw, and large ears (DeArce, 1984). The genomic region associated with this disorder has recently been identified and a partial cDNA clone from this region (FMR-1) has been sequenced and found to contain a variable number of CGG repeats (Verkerk et al., 1991).

The FraX marker has been reported to be significantly associated with the syndrome of autism. Studies have reported rates of FraX in autistic samples ranging from 0 to 16 percent (Blomquist et al., 1985; Goldfine et al., 1985; Brown et al., 1986; Wahlstrom et al., 1986; Payton et al., 1989; Piven et al., 1991b). The pooled prevalence estimate based on the screening of 614 autistic males reported in twelve studies was 7.7 percent (Brown et al., 1986). The prevalence of autism in samples of individuals with FraX has also been reported. Hagerman et al. (1986) studied fifty males with FraX and noted twenty-two (44 percent) to have a current DSM III diagnosis of autism or autism, residual state. Reiss et al. (1990), in a study of seventeen FraX males, noted that three met DSM III-R criteria for autism and ten met criteria for pervasive developmental disorder. Bregman et al. (1988) reported pervasive developmental disorder in only one in fourteen FraX males (none with autism) using DSM-III criteria. Finally, there have been a number of case reports of the FraX anomaly and autism co-occurring in siblings (Gillberg and Gillberg, 1983; August and Lockhar, 1984).

The nature of the relationship between autism and fragile X syndrome is confounded by the association of both disorders with mental retardation. In most reports that include information about IQ, the autistic subjects with FraX are among the more mentally retarded members of the sample. In a large Scandinavian study by Blomquist (1982, 1983, 1985), the FraX anomaly was found in 16 percent of autistic males, 6 percent of severely retarded, and 4.5 percent of mildly retarded males. Einfeld et al. (1989) examined both FraX individuals and a non-FraX IQ-matched control group and found no difference in the rate of autism between the two groups. He concluded that autism was not associated with FraX. Fisch et al. (1986) reported the FraX anomaly in 12.5 percent of autistic individuals ($N = 144$), compared with 20.6 percent of nonautistic mentally retarded or learning-disabled subjects ($N = 254$).

There are several possible explanations for the wide variation in reported rates of FraX in autistic individuals. First, sample characteristics vary between studies. Studies to date have not used standardized assessments and have employed varying diagnostic criteria for autism. Autistic individuals screened for FraX have come from a variety of sources (e.g., residential centers, hospital clinics, population-based samples) and have included individuals with varying distributions of IQ. Second, the cytogenetic diagnosis of the FraX anomaly is variable and subject to error. Thresholds for the diagnosis of FraX have varied across studies between 1 and 4 percent and laboratory procedures differ between centers. In addition, recent reports have described a common fragile site at Xq27.2 that may lead to frequent false positives in individuals with low levels of FraX expression (1–3 percent) (Ramos et al., 1989; Sutherland and Baker, 1990).

With the availability of a direct test for the presence of the FMR-1 gene, a number of these methodologic issues will clearly be resolved. In addition, knowledge of qualitative and quantitative differences in this gene and their correlations with phenotypic variations (in particular, autistic characteristics) are likely to provide important insights into the genetics of autism.

Disorders with Mendelian Patterns of Inheritance.   Associations have been described between autism and several disorders demonstrating Mendelian patterns of inheritance, including phenylketonuria, tuberous sclerosis, and possibly neurofibromatosis. These disorders are presumably the result of single-gene defects. Other disorders thought to be genetic on the basis of their aggregation within families have also been reported to present with autistic behaviors: De Lange syndrome (Nyhan, 1972; Johnson et al., 1976), Leber hereditary optic neuropathy (Rogers, 1989; McKusick, 1992), histidinemia (Rutter and Bartak, 1971; Kotsopoulos, 1977), and Williams syndrome (Reiss et al., 1985). For the most part, samples in these reports are small and have not been systematically collected, and assessment and diagnosis have not been standardized. Taken together, the proportion of cases of autism that are accounted for by the aggregate of these specific genetic etiologies is small. Nevertheless, understanding the etiology and mechanisms underlying these genetic disorders may lead to clues regarding the pathophysiology of autism.

Phenylketonuria (PKU), an autosomal recessive disorder resulting from an absence of the enzyme phenylalanine hydroxylase, was the first genetic disorder reported to be associated with autism. Infants are currently screened for this disorder at birth. If detected, PKU is treated with a phenylalanine-restricted diet. In addition to the frequent mental retardation of the subjects, case reports of children with untreated PKU often describe autistic-like behaviors (e.g., withdrawal, lack of speech, and repetitive behaviors) (Blainey and Guilford, 1956; Armstrong et al., 1957; Berry et al., 1958; Sutherland et al., 1960; Bjornson, 1964). Hackney et al. (1968) reported in one case series that 20 percent (9/44) of children with untreated PKU demonstrated autistic-like behaviors. Not all of those showing these behaviors had severe cognitive impairments (Blainey and Guilford, 1956; Sutherland, 1960; Bjornson, 1964). Improvement in behavior, often more dramatic than changes in IQ, has been noted with the early (i.e., between several months and three years of age) institution of a phenylalanine-restricted diet (Armstrong et al., 1955, 1957; Woolf et al., 1955; Blainey and Guilford, 1956; Berry et al., 1958). More recently, Lowe et al. (1980) screened sixty-five subjects with pervasive developmental disorder (using DSM-III criteria) and found three with PKU. However, Pueschel et al. (1985) screened fifty-eight autistic subjects (using Rutter criteria) and did not find any with PKU.

Tuberous sclerosis is an autosomal dominant neurocutaneous disorder, also frequently presenting with mental retardation. Genetic heterogeneity is evident in tuberous sclerosis from molecular studies suggesting linkage of this disorder to the distal long arm of chromosome 9 (Connor et al., 1987; Fryer et al., 1987; Northrup et al., 1987), as well as possible linkage to chromosomes 11 (Smith et al., 1990) and 16 (Kandt et al., 1992). One case series and a number of case reports have linked tuberous sclerosis and autism, although the association may be mediated by an association of both disorders with infantile spasms. Taft and Cohen (1971) and Riikonen (1981) described an association between infantile spasms and autism. In a subsequent study of eighty-nine subjects with tuberous sclerosis, Hunt and Dennis (1987) reported sixty-nine with infantile spasms. Of those sixty-nine, 58 percent were autistic. The onset of developmental abnormalities was noted in most cases to coincide with the onset of infantile spasms. These investigators also diagnosed autism in 25 percent (5/20) of those with tuberous sclerosis but without infantile spasms. Others have also observed the occasional occurrence of individuals with both autism and tuberous sclerosis (Lotter, 1974; Wing, 1975; Mansheim, 1979).

More recently, Smalley et al. (1992a) reported that seven of thirteen subjects with tuberous sclerosis, directly examined using a standardized interview for autism, met criteria for autism. Autistic individuals with tuberous sclerosis differed from fourteen autistic subjects without tuberous sclerosis in showing fewer repetitive rituals and higher rates of seizures and mental retardation. In addition, all five males with tuberous sclerosis were diagnosed as autistic, whereas only two of eight females with tuberous sclerosis were determined to be autistic. This sex-specific difference varies from the 1:1 rate expected in an autosomal disorder and suggests the possibility of sex-influenced expression of autistic behaviors.

Neurofibromatosis, another autosomal dominant neurocutaneous disorder associated with mental retardation in 10–20 percent of cases and a variable expression of symptoms, has been associated with autism in one study. Gillberg and Forsell (1984), in a population study of autism in Scandinavia, found three of fifty-one children to have both autism and neurofibromatosis. The chance that one child would have both of these relatively rare disorders is extremely unlikely. Thus, the finding of three subjects concurrently affected with both disorders in an epidemiologically collected sample warrants further study of a possible association between autism and neurofibromatosis.

Chromosomal Anomalies.   Several case reports (Hansen et al., 1977; Burd et al., 1985; Mariner et al., 1986) and case series (Nielsen et al., 1973; Hoshino et al., 1979; Gillberg and Wahlstrom, 1985) described autistic individuals with a number of autosomal and sex chromosomal anomalies. Others reported a variety of fragile sites (other than fragile

Xq27.3) in autistic individuals (Gillberg and Wahlstrom, 1985; Jayakar et al., 1986). Other than fragile Xq27.3, however, no significant association between a particular chromosomal abnormality and the autism phenotype has been consistently reported.

ENVIRONMENTAL FACTORS

In examining the importance of genetic factors in the etiology of autism, evidence for environmental factors should be reviewed as well. Unfavorable pre-, peri-, and neonatal factors have been shown to occur more commonly in autistic individuals than normal controls (Finnegan and Quarrington, 1978; Deykin and MacMahon, 1980; Gillberg and Gillberg, 1983) and more severe perinatal complications have been shown to occur in autistic than nonautistic co-twins concordant for cognitive disorder (Folstein and Rutter, 1977). In addition, concordance of autism in less than 100 percent of monozygotic twin pairs supports the role of environmental factors in the etiology of autism in twins. Finally, while the finding of significant differences in monozygotic–dizygotic concordance rates for autism is evidence for the importance of hereditary factors, the excess of unfavorable perinatal hazards known to occur in monozygotic twins (compared to dizygotic twins) may exaggerate differences in monozygotic–dizygotic concordance rates (Benirske and Kim, 1973; Hanson and Gottesman, 1976).

Several lines of evidence, however, suggest that pre-, peri-, and neonatal factors are probably not the principal cause of autism. First, the unfavorable factors in singletons found to be associated with autism are nonspecific (i.e., no particular complication is consistently associated with autism) and are considered minor complications of uncertain significance (e.g., first-trimester bleeding) (Rutter et al., 1990). While these complications may be the result of environmental events occurring during pregnancy and delivery, an alternative explanation is that they are related to genetic abnormalities of the fetus. Second, although perinatal complications have been shown to occur more commonly in autistic than nonautistic co-twins, they did not account for the concordance of autism in any of the three twin studies to date (Rutter et al., 1990). Finally, based on a proband-wise concordance rate for monozygotic twins of 53 percent (Folstein and Rutter, 1977), the heritability of autism is estimated at more than 90 percent (Rutter, 1990). The heritability statistic is an estimate of the proportion of phenotypic variance that is attributable to the average effects of genes. This estimate takes population frequency of the disorder into account (Smith, 1974). In rare disorders such as autism, concordance rates convert to higher heritability estimates. A heritability estimate of more than 90 percent suggests that few cases are likely to be due entirely to environmental causes (Rutter et al., 1990).

While the evidence suggests that pre-, peri-, and neonatal factors are not the principal or only cause of autism, they may nevertheless play an important role. In a study of the offspring of schizophrenic mothers, Canon et al. (1989) noted an association between periventricular abnormalities detected on CAT scans and the number of complications suffered at delivery, but only among subjects with an elevated genetic risk for schizophrenia (i.e., schizophrenia spectrum disorder in the father). These findings suggest an interaction between genetic risk for schizophrenia and complications at delivery. Similarly, autism may be the result of an increased vulnerability to relatively minor pre-, peri-, and neonatal complications in individuals with a high genetic liability for the disorder.

MODES OF INHERITANCE

ETIOLOGIC HETEROGENEITY

Although the importance of hereditary factors in the etiology of idiopathic autism is well established, particular genetic mechanisms have not yet been identified. Before considering possible genetic mechanisms in autism, it is necessary to address the issues of etiologic and genetic heterogeneity.

The search for a single underlying genetic mechanism in autism assumes homogeneity of genetic and environmental influences (Vandenberg et al., 1986). However, autism is a behavioral syndrome defined by clinical features, not by etiology. Although validity at a syndromic level is well established, it is almost certain that autism is an etiologically heterogeneous disorder. It is known, for example, that autism can develop in association with etiologies as diverse as congenital rubella (Chess, 1971), tuberous sclerosis (Hunt and Dennis, 1987), and the fragile X anomaly (Brown et al., 1986), as well as in the absence of any identifiable, co-occurring, etiologically defined condition.

Among autistic individuals without identifiable, associated etiologic conditions, several points suggest that there may also be genetic heterogeneity. First, the possibility that the wide variation in intelligence of autistic individuals is evidence of genetic diversity was discussed at the beginning of this chapter. In addition, the evidence suggests that the causes of profound and mild mental retardation are different. Individuals with profound mental retardation are likely to have siblings of normal intelligence, suggesting exogenous (e.g., encephalitis) or recessive (e.g., PKU) etiologies; whereas, those with mild mental retardation conform to patterns seen in polygenic inheritance (i.e., the IQ of siblings and parents is also more likely to be in the mildly retarded range) (Bouchard and McGue, 1981; Nichols, 1984).

Second, differing sex ratios in high and low IQ autism subgroups also supports the hypothesis that autism is heterogeneous. A number of studies have demonstrated that the ratio of males to females in probands of higher IQ (> 50) is approximately 3–4:1, whereas the ratio in lower IQ groups (< 50) approaches 1:1 (Lotter, 1974; Wing, 1981; Tsai and Madsen-Beisler, 1983; Lord and Schopler, 1985).

Third, heterogeneity is often more apparent in disorders previously thought to be due to a single etiology as new "phenotypic levels" are identified. For example, homocystinuria, a disorder of methionine metabolism, was originally grouped together with Marfan syndrome as one disorder defined on the basis of similar physical characteristics. These disorders were eventually differentiated into two distinct diagnostic categories following the finding of homocystine in the urine of a subgroup of patients. After the biologic distinction was made, several phenotypic distinctions became apparent. In autism, the finding of high levels of platelet serotonin in autistic probands of multiple-incidence families (i.e., at least two autistic children) compared to those of single-incidence families, as well as higher levels in single-incidence probands when compared to normal controls, similarly suggests heterogeneity in genetic liability to autism (Piven et al., 1991). In this way, selection of subjects on the basis of a "biochemical phenotype" has been suggested as one way to enhance homogeneity (Buschbaum, 1979).

Finally, some studies have presented evidence that probands defined by varying behavioral criteria differ in rates of familial aggregation of autistic-like and related disorders. Gillberg (1989) identified a significantly higher number of parents with severe social deficits and restricted interests among the parents of children with Asperger syndrome when compared to children with autism (defined by DSM-III criteria). Piven et al. (1990) similarly found differences in the familial aggregation of neuropsychiatric disorders in the adult siblings of a group of probands diagnosed by Kanner's criteria when compared to autistic probands meeting DSM III criteria. These differences were not explained by differences in IQ between the two groups.

INHERITANCE AT A SINGLE MAJOR LOCUS

It has been difficult to test the hypothesis that a single major locus could explain the inheritance patterns in autism. Two issues have complicated the analysis. First, there is no vertical transmission of the disorder, as autistic individuals, for the most part, do not marry or have children. There is only one report of an autistic individual that had children (Ritvo et al., 1988). Second, the use of "stoppage rules" decreases the likelihood that further siblings of an affected child will have autism. This tends to decrease the size of sibships and underestimate familial aggregation, but it also poses a problem in demonstrating autosomal recessive inheritance (Brookfield et al., 1988). Nevertheless, inheritance at a single major locus has been considered in autism. Because of the male excess (at least in the higher IQ groups) and the report of a possible association between the FraX anomaly and autism, X-linked inheritance has been postulated (Gurling, 1986). Smalley et al. (1988), in a review of the genetics of autism, excluded the possibility of X-linked inheritance, noting that the prevalence of autism in females (approximately 1×10^{-4}) is 1000-fold greater than would be expected (i.e., the square of the rate of autistic males in the population) if autism were X-linked. However, the disorder is highly likely to be genetically heterogeneous, and X-linkage may be responsible for only a portion of autism cases, perhaps more commonly in high IQ males. Against this possibility is the finding by Tsai et al. (1988) of an absence of DNA deletions in the Xq26–28 region in twenty autistic boys (two with the FraX anomaly) using DNA probes. However, fragile X cases alone do not begin to account for the excess of males in the whole autism population, and there could be other mutations on the X chromosome, related to autism, that have not yet been discovered. Other investigators have postulated different genetic mechanisms for males and females. For example, the etiology of autism in females may be a result of an autosomal abnormality, whereas the etiology in males may involve a mixture of both autosomal and X-linked (the majority) defects (Szatmari and Jones, 1991).

For several reasons, inheritance patterns are also inconsistent with simple autosomal dominant and recessive inheritance. First, the recurrence risk to siblings of 3–8 percent (Smalley et al., 1988; Ritvo et al., 1989a) is less than would be expected in dominant and recessive inheritance (50 percent and 25 percent, respectively). Second, monozygotic concordance for autism is less than the expected 100-percent rate (in the studies by Folstein and Rutter, 1977, and LeCouteur et al., 1989) for a single locus condition. Dizygotic concordance is less than the 50-percent and 25-percent rates expected in autosomal dominant and recessive conditions, respectively. Third, the 1:1 ratio of males to females predicted in an autosomal disorder is not found in autism. Finally, a recent complex segregation analysis of autism in a population sample, using only the diagnosis of autism as affected, was not consistent with a single major locus model of inheritance (Jorde et al., 1991).

In contrast, one study suggested that autosomal recessive inheritance may operate in a subgroup of autistic individuals. Ritvo et al. (1985), in a segregation analysis of forty-six families with multiple cases of autism, found results consistent with autosomal recessive inheritance and inconsistent with the multifactorial model. However, several problems have been noted with this study. Although Ritvo et al. reported adjusting for a bias of ascertainment of multiple-incidence families, they acknowledge that other unknown biases limited the interpretation of their results. They also pointed out that autosomal recessive inheritance is inconsistent with the excess of males observed in autism. The possibility that autosomal recessive inheritance is operating in a subgroup of multiple-incidence families, however, is not inconsistent with the finding by Piven et al. (1991) that platelet serotonin levels are highest in autistic probands from multiple-incidence families.

Considerable evidence indicates that a number of abnormalities (i.e., cognitive deficits, personality characteristics, language abnormalities, psychiatric disorder) aggregate in the families of autistic individuals. The aggregation of these abnormalities may be a result of the variable expression in relatives of an underlying genetic liability to autism and suggests that future genetic analyses in autism should broaden the definition of affected to include these milder abnormalities. The situation is similar to that seen in Tourette syndrome, where, in addition to Tourette syndrome, chronic motor tics and obsessive compulsive disorder aggregate in families. Genetic analysis of this more broadly defined phenotype was consistent with an autosomal dominant pattern of inheritance (Pauls and Leckman, 1986). A similar approach may reveal patterns consistent with single major locus inheritance in autism.

MULTIFACTORIAL POLYGENIC INHERITANCE

The multifactorial model of inheritance postulates that a number of genetic and environmental effects contribute to a continuous and normally distributed liability to autism in the population (Falconer, 1965). This model is most easily applied to quantitative traits such as IQ, but it has also been applied to non-Mendelian "all or none" attributes. Only those individuals whose liability falls beyond a certain threshold manifest the disorder. The relatives of affected individuals have a higher mean liability (and are thus more commonly affected with the disorder) than do the general population. In addition, those individuals more severely affected presumably have a higher liability for the disorder. Under the multifactorial model, the distribution of genetic liability among the sexes is usually considered to be equal. When a sex difference exists in the incidence of a disorder, it is hypothesized to be the result of a higher sex-specific threshold for expression. Therefore, probands of the more rarely affected sex are presumed to have a higher liability for the disorder.

The absence of simple Mendelian patterns in autism coupled with the low sibling recurrence risk has prompted some investigators to consider the multifactorial model in autism (Spence, 1976; Tsai et al., 1981). This model is also consistent with the excess of a variety of minor pre- and perinatal complications in autistic individuals and with the high rate of these complications observed in the autistic co-twins discordant for autism but concordant for cognitive disorder. The demonstration by some researchers that autistic females are "more severely affected" with autism has been seen as evidence for the multifactorial model (Tsai et al., 1981). The interpretation that females are more severely affected is based on the finding that autistic females generally have a lower IQ and higher rate of neurologic abnormalities than do autistic males. However, whether IQ or the presence of neurologic deficits can be used as an index of the severity of genetic liability for autism, or whether they are simply indications of genetic heterogeneity, is not clear.

More direct evidence in support of a multifactorial model comes from family and twin studies. Tsai et al. (1981) reported a higher rate of cognitive deficits in the relatives of autistic females, and Ritvo et al. (1989a) noted a higher recurrence risk for autism in the siblings of autistic females (14.5 percent) compared to males (7 percent). Others, however, have not found sex-specific differences in the familial aggregation of autism or related disorders (August et al., 1981; Piven et al., 1990, 1991a). Finally, Penrose (1953) suggested that the greater the number of genes involved in a disorder, the higher the monozygotic and lower the dizygotic concordance (or incidence in siblings). As a general rule, he suggested that monozygotic–dizygotic concordance ratios greater than 4 are consistent with polygenic rather than single-gene inheritance (Penrose, 1953). In the twin studies of Folstein and Rutter (1977), LeCouteur et al. (1989), and Steffenburg et al. (1989), the ratio of the monozygotic–dizygotic concordance rates in autism is greater than 4 and supports the possibility that the multifactorial model underlies the inheritance of autism.

FUTURE DIRECTIONS

Future studies in the genetics of autism will need to further examine the etiologic and genetic heterogeneity in this disorder. This will require large family studies that look at the relationship between the familial aggregation of related disorders and a variety of proband characteristics, such IQ, sex, behavior, the presence of perinatal complications, neurodevelopmental abnormalities, and serotonin levels. Large family studies will also be needed to clarify the variety of abnormalities that may be expressions of the underlying genetic liability to autism (i.e., the autism phenotype). Studies of the offspring of monozygotic co-twins concordant for cognitive disorder (but not for autism) may also be helpful in this regard.

Our understanding of what is inherited in families of autistic individuals will be enhanced with further knowledge regarding whether or not there is a "core deficit" in autism. Can the variety of abnormalities found in family members and autistic individuals be explained by one fundamental psychological mechanism? For example, does a deficit in social cognition, as proposed by Baron-Cohen (1988), explain both the deficits in autism and the personality, language, and cognitive deficits in family members? Or, are these abnormalities distinct manifestations of an underlying genetic abnormality (Rutter, 1988)? Consideration of these possibilities and clarification of the autism phenotype are necessary preliminary steps to further genetic analysis.

Finally, linkage analysis may be helpful in assessing the importance of simple genetic mechanisms and clarifying genetic heterogeneity in autism. In a linkage study by Spence et al. (1985) of multiple-incidence autism families using HLA and blood group polymorphisms, the absence of linkage may have been due to the fact that the markers used spanned only a small portion of the genome. The use of a battery of closely spaced polymorphic DNA markers, in addition to employing methods for dealing with heterogeneity (e.g., multipoint mapping and simultaneous search), now make it possible to find linkages even for different genes in different families (Lander and Botstein, 1986; Donis-Keller et al., 1987). Candidate loci for these analyses may include the X chromosome at q27 (Gurling, 1986), chromosome 9 in the area of the ABO blood group (Smalley, 1988), or other loci suggested by case reports of deletions or translocations occurring in autistic individuals. This approach may prove useful in studying a large number of families, ascertained through an autistic proband, who have members with milder variants of the autistic phenotype or through the study of multiple-incidence autism families.

CONCLUSIONS

A few specific genetic conditions can occasionally be associated with autism. Among cases of unknown etiology, there is ample evidence for a higher genetic liability to autism in siblings of autistic probands than expected from the population prevalence. It appears likely that both parents and siblings have a higher liability for social, language, and cognitive deficits that are milder but conceptually similar to those found in autism. Other factors may alter this underlying genetic liability, such as sex, IQ, and pre-, peri-, and neonatal injury. In the future, genetic analyses and genetic linkage studies will need to consider using a broader definition of the autism phenotype to include not only autism but also those individuals with severe cognitive and social deficits, as well as a consideration of genetic heterogeneity in this disorder. The exact genetic mechanisms and genes involved are the subject of current investigations by several research groups. Investigations in this area are likely to continue to provide important information regarding the causes of autism.

ᴀCKNOWLEDGMENTS

Support was provided, in part, by the Autism Research Grant #1 RO1 MH39936 and by the John Merck Fund. The authors appreciate the comments of Gary Chase, Ph.D., and the assistance of Cindy Taylor and Janiece Thein with the preparation of this chapter.

REFERENCES

Abramson, R. K., Wright, H. H., Cuccaro, M. L., Lawrence, L. G., Babb, S., Pencarinha, D., Marsteller, F., Harris, E. 1992. Biological liability in families with autism. Letter to the editor. *Journal of the American Academy of Child and Adolescent Psychiatry* 31:370–71.

Allen, G., and Kallman, F. J. 1955. Frequency and types of mental retardation in twins. *American Journal of Human Genetics* 7:15–20.

Armstrong, M. D., and Tyler, F. H. 1955. Studies on phenylketonuria, I. Restricted phenylalanine intake and phenylketonuria. *Journal of Clinical Investigation* 43:565–80.

Armstrong, M. D., Low, N. L., and Bosma, J. F. 1957. Studies on phenylketonuria, IX. Further observations on the effect of phenylalanine-restricted diet on patients with phenylketonuria. *American Journal of Clinical Nutrition* 5:543–54.

August, G. J., Stewart, M. A., and Tsai, L. 1981. The incidence of cognitive disabilities in the siblings of autistic children. *British Journal of Psychiatry* 138:416–22.

August, G., and Lockhart, L. H. 1984. Familial autism and the fragile-X chromosome. *Journal of Autism Developmental Disorders* 14:197–204.

Baird, T. D., and August, G. J. 1985. Familial heterogeneity in infantile autism. *Journal of Autism and Developmental Disorders* 15:315–21.

Baron-Cohen, S. 1988. Social and pragmatic deficits in autism: Cognitive or affective? *Journal of Autism and Developmental Disorders* 18:379–401.

Bartak, L., Rutter, M., and Cox, A. 1975. A comparative study of infantile autism and specific developmental receptive language disorder. 1. The children. *British Journal of Psychiatry* 126:127–45.

Berry, H. K., Sutherland, B. S., Guest, G. M., and Umbarger, B. 1958. Chemical and clinical observations during treatment of children with phenylketonuria. *Pediatrics* 21:929–40.

Bjornson, J. 1964. Behavior in phenylketonuria: Case with schizophrenia. *Archives of General Psychiatry* 10:65–70.

Blainey, J. D., and Guilford, R. 1956. Phenylalanine-restricted diets in the treatment of phenylketonuria. *Archives of Disease in Childhood* 31:452–566.

Blomquist, H. K., Bohman, M., Edvinsson, S. O., Gillberg, C., Gustavson, K-H., Holmgren, G., and Wahlstrom, J. 1985. Frequency of the fragile X syndrome in infantile autism. *Clinical Genetics* 12:303–8.

Blomquist, H. K., Gustavson, K-H., Holmgren, G., Nordenson, I., and Palsson-Strae, U. 1983. Fragile X syndrome in mildly mentally retarded children in a Northern Swedish country: A prevalence study. *Clinical Genetics* 24:393–98.

Blomquist, H. K., Gustavson, K-H., Holmgren, G., Nordenson, I., and Sweins, A. 1982. Fragile site X-chromosomes and X-linked mental retardation in severely retarded boys in a northern Swedish county: A prevalence study. *Clinical Genetics* 21:209–14.

Bouchard, T. J., and McGue, M. 1981. Familial studies of intelligence. *Science* 212:1055–59.

Bregman, J. D., Leckman, J. F., and Ort, S. I. 1988. Fragile X syndrome: Variability of phenotypic expression. *Journal of the American Academy of Child and Adolescent Psychiatry* 26:463–71.

Brookfield, J. F. Y., Pollitt, R. J., and Young, I. D. 1988. Family size limitation: A method for demonstrating recessive inheritance. *Journal of Medical Genetics* 21:181–85.

Brown, W. T., Jenkins, E. C., Cohen, I. L., Fisch, G. S., Wolf-Schein, E. G., Gross, A., Waterhouse, L., Fein, D., Mason-Brothers, A., Ritvo, E., Ruttenberg, B. A., Bentley, W., and Castells, S. 1986. Fragile X and autism: A multicenter survey. *American Journal of Medical Genetics* 23:341–52.

Burd, L., Kerbeshian, J., Fisher, W., and Martsolf, J. T. 1985. A case of autism and mosaic trisomy 8. *Journal of Autism and Developmental Disorders* 15:351–52.

Buschbaum, M. S., and Rieder, R. O. 1979. Biologic heterogeneity and psychiatric research. *Archives of General Psychiatry* 36:1163–69.

Canon, T. D., Sarnoff, M. A., and Parnas, J. 1989. Genetic and perinatal determinants of structural brain deficits in schizophrenia. *Archives of General Psychiatry* 46:883–89.

Cantwell, D. P., Baker, L., and Rutter, M. 1978. Family factors. In M. Rutter and E. Schopler, eds., *Autism: A Reappraisal of Concepts and Treatment.* 269–96. New York: Plenum Press.

Chess, S., Korns, S. J., and Fernandez, P. B. 1971. *Psychiatric Disorders of Children with Congenital Rubella.* New York: Brunner/Mazel.

Connor, J. M., Pirrit, L. A., Yates, J. R., Fryer, A. E., and Ferguson-Smith, M. A. 1987. Linkage of the tuberous sclerosis locus to a DNA polymorphism detected by v-abl. *Journal of Medical Genetics* 24:544–46.

DeArce, M. A., and Kearns, A. 1984. The fragile X syndrome: The patients and their chromosomes. *Journal of Medical Genetics* 21:84–91.

DeLong, R. G., and Dwyer, J. T. 1988. Correlation of family history with specific autistic subgroups: Asperger's syndrome and bipolar affective disease. *Journal of Autism and Developmental Disorders* 18:593–600.

Deykin, E. Y., and MacMahon, B. 1980. Pregnancy, delivery and neonatal complications among autistic children. *American Journal of Diseases of Children* 134:860–64.

Donis-Keller, H., Green, P., Helms, C., Cartinhour, S., Weiffenbach, B., Stephens, K., Keith, T. P., Bowden, D. W., Smith, D. R., Lander, E. S., Botstein, D., Akots, G., Rediker, K. S., Gravius, T., Brown, V. A., Rising, M. B., Parker, C., Powers., J. A., Watt, D. E., Kauffman, E. R., Bricker, A., Phipps, P., Muller-Kahle, H., Fulton, T. R., Ng, S., Schumm, J. W., Braman, J. C., Knowlton, R. G., Barker, D. F., Crooks, S. M., Lincoln, S. E., Daly, M. J., and Abrahamson, J. 1987. A genetic linkage map of the human genome. *Cell* 51:319–37.

Einfeld, S., Molony, H., and Hall, W. 1989. Autism is not associated with fragile X syndrome. *American Journal of Medical Genetics* 34:187–93.

Falconer, D. S. 1965. The inheritance of liability to certain disease, estimated from the incidence among relatives. *Annals of Human Genetics* 29:51–76.

Fisch, G. S., Cohen, I. L., Wolf, E. G., Brown, W. T., Jenkins, E. C., and Gross, A. 1986. *American Journal of Psychiatry* 143:71–73.

Folstein, S. E., and Rutter, M. L. 1977. Infantile autism: A genetic study of 21 twin pairs. *Journal of Child Psychology and Psychiatry* 18:297–321.

Folstein, S. E., and Rutter, M. L. 1988. Autism: Familial aggregation and genetic implications. *Journal of Autism and Developmental Disorders* 18:3–30.

Freeman, B. J., Ritvo, E. R., Mason-Brothers, A., Pingree, C., Yokota, A., Jensen, W. R., McMahon, W. M., Petersen, P. B., Mo, A., and Schroth, P. 1989. Psychometric assessment of first-degree relatives of 62 autistic probands in Utah. *American Journal of Psychiatry* 146:361–64.

Fryer, A. E., Connor, J. M., Povey, S., Yates, J. R. W., Chalmers, A., Fraser, I., Yates, A. D., and Osborne, J. P. 1987. Evidence that the gene for tuberous sclerosis is on chromosome 9. *Lancet* 1:659–60.

Gillberg, C., and Wahlstrom, J. 1985. Chromosome abnormalities in infantile autism and other childhood psychoses: A population study of 66 cases. *Developmental Medicine and Child Neurology* 27:293–304.

Gillberg, C., and Gillberg, I. C. 1983. Infantile autism: A total population study of nonoptimal, pre-, peri-, and neonatal conditions. *Journal of Autism and Developmental Disorders* 13:153–66.

Gillberg, C., Ohlson, V. A., Wahlstrom, J., Steffenburg, S., and Blix, K. 1988. Monozygotic female twins with autism and the fragile-x syndrome. *Journal of Child Psychology and Psychiatry* 29:447–51.

Gillberg, C., and Forsell, C. 1984. Childhood psychosis and neurofibromatosis: More than a coincidence? *Journal of Autism and Developmental Disorders* 14:1–8.

Gillberg, C. 1989. Asperger syndrome in 23 Swedish children. *Developmental Medicine and Child Neurology* 31:520–31.

Gillberg, C., Gillberg, I. C., and Steffenburg, S. 1992. Siblings and parents of children with autism: a controlled population-based study. *Developmental Medicine and Child Neurology* 34:389–98.

Goldfine, P. E., McPherson, P. M., Heath, G. A., Hardesty, V. A., Beauregard, L. J., and Gordon, B. 1985. Association of fragile x syndrome with autism. *American Journal of Psychiatry* 142:108–10.

Gurling, H. 1986. Candidate genes and favoured loci: Strategies for molecular genetic research into schizophrenia, manic depression, autism, alcoholism and Alzheimer's disease. *Psychiatric Developments* 4:289–309.

Hackney, L. M., Hanley, W. B., Davidson, W., and Lindsao, L. 1968. Phenylketonuria: Mental development, behavior, and termination of low phenylalanine diet. *Journal of Pediatrics* 72:646–55.

Hagerman, R. J., Jackson, A. W., Levitas, A., Rimland, B., and Braden, M. 1986. An analysis of autism in fifty males with the fragile X syndrome. *American Journal of Medical Genetics* 25:359–74.

Hansen, A., Brask, B. H., Nielsen, J., Rasmussen, K., and Sillesen, I. 1977. A case report of an autistic girl with an extra bisatellited marker chromosome. *Journal of Autism and Developmental Disorders* 7:263–67.

Hanson, D. R., and Gottesman, I. I. 1976. The genetics, if any, of infantile autism and childhood schizophrenia. *Journal of Autism and Developmental Disorders* 6:209–34.

Hay, D. A., Prior, M. R., Collett, S., and Williams, M. 1987. Speech and language development in preschool twins. *Acta Geneticae Medicae et Gemellologicae: Twin Research* 36:213–23.

Hay, D. A., O'Brien, P. J., Johnston, C. J., and Prior, M. R. 1984. The high incidence of reading disability in twin boys and its implications for genetic analyses. *Acta Geneticae Medicae et Gemellologicae: Twin Research* 33:223–36.

Hertzig, M. E., Snow, M. E., New, E., and Shapiro, T. 1990. DSM-III and DSM-III-R diagnosis of autism and pervasive developmental disorder in nursery school children. *Journal of the American Academy of Child and Adolescent Psychiatry* 29:123–26.

Hoshino, Y., Yashima, Y., Tachibana, R., Kaneko, M., Watanabe, M., and

Kumashiro, H. 1979. Sex chromosome abnormalities in autistic children. *Fukishima Journal of Medicine* 26:31–42.

Hunt, A., and Dennis, J. 1987. Psychiatric disorders among children with tuberous sclerosis. *Developmental Medicine and Child Neurology* 29:190–98.

Jayakar, P., Chudley, A. E., Ray, M., Evans, J. A., Perlov, J., and Wand, R. 1986. Fra 2 (q13) and Inv (9) (p11q12) in autism: Causal relationship? *American Journal of Medical Genetics* 23:381–92.

Johnson, H. G., Eckman, P., Friesen, W., Nyhan, W. L., and Shear, C. 1976. A behavioral phenotype in the de Lange syndrome. *Pediatric Research* 10:843–50.

Jones, M. B., and Szatmari, P. 1988. Stoppage rules and genetic studies of autism. *Journal of Autism and Developmental Disorders* 18:31–40.

Jorde, L. B., Hasstedt, S. J., Ritvo, E. R., Mason-Brothers, A., Freeman, B. J., Pingree, C., McMahon, W. M., Peterson, B., Jenson, W. R., and Moll, A. 1991. Complex segregation analysis of autism. *American Journal of Human Genetics* 49:932–38.

Kanner, L. 1943. Autistic disturbances of affective contact. *Nervous Child* 12:217–50.

Kanner, L., and Eisenberg, L. 1957. Early infantile autism, 1945–1955. In: *A Psychiatric Research Reports.* Volume 7, 55–65. Washington, D.C.: American Psychiatric Association.

Kandt, R. S., Haines, J. L., Smith, M., Northrup, H., Gardner, R. J. M., Short, M. P., Dumars, K., Roach, E. S., Steingold, S., Wall, S., Blanton, S. H., Flodman, P., Kwiatkowski, D. J., Jewell, A., Weber, J. L., Roses, A. D., and Pericak-Vance, M. A. 1992. Presentation at the meeting of the American Society of Human Genetics. San Francisco, California. Nov. 9–13, 1992.

Kotsopoulos, S., and Kutty, K. M. 1979. Histidinemia and infantile autism. *Journal of Autism and Developmental Disorders* 9:55–60.

Landa, R., Folstein, S., and Issacs, C. 1991. Spontaneous narrative-discourse performance of parents of autistic individuals. *Journal of Speech and Hearing Research* 34:1339–45.

Landa, R., Piven, J., Wzorek, M., Gayle, J., Chase, G., and Folstein, S. 1992. Social language use in parents of autistic individuals. *Psychological Medicine* 22:945–54.

Lander, E. S., and Botstein, D. 1986. Strategies for studying heterogeneous genetic traits in humans by using a linkage map of restriction fragment length polymorphisms. *Proceedings of the National Academy of Science, USA* 83:7353–57.

LeCouteur, A., Rutter, M., Summers, D., and Butler, L. 1988. Letter: Fragile X in female autistic twins. *Journal of Autism and Developmental Disorders* 18:458–60.

LeCouteur, A., Bailey, A. J., Rutter, M., and Gottesman, I. An epidemiology based twin study of autism. Presentation at the **First World Congress on Psychiatric Genetics**, Churchill College, Cambridge, August 3–5, 1989.

LeCouteur, A., Rutter, M., Lord, C., Rios, P., Robertson, S., Holdgrafer, M., and McLennan, J. 1989. Autism diagnostic interview: A standardized investigator-based instrument. *Journal of Autism and Developmental Disorders* 19:363–87.

Lord, C., and Schopler, E. 1985. Brief report: Differences in sex ratios in autism as a function of measured intelligence. *Journal of Autism and Developmental Disorders* 15:185–93.

Lord, C., Rutter, M., Goode, S., Heemsbergen, J., Mawhood, L., and Schopler, E. 1989. Autism diagnostic observation schedule: A standardized observation of communicative and social behavior. *Journal of Autism and Developmental Disorders* 19:185–212.

Lotter, V. 1966. Epidemiology of autistic conditions in young children: I. Prevalence. *Social Psychiatry* 1:124–37.

Lotter, V. 1974. Factors related to outcome in autistic children. *Journal of Autism and Childhood Schizophrenia* 4:263–77.

Lowe, T. L., Tanaka, K., Seashore, M. R., Young, J. G., and Cohen, D. J. 1980. Detection of phenylketonuria in autistic and psychotic children. *Journal of the American Medical Association* 243:126–28.

Macdonald, H., Rutter, M., Rios, P., and Bolton, P. Cognitive and social abnormalities in the siblings of autistic and Down's syndrome probands. Paper presentation at the **First World Congress on Psychiatric Genetics**, Churchill College, Cambridge, August 3–5, 1989.

Mansheim, P. 1979. Tuberous sclerosis and autistic behavior. *Journal of Clinical Psychiatry* 40:97–98.

Mariner, R., Jackson, A. W., Levitas, A., Hagerman, R. J., Braden, M., McBogg, P. M., Smith, A. C. M., and Berry, R. 1986. Autism, mental retardation and chromosomal abnormalities. *Journal of Autism and Developmental Disorders* 16:425–40.

McKusick, V. A. 1992. *Mendelian Inheritance in Man: Catalogs of Autosomal Dominant, Autosomal Recessive, and X-Linked Phenotypes, Tenth Edition.* Baltimore: Johns Hopkins University Press, pp. 1893–1894.

Minton, J., Campbell, M., Green, W., Jennings, S., and Samit, C. 1982. Cognitive assessment of siblings of autistic children. *Journal of the American Academy of Child and Adolescent Psychiatry* 213:256–61.

Nichols, P. L. 1984. Familial mental retardation. *Behavioral Genetics* 14:161–70.

Nielsen, J., Christensen, K. R., Friedrich, U., Zeuthen, E., and Ostergaard, O. 1973. Childhood of males with the XYY Syndrome. *Journal of Autism and Childhood Schizophrenia* 3:5–26.

Northrup, H., Beaudet, A. L., O'Brien, W. E., Herman, G. E., Lewis, R. A., and Pollack, M. S. 1987. Linkage of tuberous sclerosis to ABO blood group. *Lancet* 2:804–5.

Nyhan, W. L. 1972. Behavioral phenotypes in organic genetic disease. *Psychiatric Research* 6:1–9.

Ozonoff, S., Pennington, B. F., and Rogers, S. J. 1991. Executive function deficits in high-functioning autistic individuals: Relationship to theory of mind. *Journal of Child Psychology and Psychiatry* 32:1081–1105.

Pauls, D. L., and Leckman, J. F. 1986. The inheritance of Gilles de la Tourette syndrome and associated behaviors: Evidence for autosomal dominant transmission. *New England Journal of Medicine* 315:993–96.

Payton, J. B., Steele, M. W., Wenger, S. L., and Minshew, N. J. 1989. The fragile X marker and autism in perspective. *Journal of the American Academy of Child and Adolescent Psychiatry* 28:417–21.

Pennington, B. F. 1986. Issues in the diagnosis and phenotype analysis of dyslexia: Implications for family studies. In *Genetics and Learning Disabilities.* Edited by S. D. Smith. San Diego: College Hill Press.

Penrose, L. S. 1953. The genetical background of common diseases. *Acta Geneticae* 4:257–65.

Piven, J., Gayle, J., Chase, G., Fink, B., Landa, R., Wzorek, M., and Folstein, S. 1990. A family history study of neuropsychiatric disorders in the adult siblings of autistic individuals. *Journal of the American Academy of Child and Adolescent Psychiatry* 29:177–83.

Piven, J., Landa, R., Gayle, J., Cloud, D., Chase, G., and Folstein, S. E. 1991. Psychiatric disorders in the parents of autistic individuals. *Journal of the American Academy of Child and Adolescent Psychiatry* 30:471–78.

Piven, J., Tsai, G. G., Nehme, E., Coyle, J., Chase, G. and Folstein, S. Platelet serotonin, a possible marker for familial autism. 1991a. *Journal of Autism and Developmental Disorders* 21:51–59.

Piven, J., Gayle, J., Landa, R., Wzorek, M., and Folstein, S. 1991b. The prevalence of fragile X in a sample of autistic individuals diagnosed using a standardized interview. *Journal of the American Academy of Child and Adolescent Psychiatry* 30:825–30.

Piven, J., Landa, R., Wzorek, M., Gayle, J., Costa, P., Bolton, P., Chase, G., and Folstein, S. Personality Characteristics in the Parents of Autistic Individuals. Unpublished manuscript.

Prior, M., and Hoffman, M. 1990. Brief Report: Neuropsychological testing of autistic children through an exploration with frontal lobe tests. *Journal of Autism and Developmental Disorders* 20:581–90.

Propping, P., and Vogel, F. 1976. Twin studies in medical genetics. *Acta Geneticae Medical et Gemellologiae* 25:249–58.

Pueschel, S. M., Herman, R., and Groden, G. 1985. Brief report: Screening children with autism for Fragile X and phenylketonuria. *Journal of Autism and Developmental Disorders* 15:335–38.

Ramos, F. J., Emanuel, B. S., and Spinner, N. B. 1992. Frequency of the common fragile site at Xq27.2 under conditions of thymidylate stress: Implications for cytogenetic diagnosis of the fragile X syndrome. *American Journal of Medical Genetics* 42:835–38.

Reiss, A. L., and Freund, L. 1990. Fragile X syndrome, DSM III-R and autism. *Journal of the American Academy of Child and Adolescent Psychiatry* 29:885–91.

Reiss, A. L., Feinstein, C., Rosenbaum, K. N., Borengasser-Caruso, M. A., and Godsmith, B. M. 1985. Autism associated with Williams syndrome. *Journal of Pediatrics* 106:247–49.

Richardson, S. A., Koller, H., Katz, M., and McLaren, J. 1980. Seizures and epilepsy in a mentally retarded population over the first 22 years of life. *Applied Research in Mental Retardation* 1:123–38.

Riikonen, R., and Amnell, G. 1981. Psychiatric disorders in children with early infantile spasms. *Developmental Medicine and Child Neurology* 23:747–60.

Ritvo, E. R., Spence, M. A., Freeman, B. J., Mason-Brothers, A., Mo, A., and Mazarita, M. L. 1985. Evidence for autosomal recessive inheritance in 46 families with multiple-incidences of autism. *American Journal of Psychiatry* 142:187–92.

Ritvo, E. R., Freeman, B. J., Mason-Brothers, A., Mo, A., and Ritvo, A. M. 1985a. Concordance for the syndrome of autism in 40 pairs of afflicted twins. *American Journal of Psychiatry* 142:74–77.

Ritvo, E., Brothers, A. M., and Freeman, B. J. 1988. Eleven possibly autistic parents [letter]. *Journal of Autism and Developmental Disorders* 18:139–43.

Ritvo, E. R., Freeman, B. J., Pingree, C., Mason-Brothers, A., Jorde, L., Jenson, W., McMahon, W. M., Petersen, W., Mo, A., and Ritvo, A. 1989. The UCLA–University of Utah epidemiologic survey of autism: Prevalence. *American Journal of Psychiatry* 146:194–99.

Ritvo, E. R., Jorde, L. B., Mason-Brothers, A., Freeman, B. J., Pingree, C., Jones, M. B., McMahon, W. M., Petersen, P. B., Jenson, W. R., and Mo, A. 1989. The UCLA–University of Utah epidemiologic survey of autism: Recurrence risk estimates and genetic counseling. *American Journal of Psychiatry* 146:1032–36.

Rogers S. J., and Newhart-Larson, S. 1989. Characteristics of infantile autism in five children with Leber's congenital amaurosis. *Developmental Medicine and Child Neurology* 31:598–608.

Rumsey, J. M., and Hamburger, S. D. 1988. Neuropsychological findings in high-functioning men with infantile autism, residual state. *Journal of Clinical and Experimental Neuropsychology* 10:201–21.

Rutter, M. 1968. Concepts of autism: A review of research. *Journal of Child Psychology and Psychiatry* 9:1–25.

Rutter, M., and Bartak, L. 1971. Causes of infantile autism: Some considerations from recent research. *Journal of Autism and Childhood Schizophrenia* 1:20–32.

Rutter, M. 1988. Biological basis of autism:Implications for intervention. In F. J. Menolascino and J. A. Stark, eds. *Preventive and Curative Intervention in Mental Retardation.* Baltimore: P.H. Brookes Publishing, pp. 265–294.

Rutter, M., Macdonald, H., Le Couteur, A., Harrington, R., Bolton, P., and Bailey, A. 1990. Genetic factors in child psychiatric disorders-II: Empirical findings. *Journal of Child Psychology and Psychiatry* 31:39–83.

Smalley, S. L., Asarnow, R. F., and Spence, A. 1988. Autism and genetics: A decade of research. *Archives of General Psychiatry* 45:953–61.

Smalley, S. L., Von Stultz, J. M., Washington, K. M., and Tanguay, P. E. 1992. Autism and affective disorders. Poster presentation at the Meeting of the American Society of Human Genetics, San Francisco, California. Nov. 9–13, 1992.

Smalley, S. L., Tanguay, P. E., Smith, M., and Gutierrez, G. 1992a. Autism and tuberous sclerosis. *Journal of Autism and Developmental Disorders* 22:339–55.

Smith, M., Smalley, S., Cantor, R., Pandolfo, M., Gomez, M. I., Bauman, R., Flodman, P., Yoshiyama, K., Nakamura, Y., Julier, C., Dumars, K., Haines, J., Trofalter, J., Spence, M. A., Weeks, D., and Conneally, M. 1990. Mapping of a gene determining tuberous sclerosis to human chromosome 11q14–11q23. *Genomics* 6:105–14.

Spence, M. A. 1976. Genetic Studies. In E. R. Ritvo, ed. *Autism: Diagnosis, Current Research and Management.* New York: Spectrum Publishers, pp. 169–174.

Spence, M. A., Ritvo, E. R., Marazota, M. L., Funderburk, S. J., Sparkes, R. S., and Freeman, B. J. 1985. Gene mapping studies with the syndrome of autism. *Behavioral Genetics* 15:1–13.

Steele, M. W., Rosser, L., Rodnan, J. B., and Bryce, M. 1986. Effect of sibship position on reproductive behavior of couples after the birth of a genetically handicapped child. *Clinical Genetics* 30:328–34.

Steffenberg, S., Gillberg, C., and Holmgren, L. 1989. A twin study of autism in Denmark, Finland, Iceland, Norway, and Sweden. *Journal of Child Psychology and Psychiatry* 30:405–16.

Steffenburg, S., and Gillberg, C. 1986. Autism and autistic-like conditions in Swedish rural and urban areas: A population study. *British Journal of Psychiatry* 138:416–22.

Sutherland, B. S., Berry, H. K., and Shirkey, H. C. 1960. A syndrome of Phenylketonuria with normal intelligence and behavior disturbances. *Journal of Pediatrics* 57:521–25.

Sutherland, G. R., and Baker, E. 1990. The common fragile site in band q27 of the human x chromosome is not coincident with the fragile X. *Clinical Genetics* 37:167–72.

Szatmari, P., and Jones, M. B. 1991. IQ and the genetics of autism. *Journal of Child Psychology and Psychiatry* 32:897–908.

Taft, L. T., and Cohen, H. J. 1971. Hypsarrhythmia and infantile autism: A clinical report. *Journal of Autism and Childhood Schizophrenia* 1:327–36.

Tsai, L. Y., Stewart, M. A., and August, G. 1981. Implication of sex differences in the familial transmission of infantile autism. *Journal of Autism and Developmental Disorders* 11:165–73.

Tsai, L. 1991. Autistic disorder. In J. M. Wiener, ed. *Textbook of Child and Adolescent Psychiatry.* Washington, D.C.: American Psychiatric Press, pp. 169–191.

Tsai, L. Y., and Madsen–Beisler, J. 1983. The development of sex differences in infantile autism. *British Journal of Psychiatry* 142:373–78.

Tsai, L. Y., Crowe, R. R., Patil, S. R., Murray, J., and Quinn, J. 1988. A study of autism using X chromosome DNA probes. *Biological Psychiatry* 24:473–79.

Turner, G., Robinson, H., Laing, S., and Purvis-Smith, S. 1986. Preventive screening for the fragile-X syndrome. *New England Journal of Medicine* 315:607–9.

Vandenberg, S. G., Singer, S. M., and Pauls, D. L., eds. 1986. *The Heredity of Behavior Disorders in Adults and Children.* New York: Plenum, pp. 201–207.

Verkerk, A. J. M. H., Pieretti, M., Sutcliffe, J. S., Fu, Y.-H., Kuhl, D. P. A., Pizotti, A., Reiner, O., Richards, S., Victoria, M. F., Ahang, F., Eussen, B. E., Van Ommen, G. J. B., Blonden, L. A. J., Riggins, G. J., Ghastain, J. C., Kunst, C. B., Galjaard, H., Caskey, C. T., Nelson, D. C., Oostra, B. A., and Warren, S. T. 1991. Identification of a gene (FMR-1) containing a CGG repeat coincident with a breakpoint cluster region exhibiting length variation in fragile X syndrome. *Cell* 65:905–14.

Volkmar, F. R., Bregman, J., Cohen, D. J., and Cicheetti, D. V. 1988. DSM-III and DSM-III-R diagnosis of autism. *American Journal of Psychiatry* 11:1404–8.

Volkmar, F. R., and Nelson, D. S. 1989. Seizure disorders in autism. *Journal of the American Academy of Child and Adolescent Psychiatry* 29:127–29.

Wahlstrom, J., Gillberg, C., Gustavson, K. H., and Holmgren, G. 1986. Infantile autism and the fragile X: A Swedish multicenter study. *American Journal of Psychiatry* 23:403–8.

Wing, L., Yeates, S. R., Brierley, L. M., and Gould, J. 1976. The prevalence of early childhood autism: Comparison of administrative and epidemiological studies. *Psychological Medicine* 6:89–100.

Wing, L. 1981. Sex ratios in early childhood autism and related conditions. *Psychiatry Research* 5:129–37.

Wolff, S., Narayan, S., and Moyes, B. 1988. Personality characteristics of parents of autistic children. *Journal of Child Psychology and Psychiatry* 29:143–53.

Woolf, L. I., Griffiths, R., and Moncrief, A. 1955. Treatment of phenylketonuria with a diet low in phenylalanine. *British Medical Journal* 1:57–64.

Wzorek, M., Landa, R., Piven, J., and Folstein, S. 1991. Cognition in parents and siblings of autistic probands. Presentation at the meeting of the American Psychiatric Association, New Orleans, Louisiana. May 11–16, 1991.

3

NEUROPHYSIOLOGIC OBSERVATIONS IN AUTISM AND IMPLICATIONS FOR NEUROLOGIC DYSFUNCTION

Michelle Dunn, Ph.D.

Autism is a behavioral syndrome of early childhood (DeMeyer et al., 1981; Rutter and Schopler, 1987) characterized by impaired socialization and communication in the presence of perseveration and poor cognitive flexibility. At one time thought to be determined by psychodynamic factors, autism is now widely held to reflect the dysfunction of as-yet-unidentified brain systems. The neurologic hypothesis of autism was originally advanced based on the observation that symptoms began very early in life and could not be consistently associated with defective parenting or other severe environmental stressors. Although mental deficiency, attention deficit, and seizures are commonly present, they are not core symptoms and may indicate the dysfunction of additional brain systems.

Intelligence in autistic individuals may range from profoundly retarded to superior. It is estimated that between 5 and 30 percent of autistic individuals have intelligence in the normal range (DeMeyer, 1979).

The mean or typical cognitive profile (Rutter, 1978; Lincoln et al., 1988) in the autistic population indicates that nonverbal abilities are significantly stronger than verbal abilities. Particularly remarkable is a very impaired ability to answer wh-questions, which require higher-level language comprehension, expression, and social problem solving, in the face of especially strong visuospatial abilities.

There is a range of individual variation in the cognitive profiles. Lincoln et al. (1988) found that twenty-seven of thirty-three autistic individuals showed the typical profile. Fein et al. (1985) found that while approximately 60 percent of their sample showed the classic profile, 20 percent showed a flat profile and 20 percent showed a reversed profile with language superiority.

Autism is thought to reflect nonprogressive brain impairment. Deficits are lifelong, even in the highest-functioning individuals. The presence of brain abnormalities has been supported by brain imaging (Courchesne et al., 1987; Piven et al., 1990; Courchesne, 1991), pathologic studies (Bauman, 1991), and neurophysiologic studies (Novick et al., 1980; Courchesne, 1987).

There are three major methodologic approaches to research addressing the identification of affected brain systems in autism: (1) cognitive and behavioral evaluations attempt to discover those deficits that are specific to autism; (2) structural abnormalities are identified through magnetic resonance imaging and pathologic studies; and (3) electrophysiologic studies attempt to identify brain systems that function aberrantly and relate brain and behavioral abnormalities. In the first case hypotheses concerning the brain systems responsible for the core deficits in autism are based largely on the pattern of spared and impaired cognitive, behavioral, and motor functions. To date, the findings of imaging, pathologic, and electrophysiologic studies are preliminary and are based on a small number of individuals.

A major goal for the field is to relate structural abnormalities and aberrant neural processing to the cognitive and behavioral deficits specific to autism. Neuropsychological evaluation is useful for detailing cognitive and behavioral functioning and, in individuals with acquired lesions, for identifying the location of brain abnormality. However, in developmentally impaired populations, patterns of neuropsychological findings can establish functional integrity, but, due to issues of neural plasticity in the developing brain, may not indicate the locus of neurologic dysfunction (Fletcher and Taylor, 1984).

New electrophysiologic techniques of topographic analysis provide a powerful tool for studying the relationship between cognition/behavior and brain activity. By recording brain electrical activity while a person is actively engaged in a task, it is possible to identify a spatial pattern of neural activation during the time that is associated with the performance of that task. Behavioral task requirements are established to engage aspects of processing subserved by specific functional brain systems. By comparing the spatiotemporal patterns seen in autistic individuals with those of normal subjects, investigators can identify abnormal patterns of activation of brain regions.

NEUROPHYSIOLOGIC OBSERVATIONS

ELECTROENCEPHALOGRAPHY

Electroencephalography (EEG) was the first neurophysiologic technique used to investigate the neurobiology of autism. There is a high prevalence of EEG abnormalities and seizure disorders in the autistic population. This provided some of the earliest support for the notion that autism has a biologic basis. Most EEG abnormalities seen in autism include diffuse or focal spikes or slowing and paroxysmal spike-and-wave activity. The abnormalities have involved all regions of cortex, not one specific brain region (Minshew, 1991). There is a significant relationship between the presence of EEG abnormality and IQ in autism. Seventy-five percent of autistic persons with abnormal EEGs have IQs in the moderate range of mental deficiency (IQ=35–49), while 58 percent of autistic persons with normal EEGs have IQs in this range (Small, 1975). A similar relationship exists between cognitive level and epilepsy. The onset of seizures occurs most often in early childhood or in adolescence (Volkmar and Nelson, 1990), although epilepsy may begin at any age in autism (Lockyer and Rutter, 1970; Gillberg and Steffenburg, 1987).

Research on EEG abnormalities and epilepsy in autism has included both idiopathic cases as well as individuals whose autism was secondary to acquired damage. Until recently, it was not recognized that a single recording might not detect EEG abnormalities. Further, complex partial and minor motor seizures might go undetected unless telemetric EEG monitoring is used. Awareness of these issues will no doubt improve our understanding of the relation of EEG abnormalities and epilepsy to autism.

EEG in the 8- to 12-Hz frequency band, otherwise known as alpha activity, is selectively attenuated in brain areas activated during different cognitive tasks. Alpha supression is seen as grossly indicative of the general neural regions activated in information processing (Butler and Glass, 1974; Doyle, Galin, and Ornstein, 1974) and has been utilized to gain a preliminary understanding of the hemispheric lateralization and intrahemispheric topography of information processing in autistic persons. Small (1975) recorded the resting EEG over right- and left-occipital lobes in normal and autistic subjects. Normal subjects showed higher mean integrated voltage values for the left hemisphere than they did for the right hemisphere, while autistic subjects showed no asymmetry. Ogawa et al. (1982) recorded EEG activity during the delivery of clicks and flashes in two- through eight-year-old autistic and normal children. Forty-two percent of the normal subjects showed an asymmetry for the clicks; none of the autistic children did ($N = 21$). For the flashes, 64 percent of normal subjects showed an asymmetry, while only 28 percent of autistic subjects showed any asymmetry. Dawson, Warrenburg, and Fuller recorded right- and left-hemisphere parietal alpha activity in nine- to thirty-four-year-old subjects during verbal and spatial cognitive tasks (1982) and during manual and oromotor imitation tasks (1983). Autistic subjects showed greater activation over the right hemisphere during the verbal tasks than did normal subjects. Seven of ten autistic subjects showed this right-hemihere dominance. In the autistic sample, greater asymmetry was directly related to IQ and age. There was no difference in activation over the two hemispheres between the autistic and normal samples during spatial activities. Again, autistic subjects showed greater activity over the right hemihere during the motor tasks, particularly during oromotor imitation. Older autistic subjects tended to show patterns of asymmetry more like those of the normal subjects for all tasks.

EVENT-RELATED POTENTIALS

Event-related potentials (ERPs) reflect brain electrical activity, which is time-locked to a discrete event such as a stimulus or motor act. Averaged over many trials, the stimulus-specific response emerges from the background EEG, which is not time-locked to the event. The auditory brainstem response, early cortical potentials, and some cognitive/endogenous potentials have been studied in the autistic population. Sensory evoked potentials (EPs) are obligatory brain responses to the physical attributes of a stimulus. They are influenced by intensity, duration, and frequency characteristics. The waveform reflects the sequential activation of brain structures underlying sensory processing from the periphery through primary sensory cortex. Cognitive or endogenous potentials are associated with the cognitive processing of stimuli. A variety of endogenous components follow or overlap with the obligatory ERPs. ERP recording is used clinically to determine the integrity of a neural system from periphery to cortex. It is also a powerful research tool for determining the location and timing of neural activation associated with specific aspects of cognitive processing.

FINDINGS ON AUDITORY BRAINSTEM RESPONSE IN AUTISM

The auditory brainstem response (ABR) is a short-latency EP generated within the subcortical auditory pathways from the ear through the brainstem. It is elicited by a brief auditory stimulus (i.e., clicks or tones), which is comprised of five positive waves occurring within 10–15 msec of the onset of the stimulus. Waves I and II represent activity of the eighth cranial nerve. Wave III is the result of activity in the lower pons and in the area of the superior olive, while Wave V is related to activity in the upper pons and in the area of the inferior colliculus. The latencies and amplitudes of the peaks of these waves relative to norms and to each other indicate the presence or absence of dysfunction at different levels of the system being assessed. However, each component has multiple generators, thereby making it difficult to assess locus of dysfunction (Stockard et al., 1986). The ABR assesses auditory sensitivity in infants and in others in whom behavioral audiometric testing is precluded by cognitive/behavioral impairment. The ABR is also used to assess the integrity of the brainstem auditory pathway.

Although not a symptom included in current diagnostic criteria for autism, a frequently associated feature is inadequate modulation of sensory input (Ornitz, 1989). Autistic people may overreact to certain sounds in their environment (such as the sounds of hair dryers and vacuum cleaners) and completely disregard other loud noises or the human voice. This observation, implicating brainstem dysfunction in autism, prompted a series of studies exploring the integrity of the auditory brainstem pathways through examination of ABRs. ABR studies in autistic subjects have yielded inconsistent results. Some have reported a high prevalence of prolonged brainstem transmission times, while others have reported shortened transmission times, and still others have shown no abnormalities (Tanguay et al., 1982; Rumsey et al., 1984; Courchesne et al., 1987). It is difficult to interpret these studies due to failure to exclude subjects with frank neurologic disease from the sample to be studied, and questionable diagnostic criteria for autism. Tanguay et al. (1982) found no differences in ABRs between autistic and normal children when they were matched for age and gender and the autistic children selected had normal hearing and no other sign of neurologic disorder. Both Courchesne et al. (1985) and Grillon et al. (1989) found no brainstem transmission abnormalities when they controlled for mental retardation and associated neurologic disorders. Rumsey et al. (1984) reported normal ABRs in all but one of their subjects, who ranged in intelligence from profoundly retarded to above average. Their exclusionary criteria included infectious, metabolic, and neurologic disease, and severe sensory impairment. Their subjects were matched for gender. The presence of peripheral hearing loss appears to account for the abnormal ABR results in two studies (Skoff et al., 1980; Tanguay et al., 1982).

Whereas ABR studies were intended to assess the integrity of the auditory brainstem pathways and not to assess peripheral sensitivity, taken together they reveal that a relatively high percentage of autistic individuals have peripheral hearing impairment. Fourteen of thirty-two subjects studied by Taylor et al. (1982) were moderately to profoundly hearing impaired as assessed by ABR thresholds. All of Student's and Sohmer's (1978) subjects and 46 percent of those examined by Skoff et al. (1986) exhibited peripheral hearing impairment. Because autistic persons can be very difficult to test behaviorally, some reaction to sound is often interpreted as ruling out deafness. Hearing impairment may be widely overlooked in autistic individuals; in fact, the prevalence of sensorineural hearing loss may be higher than it is in the normal population and higher than previously thought. A retrospective study done by Konstantareas and Homatidis (1987) has indicated a greater prevalence of otitis media in autistic than in normal subjects. Otitis media is a frequent cause of conductive hearing loss (Friel-Patti and Finzo, 1990). Hearing sensitivity influences language development (Gravel et al., 1990; Gravel and Wallace, 1992). Therefore, it is important, especially in developmentally impaired populations, that hearing impairment be detected and treated early.

While behavioral audiometry is frequently unreliable in young and low-functioning autistic persons, the ABR (which is not sensitive to state, attentional variation, or sedative medication) is useful in assessing individuals who are extremely difficult or impossible to test behaviorally.

There is little support for dysfunction in the brainstem systems subserving auditory processing in all autistic individuals. However, a few studies found interpeak latency abnormalities that cannot be questioned on methodologic grounds (Skoff et al. 1980, 1986; Gillberg et al., 1983). It appears that prolonged brainstem transmission times may exist in a subset of autistic individuals.

FINDINGS ON ERPS IN AUTISM

Before addressing the findings of the cortical ERP studies in autism, a brief description of the relevant ERP components and the conditions under which they are elicited is in order.

A common way to label ERP components is by polarity at the scalp electrode, and latency measured in milliseconds after stimulus onset. For example, N1 or N100 is a negativity peaking at about 100 msec after stimulus onset. P300 or P3, which has been most extensively studied in autism, is a positive potential peaking at 300 msec, although the latency of P3 varies as a function of task difficulty. Some components are not labeled according to this convention. The two that have been studied in autism are Nc, which is a frontally distributed negativity, and Nd, which is a negative waveform, derived through the subtraction method, which is seen in normal subjects during selective attention.

CORTICAL AUDITORY EPS

In adults the cortical auditory EP is comprised of the N1 component, which is a negativity occurring at a latency of about 100 msec, and the P2 component, which is a positivity peaking at approximately 200 msec. These components, also called *obligatory responses*, are generated in primary and secondary auditory cortex in the superior and lateral surfaces of the superior temporal gyrus (Vaughan and Ritter, 1970; Scherg et al., 1989). The latency and amplitude of these components vary as a function of the subject's age and the physical parameters of the stimuli. Kurtzberg et al. (1986) observed differences in wave morphology and topography associated with differences in the place of articulation and voice-onset time in infants and children.

ENDOGENOUS/COGNITIVE ERPS

Endogenous potentials are associated with the cognitive processing of stimuli. A variety of endogenous components overlap with or follow the obligatory EPs. Not all ERP components are directly observable in the waveform. When endogenous and exogenous/obligatory components overlap, it is necessary to uncover the endogenous component through the subtraction method, wherein the ERP to stimuli requiring a discriminative response is subtracted from the ERP to stimuli where no discrimination was required. The entire spectrum of components will not be reviewed in this chapter (see Picton and Hillyard, 1988, for a review); only the components that have been studied in the autistic population will be described.

Attentional control and modulation have been the focus of ERP research in autism. A number of comparisons in attention-related cognitive ERP components have been made between autistic and normal subjects and in some cases specifically developmentally language-disordered individuals. These include P3a, P3b, Nd, N270, Nc, and P700. Each is thought to reflect neural mechanisms underlying different aspects of attention.

The so-called P3a appears to be related to orientation to unexpected, salient stimulation and is elicited by novel, random, infrequent stimuli presented in a background of frequently occurring nontargets (which are expected and attended to) and infrequent targets. The subject is required to respond to the targets. The point of the task is to see how well an individual orients to novel, unexpected material while he or she is concentrating on doing a task. P3a is present in normal subjects in response to an unexpected visual or auditory event. Visual P3a is sometimes termed P400. In normal subjects the auditory P3a and the visual P400 are larger in amplitude for targets than they are for nontargets. Couchesne (1992) has conceptualized this component as being related to the capturing of attention.

The most extensively studied component in autism is P3b. P3b is typically elicited in a paradigm that involves identifying a rarely presented target that is embedded within a train of frequently occurring background stimuli. This task requires subjects to sustain their attention to and to identify accurately and consistently the rare target. P3b is present when a passive or active discrimination is made. It represents the outcome of the discriminative process. There are a number of hypotheses concerning the processes that P3b reflects. It may be related to resolution of uncertainty, working memory, or stimulus significance. It is likely that P3b has multiple generators that reflect more than one psychological process.

The parietally maximal P3b as well as the frontally distributed Nc, Nd, and N270 appear to be related to maintaining selective attention. An example of the type of task in which these components are elicited is one in which subjects were presented with a stream of auditory and visual stimuli where targets are presented randomly and infrequently in a background of frequent stimuli ("standards"). The subjects are asked either to respond to auditory targets while not responding to auditory standards and ignoring all visual stimuli, or to respond to visual targets and ignore the auditory stimuli. In normal subjects, frequent/background standard stimuli in an attended channel elicit frontal Nd (for auditory stimuli) or N270 (for visual stimuli), and auditory and visual targets elicit both Nc and P3b components. Nc and P3b have been elicited by omitted targets as well as present targets in normal subjects (Courchesne et al., 1989).

P700, a parieto-occipital positive waveform, is elicited by stimuli that signal the need for a shift in attention and appears to be related to the ability to redirect attention rapidly and accurately (Courchesne, 1992).

The relationship between information processing and changes in ERP components in normal adults has been studied extensively (Courchesne, 1983; Hillyard and Picton, 1979; Kutas and Hillyard, 1980; Ruchkin, 1980a, 1980b; Friedman et al., 1981). These data have guided research and interpretation of ERP findings in autistic subjects.

Although the general neuropsychological profile of processing strengths and weaknesses in the autistic population is known, neither neuropsychological profile nor current diagnostic criteria for autism have guided ERP research in the autistic population. As stated earlier, language impairment is a well-known and integral part of the picture of autism (Rutter, 1974). Yet, there are very few electophysiologic investigations of language deficits in autistic individuals.

Deficits in attention (James and Barry, 1980) and deficits in sensory modulation as manifested behaviorally by overreactivity and underreactivity to stimuli (Ornitz, 1992) have been explored most extensively with electrophysiologic techniques. These studies have explored responses related to orientation to novelty, as well as to sustained and selective attention. Some preliminary work has been done in directed attention and ability to shift attention appropriately.

Orienting to Novelty.   Individuals with autism do not seem to orient to novel information in a normal way. Electrophysiologic evidence supports this notion, at least for certain classes of stimuli.

Small, DeMyer, and Milstein (1971) observed no difference in the ERPS to familiar versus unfamiliar faces in their autistic sample, while clear differences in ERPs to the two sets of stimuli were seen in normal subjects: Normal subjects' responses to unfamiliar faces were more negative in polarity between 100 and 300 msec after stimulus onset than were their responses to familiar faces.

Courchesne et al. (1984, 1985) addressed this question by presenting autistic subjects of normal intelligence and normal subjects with lists of auditory or visual stimuli where 80 percent of the stimuli were background, 10 percent targets (to which a response was required), and 10 percent novels. Novel stimuli were nonsense sounds or forms. They observed an attenuation of P3a in the autistic subjects on the auditory task. In a similar visual paradigm there was no significant difference between autistic and normal subjects in P400 to novel stimuli. The differences in the P3a in the auditory task cannot be accounted for by generally impaired arousal or lack of motivation because the autistic and normal subjects did not differ with respect to behavioral performance. Of note, the attenuation of the auditory P3a resulted from averaging highly variable responses, which were of normal to below-normal amplitude and did not result from the average of consistently small responses.

Niwa et al. (1983) provided convergent evidence finding that even in "no task" conditions, where the subject was merely required to listen to auditory stimuli, were the autistic subjects' responses smaller than were the normal subjects' for rare novel stimuli.

Sustained and Selective Attention. Maintaining selective attention to specific stimuli is associated with certain ERP responses, including Nc, Nd, N270, and P3b. In autistic subjects these responses are abnormally reduced in amplitude or are absent.

The first studies of sustained attention in autistic persons were carried out by Novick et al. (1979). They utilized a paradigm where subjects were required to detect missing stimuli in a regular series of stimuli (tones or flashes). Despite normal task performance, their three autistic subjects had small or absent P3bs in both the auditory and the visual paradigms, although P3b was not as severely attenuated in the visual paradigm. Novick et al. (1980) employed an auditory paradigm in which both rare target tones differing in pitch from background stimuli and stimulus deletions were to be detected by subjects. In their five autistic adolescents, both the P2 and P3b components of the ERP were significantly smaller than were those of normal controls, once again despite normal task performance. Courchesne et al. (1984, 1985) replicated the findings with auditory stimuli, but unlike Novick et al. (1979) did not observe attenuation of P3b in the visual tasks in autistic subjects. In the Courchesne et al. (1985) study, the visual P3b was elicited by target stimuli whereas the attenuated P3b in the visual task in the Novick et al. (1979) study was elicited by stimulus omissions. It is also important to note that the auditory and visual stimuli employed by Courchesne et al. were not analogous. In the visual paradigm the target and background stimuli were letters. In the auditory paradigm the target stimulus was the word *you* and the background stimulus was the word *me*. It is possible that the differences observed were related to content as opposed to modality of presentation. The visual stimuli could have been inherently more salient for the autistic subjects than these auditory stimuli. It is widely known that many autistic persons are particularly interested in, even preoccupied with, letters. In addition, many autistic persons have difficulty discriminating pronouns. Since the degree to which information about a stimulus is used is directly related to the amplitude of P3b (Hillyard, 1985), interest level of the materials may be a potential confound. There is also other evidence that will be discussed shortly that lends support to the notion of modality-specific processing impairment in autism.

Autistic individuals have been hypothesized to have impaired selective attention (Rimland, 1964; Ornitz, 1978; Courchesne, 1987). There is a large literature concerning the use of ERPs to study selective attention (for reviews, see Harter and Aine, 1984; Hillyard and Picton, 1987; Naatanen and Picton, 1987; Woods, 1989). Ciesielski et al. (1990) employed tasks requiring focused selective attention to visual and auditory stimuli to investigate the maintenance of selective attention in autistic subjects of normal intelligence. The stimulus trains consisted of 12.5 percent rare auditory stimuli, 37.5 percent standard auditory stimuli, 12.5 percent rare visual target, and 37.5 percent standard visual stimuli. Visual stimuli were red and green flashes; auditory stimuli were high and low "sounds." In the auditory focal attention paradigm subjects were to respond to rare auditory targets; in the visual focal attention paradigm they were to respond to rare visual stimuli. Normal subjects showed the expected enhanced frontal negativities (Nd in the auditory task, N270 in the visual task, and Nc for both modalities). They also showed enhanced later positivities (P3b) at posterior electrode sites in response to all stimuli in the attended modality. In autistic subjects all visual and auditory attention-related negativities were not seen. P3b in the auditory task was significantly smaller in autistic than in normal subjects, but interestingly the visual P3b did not differ from that of the normal subjects. In similar paradigms where the target was an omitted stimulus (Courchesne, 1989) autistic subjects still did not produce the Nc and had a diminished P3b in the auditory task. These studies provide some convergent evidence for differences in processing auditory and visual material in autistic subjects.

In all of the paradigms described thus far, the behavioral performance of the autistic subjects did not differ from that of the normal controls while ERPs were clearly different. Novick et al. (1980) interpreted the attenuation of P3b as inefficient information processing. It is possible that this inefficiency is subclinical and is not reflected in deficient clinical performance until the subject is sufficiently stressed by the task demands.

Modulation of Attention.   Evidence from neuropsychological testing and behavioral observation indicates that autistic individuals have perseverative tendencies and are impaired with respect to their ability to shift their attention quickly, accurately and appropriately. Some ERP evidence (Courchesne, 1992) suggests impaired ability to shift attention is seen in the ERP. Subjects were administered a series of auditory and visual stimuli and were told to respond to targets in one of the modalities. Embedded in the train of stimuli was an attention-directing cue that signaled the subject to shift attention to the stimuli presented in the other modality and then respond to targets in the new modality. The autistic subjects were behaviorally slow to shift their attention, continuing to respond to stimuli in the first modality, although finally shifting after several seconds. In normal subjects, the cue to shift attention elicited a parietally maximal positivity peaking at about 700 msec after stimulus onset (P700). This response was much smaller in the autistic subjects.

ERPS: TOPOGRAPHY/HEMISPHERIC LATERALIZATION

Few studies have attempted to map the brain areas involved in information processing in autism. Alpha supression studies provided gross evidence for some difference in the brain regions underlying cortical information processing in autistic and normal persons. ERP studies have provided some very preliminary evidence regarding the neural substrates for nonverbal, visuospatial, and linguistic information processing in autistic individuals. Tanguay (1975) recorded auditory evoked potentials (AEP) during sleep. Normal subjects displayed larger right- than left-hemiphere potentials during REM sleep. The autistic subjects showed no differences between right- and left-hemisphere potentials. Dawson et al. (1986) examined right and left hemiphere cortical AEPs to linguistic stimuli (da). The N1 component of the AEP was larger over the right hemisphere in eleven of seventeen autistic subjects. The latency of N1 over right and left hemispheres differed from normal in their autistic group. While the N1 peak latency was earlier over the left hemiphere than it was over the right in their normal subjects, the reverse was true in the autistic subjects. It is interesting that there was no difference between the groups in N1 latency over the left hemisphere. N1 latency over the right hemisphere was much earlier in autistic than it was in normal subjects. This reversed pattern of asymmetry from normal was true of younger autistic subjects and those with poorer language abilities. Older autistic subjects with better language tended to show the normal direction of asymmetry. Taken together, the alpha supression and ERP studies appear to support the notion that the majority of autistic persons show either absent or reversed hemispheric asymmetry, at least in an earlier stage of cortical processing, for tasks requiring the processing of simple nonlinguistic stimuli (i.e., tones and flashes) and simple language stimuli (e.g., da) when compared with normal subjects.

Very few studies have explored the relationship between ability within a neuropsychological domain indexed by formal test data (e.g., language, motor, visuospatial abilities) and the pattern of hemispheric lateralization during related tasks. As alluded to earlier, there are preliminary findings regarding the relationship between the pattern of lateralization for language-related tasks and language ability. Dawson et al. (1986) found that the difference in the latency of the N1 component of the evoked response over right and left hemipheres was related to language level in their autistic sample, but not in normal subjects. Poorer language ability was associated with shorter latency for N1 over the right hemisphere than over the left. These investigators administered a variety of formal language measures to their subjects including indices of receptive and expressive vocabulary, syntax and semantics. Differences in the amplitude and latency (right minus left) of the N1 component between the two hemispheres were most strongly related to receptive vocabulary and mean length of utterance. In a later study, Dawson (1989) compared autistic children and children with specific developmental language disorder. Their results indicated that both dysphasic and autistic children had a reversed pattern of asymmetry compared to normal subjects for amplitude and latency of the N1 component of the ERP. While severity of language impairment and reversal of asymmetry were strongly related in the autistic group, this relationship did not hold in the dysphasic children.

There are some important reservations in the interpretation of most of these studies. Autistic and nonautistic subjects were not always matched for chronological age and were not consistently matched for IQ. In the Tanguay (1976) study, the autistic subjects were two-to-five-years old, while the normal subjects were four-to-five-years old. It is well known that considerable changes in the ERP accompany development; therefore, comparison of groups of children differing in age is invalid. In the studies where IQs were reported, they ranged from 40 to 113 in the autistic subjects and fell in the average to high average range in the nonautistic subjects. If one is to come to an understanding of deficits specific to autism, potential confounds such as mental deficiency and the need for appropriate control subjects must be taken into account (Prior, 1979; Rutter, 1983). In addition a limitation of the findings of the few ERP studies aimed at elucidating brain topography underlying information processing is that very few recording sites were used. These studies typically included one electrode at the vertex (Cz), one over the left temporal area, and one over the right temporal area.

IMPLICATIONS FOR NEUROLOGIC DYSFUNCTION

There are several hypothesized anatomic and neurophysiologic explanations for autism (Rimland, 1964; Damasio and Maurer, 1978; DeLong, 1978; Ornitz, 1985; Courchesne, 1987). The brainstem hypothesis of autism proposes that the etiology is related to compromised brainstem and diencephalic structures. There is little evidence from ABR studies for the involvement of structures underlying early auditory processing, save perhaps in a small subset of autistic persons. This does not rule out the involvement of other subcortical structures. Courchesne's (1987) findings appear to implicate neurophysiologic abnormalities in parietal and frontal association cortex. This is probably an oversimplified interpretation (see Courchesne, 1987, for a thoughtful treatment of this issue). A number of studies support the notion that the majority of autistic persons have either absent or reversed hemipheric asymmetry from normal for tasks requiring the processing of simple linguistic stimuli, whereas they exhibit normal patterns of hemispheric activation during spatial tasks. There is some indication that degree and direction of asymmetry for language tasks is related to chronological age and language level, with older, less-impaired autistic subjects evidencing normal or near normal patterns. In high-functioning autistic subjects, ERP abnormalities are reportedly bilaterally symmetric (Courchesne, 1987).

DIRECTIONS FOR FUTURE RESEARCH

There are a number of methodologic and conceptual considerations for future research in this area.

First, subject selection must be considered. Handedness is rarely reported for any of the subjects enrolled in these studies. This is an important consideration in evaluating possible differences in hemispheric functioning, especially for language.

High-functioning autistic persons as well as autistic individuals with mental deficiency, who comprise the largest proportion of the population, have been subjects in neurophysiologic studies. There is strong justification for having high-functioning autistic persons as subjects. They afford the possibility of discovering differences in functioning that are unique to autism without the confound of mental deficiency. If retarded autistic persons are to be subjects, then pains should be taken to recruit appropriate nonautistic, mentally deficient controls.

Most autistic subjects have been adolescents or young adults. There are few studies of children, and there are no longitudinal studies. Although autistic children are particularly difficult to assess with neurophysiologic techniques, it is possible to assess them if the session length, structuring, and reinforcement are appropriate. Through the use of longitudinal designs it is possible to identify developmental patterns, specific outcomes, and prognostic indicators.

To date, the identification of brain structures involved in information processing in the autistic population has relied on global measures such as alpha supression. ERP studies have used a very limited number of recording sites. Recently, brain electrical source analysis, a new non-invasive electrophysiologic method for localizing brain activity linked with magnetic resonance imaging (MRI) has become available for the dynamic colocalization of brain activity associated with task performance over time (Scherg et al., 1989). This technique offers converging evidence with that provided by positron emission tomography (PET) and blood flow studies to provide more specific localization of brain activity during a variety of tasks involving cognitive and linguistic processing in the auditory and visual modalities.

A major goal in the study of autism is to determine which brain systems are affected. To achieve this, it is important to specify the behavioral and cognitive deficits that are specific to autism and to identify the pathophysiology directly related to those deficits.

To date, most ERP studies in autism have focused on various aspects of attentional processing. Many behavioral and cognitive/linguistic processing deficits, specifically those enumerated in the diagnostic criteria for autism, have remained virtually unaddressed in the ERP literature.

Language impairment is one of the defining features of autism. The literature indicates a developmental asynchrony between the structural and semantic aspects of language. Autistic children may or may not exhibit deficits in the structural aspects but are invariably deficient in the semantic and pragmatic aspects. It has been proposed by some that the semantic deficit is essential to autism (Hermelin and O'Connor, 1970; Menyuk, 1978; Fay and Schuler, 1980; Tager-Flusberg, 1981a). Evidence for this view comes from autistic subjects' failure to use relational meaning in comprehending language (Tager-Flusberg, 1981b) and to aid in memorizing and learning new material (Hermelin and O'Connor, 1967). However, studies do not elucidate whether the basis of this failure lies in the structure of semantic categories or in language use. ERP semantic priming paradigms provide optimal ways for looking at the structure of semantic categories (Holcomb and Neville, 1990).

Deficits in sustained and selective attention are not specific to autism, but impairment in aspects of attentional modulation such as orienting to novelty and shifting the attentional spotlight may be characteristic. Recent ERP research has moved in the direction of assessing what appear to be characteristic attentional deficits in autism. Continued research in this area is clearly warranted. Modulation of attention is a critical issue for autistic individuals. Specifically, the ability to shift attention is impaired even in the highest-functioning autistic adults. This may be one of the deficits in autism that is most resistant to remediation. It would be important to look at the relationship between ERP findings and performance on tests and checklists that assess ability to shift set in different situations. It would also be interesting to do ERP testing under conditions where the set shifting task is so easy that the subject's performance could fall within the normal range as well as testing under conditions where behavioral performance is poor.

Differences between auditory and visual information processing in high-functioning autistic subjects reported in the literature are of great interest, especially since there is a higher prevalence of hyperlexia in the autistic population. These differences should be explored further with a variety of stimuli where content and salience to the subject are controlled or intentionally manipulated.

Although autistic individuals as a group may have certain processing deficits in common, there are individual differences; in fact, it has been suggested that there are subgroups within the autistic population (Allen, 1988). The study of heterogeneous groups of autistic individuals can yield conflicting and contradictory results. At this time subtyping may not provide an answer to this problem. There is wide disagreement concerning the dimensions along which to subtype. Some investigators have focused on behavioral and social variables, while others have included language and /or other aspects of cognition in the subtyping scheme. Single case studies that explore the relationship between a particular subject's pattern of neuropsychological strengths and deficits in information processing and the pattern of neural activation for different tasks appear to be the optimal design at present.

Through electrophysiologic paradigms, driven by our knowledge of neuropsychological processing patterns in autistic individuals, in combination with new topographic localization techniques it is possible to greatly advance our knowledge concerning the time course and neural substrates for cognitive and linguistic processing in this remarkable population.

ACKNOWLEDGMENTS

This chapter was suported by NINCDS grant 5PO1NS20489 awarded to Isabelle Rapin. I would like to thank Isabelle Rapin, M.D., Diane Kurtzberg, Ph.D., Herb Vaughan, M.D., and Judith Flax, Ph.D., for their helpful comments on this manuscript and Hilary Gomes and Saradee Cohen for comments on an earlier version.

REFERENCES

Allen, D. A. 1988. Autistic spectrum disorders: Clinical presentation in preschool children. *Journal of Child Neurology* 3:48–56.

Allen, D. A., and Rapin, I. 1992. Autistic children are also dysphasic. In Naruse, H., and Ornitz, E.M., eds. *Neurobiology of Infantile Autism*. Amsterdam: Excerpta Medica, pp. 157–68.

Ameli, R., Courchesne, E., Lincoln, A. J., Kaufman, A., and Grillon, C. 1988. Visual memory processes in high-functioning individuals with autism. *Journal of Autism and Developmental Disorders* 18:601–15.

Bartak, L., Rutter, M., and Cox, A. 1975. A comparative study of infantile autism and specific developmental receptive language disorders. I. The children. *British Journal of Psychiatry* 126:127–45.

Bartak, L., Rutter, M., and Cox, A. 1977. A comparative study of infantile autism and specific developmental receptive language disorders. III. Discriminant function analysis. *Journal of Autism and Childhood Schizophrenia* 7:383–396.

Bauman, M.L. 1991. Microscopic neuroanatomic abnormalities in autism. *Pediatrics* 87(suppl.):791–96.

Butler, S. R., and Glass, A. 1974. Asymmetries in the electroencephalogram associated with cerebral dominance. *Electroencephalography and Clinical Neurophysiology* 36:481–91.

Cohen, D. J., Paul, R., and Volkmar, F. R. 1987. Issues in the classification of pervasive developmental disorders and associated conditions. In D. J. Cohen and A. M. Donnellan, eds. *Handbook of Autism and Pervasive Developmental Disorders.* New York: Wiley, pp. 20–40.

Courchesne, E. 1983. Cognitive components of the event-related brain potential: Changes associated with development. In A. W. K. Gaillard and W. Ritter, eds. *Tutorials in ERP Research: Endogenous Components.* North Holland: Elsevier, pp. 329–44.

Courchesne, E., Kilman, B. A., Galambos, R., and Lincoln, A. J. 1984. Autism: Processing of novel auditory information assessed by event-related brain potentials. *Electroencephalography and Clinical Neurophysiology* 59:238–48.

Courchesne, E., Lincoln, A. J., Kilman, B. A., and Galambos, R. 1985. Event-related brain potential correlates of the processing of novel visual and auditory information in autism. *Journal of Autism and Developmental Disorders* 15:55–76.

Courchesne, E., Yeung-Courchesne, R., Hicks, G., and Lincoln, A. J. 1985. Functioning of brain-stem auditory pathways in non-retarded autistic individuals. *Electroencephalography and Clinical Neurophysiology* 61:491–501.

Courchesne, E. 1987. A neurophysiological view of autism. In E. Schopler and G. Mesibov, eds. *Neurobiological Issues in Autism.* New York: Plenum Press, pp. 285–324.

Courchesne, E., Elmasian, R. O., and Yeung-Courchesne, R. 1987. Electrophysiological correlates of cognitive processing: P3b and Nc, basic, clinical and developmental research. In A. M. Halliday, R. Butler, and R. Paul, eds. *A Textbook of Clinical Neurophysiology.* Chichester: Wiley, pp. 645–76.

Courchesne, E., Hesselink, J. R., Jernigan, T. L., and Yeung-Courchesne, R. 1987. Abnormal neuroanatomy in a nonretarded person with autism: Unusual findings with magnetic resonance imaging. *Archives of Neurology* 44:335–41.

Courchesne, E., Lincoln, A. J., Yeung-Courchesne, R., Elmasian, R., and Grillon, C. 1989. Pathophysiologic findings in non-retarded autism and receptive developmental language disorders. *Journal of Autism and Developmental Disorders* 19:1–17.

Courchesne, E. 1991. Neuroanatomic imaging in autism. *Pediatrics* 87(suppl.): 781–90.

Courchesne, E., Akshoomoff, N. A., and Townsend, J. 1992. Recent advances in autism. In H. Naruse and E. M. Ornitz, eds. *Neurobiology of Infantile Autism.* Amsterdam: Excerpta Medica, pp. 111–28.

Damasio, A. R., and Maurer, R. G. 1978. A neurological model for childhood autism. *Archives of Neurology* 35:777–86.

Davidson, R. J., Schwartz, G. E., Saron, C., Bennett, J., and Goleman, D. J. 1979. Frontal versus parietal EEG asymmetry during positive and negative affect. *Psychophysiology* 16:202–3.

Dawson, G., Finley, C., Phillips, S., and Galpert, L. 1986. Hemispheric specialization and the language abilities of autistic children. *Child Development* 57:1440–53.

Dawson, G., Finley, C., Phillips, S., Galpert, L., and Lewy, A. 1988. Reduced P3 amplitude of the event-related brain potential: Its relationship to language ability in autism. *Journal of Autism and Developmental Disorders* 18:493–504.

Dawson, G., Finley, C., Phillips, S., and Lewy, A. 1989. A comparison of hemispheric asymmetries in speech-related brain potentials of autistic and dysphasic children. *Brain and Language* 37:26–41.

Dawson, G., Warrenburg, S., and Fuller, P. 1982. Cerebral lateralization in individuals diagnosed as autistic in early childhood. *Brain and Language* 15:353–68.

Dawson, G., Warrenburg, S., and Fuller, P. 1983. Hemisphere functioning and motor imitation in autistic persons. *Brain and Cognition* 2:346–54.

DeLong, G. R. 1978. A neurological interpretation of infantile autism. In M. Rutter and E. Schopler, eds. *Autism: A Reappraisal of Concepts and Treatment.* New York: Plenum Press, pp. 207–18.

DeMyer, M. K. 1979. *Parents and Children in Autism.* Washington, D.C.: Winston & Sons.

DeMyer, M. K., Hingtgen, J. L. N., and Jackson, R. K. 1981. Infantile autism reviewed: A decade of research. *Schizophrenia Bulletin* 7:390–453.

Doyle, J., Galin, D., and Ornstein, R. E. 1974. Lateral specialization of cognitive mode: EEG frequency analysis. *Psychophysiology* 11:567–78.

Fay, W., and Schuler, A. L. 1979. *Emerging Language in Autistic Children.* Baltimore: University Park Press.

Fein, D., Humes, M., Kaplan, E., Lucci, D., and Waterhouse, L. 1984. The question of left hemisphere dysfunction in infantile autism. *Psychological Bulletin* 7:447–53.

Fein, D., Pennington, B., Markowitz, P., Braverman, M., and Waterhouse, L. 1986. Toward a neuropsychological model of infantile autism: Are the social deficits primary? *Journal of the American Academy of Child Psychiatry* 25:198–212.

Fletcher, J. M., and Taylor, H. G. 1984. Neuropsychological approaches to children: Towards a developmental neuropsychology. *Journal of Clinical Neuropsychology* 6:39–56.

Flusberg-Tager, H. 1989. A psycholinguistic perspective on language development in the autistic child. In G. Dawson, ed. *Autism: Nature, Diagnosis, and Treatment.* New York: Guilford Press, pp. 92–109.

Friedman, D., Vaughan, H. G., Jr., and Erlenmeyer-Kimling, L. 1981. Multiple late positive potentials in two visual discrimination tasks. *Psychophysiology* 18:635–49.

Friel-Patti, S., and Finitzo, T. 1990. Language learning in a prospective study of otitis media with effusion in the first two years of life. *Journal of Speech and Hearing Research* 33:188–94.

Friel-Patti, S., Finitzo-Hieber, T., Conti, G., and Clinton-Brown, K. 1982. Language delay in infants associated with middle ear disease and mild, fluctuating hearing impairment. *Journal of Pediatric Infectious Disease* 1:104–9.

Gillberg, C., Rosenhall, U., and Johansson, E. 1983. Auditory brainstem responses in childhood psychosis. *Journal of Autism and Developmental Disorders* 13:181–95.

Gillberg, C., and Steffenburg, S. 1987. Outcome and prognostic factors in infantile autism and similar conditions: A population-based study of 46 cases followed through puberty. *Journal of Autism and Developmental Disorders* 17:273–87.

Gravel, J. S., and Wallace, I. F. 1992. Listening and language at 4-years of age: Effects of early otitis media. *Journal of Speech and Hearing Research* 35:588–95.

Gravel, J. S., Wallace, I. F., and Abraham, S. 1990. Communication sequelae of otitis media: Hearing, language and phonology. *ASHA* 32:119.

Grillon, C., Courchesne, E., and Akshoomoff, N. 1989. Brainstem and middle latency auditory evoked potentials in autism and developmental language disorders. *Journal of Autism and Developmental Disorders* 19:255–69.

Harter, M. R., and Aine, C. J. 1984. Brain mechanisms of visual selective attention. In R. Parasuraman and I. D. R. Davies, eds. *Varieties of Attention*. New York: Academic Press, pp. 293–321.

Hermelin, B., and O'Conner, N. 1967. Remembering words by psychotic and subnormal children. *British Journal of Psychology* 58:213–18.

Hermelin, B., and O'Conner, N. 1970. *Psychological Experiments with Autistic Children*. Oxford: Pergamon Press.

Hillyard, S. A. 1985. Electrophysiology of human selective attention. *Trends in Neuroscience* 8:400–405.

Hillyard, S. A., Hink, R. F., Schwent, V., and Picton, T. W. 1973. Electrical signs of selective attention in the human brain. *Science* 182:177–80.

Hillyard, S. A., and Picton, T. W. 1979. Event-related brain potentials and selective information processing in man. In J. E. Desmedt, ed. *Progress in Clinical Neurophysiology. Vol. 6. Cognitive Components in Event-Related Cerebral Potentials.* Basel: S. Karger, pp. 1–52.

Hillyard, S. A., and Picton, T. 1987. Electrophysiology of cognition. In V. B. Mountcastle, F. Plum, and S. R. Geiger, eds. *Handbook of Physiology: Higher Functions of the Brain.* Vol. 5, Part II. Bethesda: American Physiologic Society, pp. 519–84.

Holcomb, P. J., and Neville, H. J. 1990. Auditory and visual semantic priming in lexical decision: A comparison using event-related brain potentials. *Language and Cognitive Processes* 5:281–312.

James, A. L., and Barry, R. J. 1980. Respiratory and vascular responses to simple visual stimuli in autistics, retardates and normals. *Psychophysiology* 17:541–47.

Konstantareas, M. M., and Homatidis, S. 1987. Ear infections in autistic and normal children. *Journal of Autism and Developmental Disorders* 17:585–93.

Kutas, M., and Hillyard, S. A. 1980. Reading between the lines: Event-related brain potentials during natural sentence processing. *Brain and Language* 11:354–73.

Lincoln, A. J., Courchesne, E., Kilman, B. A., Elmasian, R., and Allen, M. 1988. A study of intellectual abilities in high-functioning people with autism. *Journal of Autism and Developmental Disorders* 18:505–24.

Lockyer, L., and Rutter, M. 1970. A five to fifteen year follow-up study of infantile psychosis: Patterns of cognitive ability. *British Journal of Social and Clinical Psychology* 9:152–62.

Menyuk, P. 1978. Language: What's wrong and why. In M. Rutter and E. Schopler, eds. *Autism: A Reappraisal of Concepts and Treatment.* New York: Plenum, pp. 105–16.

Menyuk, P., and Quill, K. 1985. Semantic problems in autistic children. In E. Schopler and G. Mesibov, eds. *Communication Problems in Autism.* New York: Plenum, pp. 127–45.

Minshew, N. 1991. Indices of neural function in autism: Clinical and biologic implications. *Pediatrics* 87:774–80.

Naatanen, R., and Picton, T. 1987. The N1 wave of the human electric and magnetic response to sound: A review and an analysis of the component structure. *Psychophysiology* 24:375–425.

Niwa, S., Ohta, M., and Yamazaki, K. 1983. P300 and stimulus evaluation process in autistic subjects. *Journal of Autism and Developmental Disorders* 13:33–42.

Novick, B., Kurtzberg, D., and Vaughan, H. G. 1979. An electrophysiologic indication of defective information storage in childhood autism. *Psychiatry Research* 1:101–8.

Novick, B., Vaughan, H. G., Kurtzberg, D., and Simon, R. 1980. An electrophysiologic indication of auditory processing defects in autism. *Psychiatry Research* 3:107–14.

Ogawa, T., Sugiyama, A., Ishiwa, S., Suzuki, M., Ishihara, T., and Sato, K. 1982. Ontogenic development of EEG-asymmetry in early infantile autism. *Brain Development* 4:439–49.

Olsson, I., Steffenburg, S., and Gillberg, C. 1988. Epilepsy in autism and autistic like conditions. *Archives of Neurology* 45:666–68.

Ornitz, E. M. 1969. Disorders of perception common to early infantile autism and schizophrenia. *Comparative Psychiatry* 10:259–74.

Ornitz, E. M. 1974. The modulation of sensory input and motor output in autistic children. *Journal of Autism and Developmental Disorders* 4:197–215.

Ornitz, E. M. 1985. Neurophysiology of infantile autism. *Journal of the American Academy of Child Psychiatry* 24:251–62.

Ornitz, E. M. 1989. Autism at the interface between sensory and information processing. In G. Dawson, ed. *Autism Nature, Diagnosis, and Treatment.* New York: Guilford Press, pp. 174–99.

Ornitz, E. M. 1992. A behavioral-based neurophysiological model for dysfunction of directed attention in infantile autism. In H. Naruse and E. M. Ornitz, eds. *Neurobiology of Infantile Autism.* Amsterdam: Excerpta Medica, pp. 89–110.

Ornitz, E. M., Atwell, C. W., Kaplan, A. R., and Westlake, J. R. 1985. Brain-stem dysfunction in autism. *Archives of General Psychiatry* 42:1018–25.

Ornitz, E. M., Guthrie, D., and Farley, A. J. 1978. The early symptoms of childhood autism. In G. Serban, ed. *Cognitive Defects in the Development of Mental Illness.* New York: Brunner/Mazel, pp. 24–42.

Picton, T. W., and Hillyard, S. A. 1988. Endogenous event-related potentials. In T. W. Picton, ed. *Handbook of Electroencephalography and Clinical Neurophysiology, Vol. 3, Human Event-Related Potentials.* Amsterdam: Elsevier, pp. 361–426.

Piven, J., Berthier, M. L., Starkstein, S. E., Nehme, E., Pearlson, G., and Folstein, S. 1990. Magnetic resonance imaging evidence for a defect of cerebral cortical development in autism. *American Journal of Psychiatry* 147:734–39.

Prior, M. R., and Bradshaw, J. L. 1979. Hemispheric functioning in autistic children. *Cortex* 15:73–81.

Rapin, I. 1991. Autistic children: Diagnosis and clinical features. *Pediatrics* 87(suppl.):751–60.

Rimland, B. 1964. *Infantile Autism: The Syndrome and Its Implications for a Neural Theory of Behavior.* New York: Appleton-Century Crofts.

Ritvo, E. R., Ornitz, E. M., Walter, R. D., and Hanley, J. 1970. Correlation of psychiatric diagnoses and EEG findings: A double-blind study of 184 hospitalized children. *American Journal of Psychiatry* 126:112–20.

Ruchkin, D. S., Sutton, S., and Stega, M. 1980. Emitted P300 and slow wave event-related potentials in guessing and detection tasks. *Electroencephalography and Clinical Neurophysiology* 49:1–14.

Ruchkin, D. S., Sutton, S., Kietzman, M. L., and Silver, K. 1980. Slow wave and P300 in signal detection. *Electroencephalography and Clinical Neurophysiology: Evoked Potentials* 50:35–47.

Rumsey, J. M., Grimes, A. M., Pikus, A. M., Duara, R., and Ismond, D. R. 1984. Auditory brain-stem responses in pervasive developmental disorders. *Biological Psychiatry* 19:1403–18.

Rumsey, J. M., and Hamburger, S. D. 1988. Neurophysiological findings in high-functioning men with infantile autism, residual state. *Journal of Clinical and Experimental Neuropsychology* 10:201–21.

Rumsey, J. M., and Hamburger, S. D. 1990. Neuropsychological divergence of high-level autism and severe dyslexia. *Journal of Autism and Developmental Disorders* 20:155.

Rutter, M. 1968. Concepts of autism: A review of the research. *Journal of Child Psychiatry* 9:1–5.

Rutter, M. 1974. The development of infantile autism. *Psychological Medicine* 4:147–63.

Rutter, M. 1978. Language disorder and infantile autism. In M. Rutter and E. Schopler, eds. *Autism: A Reappraisal of Concepts and Treatment*. New York: Plenum Press, pp. 85–104.

Rutter, M. 1983. Cognitive deficits in the pathogenesis of autism. *Journal of Child Psychology and Psychiatry* 24:513–31.

Rutter, M., and Lockyer, L. 1967. A five-to-fifteen year follow-up study of infantile psychosis: I. Description of sample. *British Journal of Psychiatry* 113:1169–82.

Scherg, M., Vajsar, J., and Picton, T. W. 1989. A source analysis of the late human auditory evoked potentials. *Journal of Cognitive Neuroscience* 1:336–55.

Skoff, B. F., Fein, D., McNally, B., Lucci, D., Humes Bartlo, M., and Waterhouse, L. 1986. Brainstem auditory evoked potentials in autism. *Psychophysiology* 23:462.

Skoff, B. F., Mirsky, A. F., and Turner, D. 1980. Prolonged brainstem transmission time in autism. *Psychiatry Research* 2:157–66.

Small, J. G. 1968. Epileptiform electroencephalographic abnormalities in mentally ill children. *Journal of Nervous and Mental Disease* 147:341–48.

Small, J. G., DeMyer, M. K., and Milstein, V. 1971. CNV responses of autistic and normal children. *Journal of Autism and Childhood Schizophrenia* 1:215–31.

Small, J. G. 1975. EEG and neurophysiological studies of early infantile autism. *Biological Psychiatry* 10:385–89.

Stockard, J. J., Stockard, J. E., and Sharbrough, F. W. 1986. Brainstem auditory evoked potentials in neurology: Methodology, interpretation, clinical application. In M. J. Aminoff, ed. *Electrodiagnosis in Clinical Neurology*. New York: Churchill Livingstone, pp. 467–503.

Student, M., and Sohmer, H. 1978. Evidence from auditory nerve and brainstem evoked responses for an organic brain lesion in children with autistic traits. *Journal of Autism and Developmental Disorders* 8:13–20.

Tager-Flusberg, H. 1981. On the nature of linguistic functioning in early infantile autism. *Journal of Autism and Developmental Disorders* 11:45–54.

Tager-Flusberg, H. 1981. Sentence comprehension in autistic children. *Applied Psycholinguistics* 2:5–24.

Tanguay, P. E. 1976. Clinical and electrophysiological research. In E. R. Ritvo, ed. *Autism: Diagnosis, Current Research and Management*. New York: Spectrum, pp. 75–84.

Tanguay, P. E., Edwards, R. M., Buchwald, J., Schwafel, J., and Allen, V. 1982. Auditory brainstem evoked responses in autistic children. *Archives of General Psychiatry* 39:174–80.

Taylor, M. J., Rosenblatt, B., and Linschoten, L. 1982. Auditory brainstem response abnormalities in autistic children. *Canadian Journal of Sci Neurol* 9:429–33.

Taylor, M. J., Rosenblatt, B., and Linschoten, L. 1982. Electrophysiological study of the auditory system in autistic children. In A. Rothenberger, ed. *Event-Related Potentials in Children.* New York: Elsevier, pp. 379–86.

Vaughan, H. G., and Ritter, W. 1978. The sources of auditory evoked responses recorded from the human scalp. *Electroencephalography and Clinical Neurophysiology* 28:360–67.

Volkmar, F. R., and Nelson, D. S. 1990. Seizure disorders in autism. *Journal of the American Academy of Child Psychiatry* 1:127–29.

Waldo, M. C., Cohen, D. J., Caparulo, B. K., Young, G., Prichard, J. W., and Shaywitz, B. A. 1978. EEG profiles of neuropsychiatrically disturbed children. *American Academy of Child Psychiatry* 17:656–70.

Wood, C. C., McCarthy, G., Squires, N. K., Vaughan, H. G., Woods, D. L., and McCallum, W. C. 1984. Anatomical and physiological substrates of event-related potentials: Two case studies. *Annals of the New York Academy of Sciences* 425:681–721.

4

IN VIVO NEUROANATOMY OF AUTISM: NEUROIMAGING STUDIES

Nancy J. Minshew, M.D.
Stephen M. Dombrowski, B.S.

With the limited availability of autopsy brain material, researchers have had to rely largely on imaging techniques to investigate the neuroanatomy of autism. Although some data were initially provided by pneumoencephalographic (PEG) studies, imaging research began in earnest with the introduction of computed tomographic (CT) scanning in the early 1970s. This era coincided with the general scientific interest in the role of brain asymmetries in disease processes, so the initial imaging studies in autism focused on brain asymmetry.

BRAIN ASYMMETRIES IN AUTISM

The investigation of brain asymmetries with CT imaging typically involved measurements of brain width and notation of the presence or absence of petalia (impressions on the inner table of the skull made by the hemispheres) in the parieto-occipital and frontal regions. In the normal population, the left parieto-occipital brain region is generally wider than the right, and the right frontal region is wider than the left. When present, frontal petalia are more commonly right-sided and occipital petalia left-sided. Brain asymmetries were initially thought to vary with handedness and gender (LeMay and Kido, 1978). However, these associations were not reproduced in the subsequent normative study of Chui and Damasio (1980), leading to the suggestion that cerebral asymmetry might be more closely related to hemispheric language dominance than handedness or gender.

The first CT study of autism reported a reversal of the normal left–right parieto-occipital asymmetry in nine of sixteen (57 percent) autistic subjects (Hier, LeMay, and Rosenberger, 1979), as compared to 23 percent of a mentally retarded comparison group and 25 percent of a neurologic control group. On the basis of these findings, it was hypothesized that the absence of the normal morphologic predominance of the left hemisphere might compromise the left hemisphere's capacity to support language acquisition in autism.

Brain asymmetry was subsequently investigated in greater detail by Damasio et al. (1980) in a CT study of seventeen cases of primary (idiopathic) and secondary (the result of an associated infectious, metabolic, or genetic disorder) autism. Measurements of parieto-occipital brain width in this sample revealed a reversal of the normal asymmetry in only 18 percent (3/17), symmetry in 35 percent (6/17), and the normal left-sided predominance in 47 percent (8/17). Measurements of the frontal lobe revealed reversed or left-sided predominance in 18 percent, symmetry in 23 percent, and the normal right-sided predominance in 59 percent. When present, frontal petalia were more often found on the right side and occipital petalia on the left side. When the measurements for this autistic sample were compared to a group of 50 right-handed normal adults (Chui and Damasio, 1980), no significant differences were found on any of the measures of asymmetry. This study, therefore, did not support the initial findings of Hier et al. (1979) of reversed asymmetry in autism.

In an attempt to resolve the disparity between these two studies, Tsai, Jacoby, and Stewart (1983) studied eighteen right-handed or ambidextrous autistic males and eighteen age-, gender-, and handedness-matched controls who had various neurologic complaints, such as headache, seizures, and skull fracture. For the total group of eighteen autistic males, the investigators reported reversed or right-sided parieto-occipital predominance in 22 percent, symmetry in 56 percent, and the normal left parieto-occipital predominance in 22 percent, compared to 22, 50, and 28 percent, respectively, for their neurologic control group. For frontal brain width, reversed or left-sided predominance was present in 5 percent, symmetry in 61 percent, and the normal right frontal predominance in 33 percent of the eighteen autistic subjects, as compared to 5, 72, and 22 percent, respectively, for the neurologic control group. There were no statistically significant differences between the autistic and either the mentally retarded or the neurologic control group in the distribution of frontal and occipital asymmetries using either of two methods of measurement. Furthermore, there were no correlations between the degree of asymmetry and the language deficit, suggesting that reversed parieto-occipital predominance was not associated with more severe language deficits as originally postulated.

When these autistic subjects were divided into two subgroups of twelve right-handed and six ambidextrous subjects and compared to the normative data from Chui and Damasio (1980), there were again no statistically significant differences in brain asymmetries. When the twelve right-handed autistic subjects were compared with the normative data from LeMay and Kido (1978), there were also no statistical differences in parieto-occipital or frontal asymmetry (L > R or R > L), but there was a statistically significant increase in the proportion of the autistic brains that were symmetric (L = R). Hence, there was a statistically significant difference on only one comparison out of many in this study, and that finding supported greater symmetry rather than asymmetry in the autistic sample. The investigators drew two conclusions from these data: (1) the frequency of reversed asymmetry in autistic subjects was comparable to that of other neurologically impaired individuals, and (2) there was no relationship between the severity of the language deficit and reversed parieto-occipital asymmetry in autism. The investigators also emphasized that small differences in the method of measurement had a significant impact on measurements of asymmetry.

A fourth study of brain asymmetry in autism was conducted by Rumsey et al. (1988) employing the methods of Chui and Damasio (1980) and Damasio et al. (1980). The subject pool consisted of fifteen autistic adults screened for associated neurologic conditions and twenty normal controls. The results for both subject groups were also compared to the normative data from the fifty right-handed adults of Chui and Damasio (1980). For parieto-occipital brain width, reversed asymmetry was present in 0 percent, symmetry in 47 percent, and the normal left-sided predominance in 53 percent. For frontal brain width, reversed asymmetry was present in 13 percent, symmetry in 60 percent, and the normal right-sided predominance in 27 percent. There were no statistically significant differences between the autistic group and the two control groups on any of the measures of brain asymmetry, which included petalia, deviation of the straight sinus, and frontal and occipital brain widths.

The data from these four asymmetry studies are compiled in Tables 4.1 (parieto-occipital brain width) and 4.2 (frontal brain width). For the parieto-occipital measurements, the most consistent data across studies were for reversed asymmetry (e.g., R > L). The proportion of subjects classified as having the normal L > R predominance and L = R symmetry varied widely from study to study. For the frontal lobe measurements, the data were fairly consistent across studies, with the exception of the autistic group from the study of Damasio et al. (1980), which included subjects with hydrocephalus, acquired brain damage, and genetic conditions.

In summary, studies have not supported differences in brain asymmetry in autism. In addition, morphologic asymmetries of the brain ultimately ceased to be a tenable basis for autism in the face of the evolving awareness of the complexity of the clinical syndrome (Rutter, 1988) and the symmetry of neuropathologic (Bauman and Kemper, 1985) and neurophysiologic (Courchesne et al., 1984, 1987) abnormalities.

Table 4.1. Parieto–Occipital Brain Width

Subjects	N	R > L (%)	R = L (%)	L > R (%)
Austistic				
Hier et al., 1979	16	57	11	31
Damasio et al., 1980	17	18	35	47
Tsai et al., 1983	18	22	56	22
Rumsey et al., 1988	15	0	47	53
Neurologic control				
Hier et al., 1978	44	23	18	59
Hier et al., 1979	100	25	18	57
Tsai et al., 1983	18	22	50	27
Normal control				
Chui and Damasio, 1980	50	20	44	36
Rumsey et al., 1988	20	10	45	45

Table 4.2. Frontal Brain Width

Subjects	N	R > L (%)	R = L (%)	L > R (%)
Autistic				
Damasio et al., 1980	17	59	23	18
Tsai et al., 1983	18	33	61	5
Rumsey et al., 1988	15	27	60	13
Neurologic control				
Tsai et al., 1983	18	22	72	5
Normal control				
Chui and Damasio, 1980	50	36	42	22
Rumsey et al., 1988	20	45	45	10

Although subsequent imaging studies shifted to the investigation of specific neuroanatomic structures in the search for the etiology of autism, the early CT study of Damasio et al. (1980) remained a landmark in the autism imaging literature. It highlighted the relationship of gross brain abnormalities to associated neurologic conditions and emphasized the need for careful discrimination in research studies between primary or idiopathic cases of autism and those due to acquired or genetic disorders involving the brain (Damasio, 1984).

VENTRICULAR ABNORMALITIES IN AUTISM

Reports of enlargement of the lateral ventricles in autism first appeared in PEG studies in the 1950s to 1970s. The final PEG study emphasized enlargement of the left temporal horn (Hauser, DeLong, and Rosman,

1975) and was linked to hypotheses of the primacy of memory, language, and the left hemisphere in the pathogenesis of autism. As a result of the CT investigations of Damasio et al. (1980), Prior et al. (1984), and Creasey et al. (1986), it was ultimately appreciated that enlargement of the lateral ventricles in autism was largely related to the inclusion of individuals with brain damage (Damasio, 1984). Hence, in studies conducted before the introduction of screening procedures to exclude autistic subjects with acquired brain damage or genetic abnormalities, lateral ventriculomegaly was often, but not always, related to hydrocephalus complicating meningitis or *ex vacuo* changes due to other forms of brain damage (Hauser et al., 1975; Damasio et al., 1980; Gillberg and Svendsen, 1983; Courchesne et al., 1987). However, some studies of carefully screened autistic populations have reported a low incidence of lateral ventricular enlargement. The size of the third and fourth ventricles has been investigated more recently, with basically negative findings in idiopathic cases of autism.

ENLARGEMENT OF THE LATERAL VENTRICLES

Of the studies that screened autistic subjects for other neurologic disorders and used quantitative measurements rather than qualitative assessment of images, most have observed no evidence of lateral ventricular enlargement in autism. However, a few studies have reported a 15–25 percent incidence of enlargement of the lateral ventricles in autism. In the first study of ventricular size, Campbell et al. (1982) evaluated forty-five carefully screened young autistic children and found mild or moderate ventricular enlargement in __ (24 percent), as judged initially by radiologic readings and then by comparisons between subgroups selected according to ventricular size. *Ventricular size, however, was not found to correlate with any clinical variable*, including language quotient, severity of withdrawal, stereotypies, developmental quotient, head circumference, obstetrical factors, birth weight, minor physical anomalies, and maternal age. Because the methods of data analysis in this study differed from those used in subsequent studies, they deserve further comment. In this study, the autistic group was divided into three subgroups before statistical analysis according to a radiologist's subjective judgment of ventricular size: (1) those judged to have normal-sized lateral ventricles, (2) those with mild enlargement of the ventricles, and (3) those with moderate or severe enlargement of the ventricles. Statistical comparisons were then made using these subgroups. No analyses were presented on the comparison between the total group of autistic subjects and the control subjects, making it difficult to determine if the presence of ventricular enlargement would have been manifested at the level of group analysis. In contrast, subsequent research studies based their analyses on the autistic group in toto. Some looked at the amount of variance to assess for outliers with ventricular enlargement, but others did not. Hence, it is not always possible to determine if there was or was not a subgroup of autistic individuals in other studies with ventricular enlargement. In addition, only an occasional study has compared subject data to clinical norms, another important consideration in assessing the significance of findings.

In a follow-up study, Rosenbloom, Campbell, and George (1984) investigated ventricular and cisternal volume in thirteen carefully selected young autistic children and ten neurologic controls. Three of the autistic subjects in this study were also in the study of Campbell et al. (1982), but it was not clear whether these three were in the normal or enlarged ventricle subgroup or how they were selected for inclusion in this follow-up study. If the three from Campbell's study had ventricular enlargement, then the findings in this study cannot be interpreted as a replication study of the prevalence of ventricular enlargement in autism. This study reported volume measurements for the lateral ventricles that were calculated by multiplying the area of cerebrospinal fluid (CSF) in each slice by the thickness of the slice (10 mm) and summing over the slices containing the structure of interest. Such measurements were referred to as volume measurements; however, they were not true volumes because of the gaps between slices and the omission of the highest slices because of poor resolution. Linear measurements of the size of the lateral and third ventricles were also derived from these scans. Although there were no statistically significant differences between the autistic group and the control subjects on the nine volumetric and four linear measurements of ventricular and cisternal volume, the measurements for net ventricular and net subarachnoid volume had an increase in variance in the autistic group due to the outlying measurements of a few autistic individuals. For each of these two parameters, two autistic subjects (15 percent) had values considerably higher than those for the other autistic and control subjects, and an additional two autistic subjects had values at the upper limits for the groups. This again suggested that there was a small subgroup with ventricular enlargement within the carefully screened population of autistic subjects.

The size of the lateral ventricles was also investigated by Hoshino et al. (1984) in twenty-four Japanese children with autism. No statistically significant differences were found in bifrontal and bicaudate ratios between the autistic group as a whole and the neurologic comparison group, but there was a tendency toward enlargement of the lateral ventricles with age in the autistic subjects when the subjects were analyzed by age subgroups. However, this age-related change in ventricular size was largely based on the presence of statistically significant findings for the oldest age group (ten to seventeen years) and their absence in the younger aged groups. Unfortunately, the description of the autistic sample did not comment on screening procedures for associated neurologic diseases and the two case studies provided were both positive for asphyxia neonatorum. These two cases constituted one-third of the oldest age group, the group with the largest values for ventricular size. In addition, the variance in ventricular measurements appeared considerably larger for this older autistic subgroup, suggesting that statistically significant findings between the older subgroup and controls could have been the result of a few outliers.

In an effort to eliminate mental retardation as a confounding variable in imaging findings in autism, Prior et al. (1984) studied ventricular size in nine high-functioning autistic boys. Evans's and bifrontal ratios were normal in all cases, and the bicaudate ratio was normal in eight of the nine and just below the normal limit in the ninth case. Lateral ventricular size and symmetry were also found to be normal in three subsequent CT studies (Harcherik et al., 1985; Creasey et al., 1986; Jacobson et al., 1988) of sixteen, twelve, and nine teenage and adult autistic individuals who spanned the entire range of IQs and were free of infectious, metabolic, and other neurologic diseases. Jacobson et al. (1988) also investigated the size of the Sylvian fissures and interhemispheric fissure and again found no difference between autistic and control subjects.

The first MRI study to investigate the size of the lateral ventricles in autism was based on area measurements from 10-mm slices (Gaffney et al., 1989). Unfortunately, the autistic subjects were not screened for associated conditions and two had neurofibromatosis, one of whom also had seizures. Similarly, two of the controls had seizure disorders and one had neurofibromatosis. This study measured ventricular area of the anterior and posterior horns and of the bodies of the lateral ventricles and found a subtle but statistically significant increase in the size of the anterior horns and bodies in the autistic group compared to the control group. No comment was made about the contribution of outliers to these findings. These findings were interpreted as evidence of subtle alterations in forebrain anatomy in autism, but they are limited by the inclusion of autistic subjects with other neurologic diseases and the 10-mm slice thickness, which results in increased volume averaging and measurement error.

In addition to assessing lateral ventricular size, most of the preceding studies also assessed symmetry between the left- and right-lateral ventricles and failed to find evidence of abnormality. Asymmetry, either L > R or R > L, was occasionally seen in the autistic subjects, but it did not represent a significant trend.

In summary, symmetric enlargement of the lateral ventricles was present in thirteen of fifty-eight, or 22 percent, of the carefully screened autistic subjects from one center. No enlargement was reported in ninety-nine cases collected at five other centers. The studies by Gaffney et al. (1989) and Hoshino et al. (1984) were not included in this summary of cases because of the inclusion of autistic subjects with associated conditions, although the findings they reported are also largely negative. Although enlargement of the lateral ventricles was not a consistent finding across centers, its presence in the largest group of carefully screened autistic subjects from any one center is not obviously attributable to any other condition besides autism and, hence, cannot be dismissed. Additional studies are needed to determine the actual prevalence of this finding in idiopathic autism and its potential significance for the pathophysiology. Thus far, when present, ventricular enlargement has not appeared to correspond to the severity of autism, eliminating the most obvious connection to pathophysiology. However, none of the studies has investigated the relationship between ventricular enlargement and the mode of presentation in autism (e.g., developmental delay versus regression), which would be the second most likely pathophysiologic relationship. The clinical regression observed in approximately one-third of autism cases has an increased likelihood of neuronal loss, which could result in *ex vacuo* changes.

ENLARGEMENT OF THE THIRD AND FOURTH VENTRICLES

Only a few studies have reported on the size of the third and fourth ventricles in autism. Of the studies that screened autistic subjects for associated conditions that cause brain abnormalities and used quantitative measurements, two of four reported enlargement of the third ventricle and one out of seven reported enlargement of the fourth ventricle.

An increase in the size of the third ventricle was observed in six of the forty-five autistic children studied by Campbell et al. (1982) and was associated with moderate enlargement of the lateral ventricles. In a second study of nine autistic adults (Jacobson et al., 1988), an increase in size of the third ventricle was also observed, but it was not associated with either an increase in variance in the third ventricle measurements or an increase in size of the lateral or fourth ventricle. In the third study of twenty-four Japanese autistic children, Hoshino et al. (1984) found no statistically significant differences in the width of the third ventricle in their autistic group as a whole, but did see an increase in the teenage subgroup. The size of the third ventricle in this subgroup was not associated with an increase in variance, but this subgroup also had the largest measurements for lateral ventricular size, and two of the seven subgroup members had a history of asphyxia neonatorum. Two other CT studies of thirteen autistic children and twelve autistic adults found no increase in the width (Rosenbloom et al., 1984) or volume (Creasey et al., 1986) of the third ventricle and no increase in the variance of these measurements.

The size of the fourth ventricle in autism has been assessed in seven studies as part of an evaluation of posterior fossa structures. Hence, the status of the rest of the ventricular system was rarely available to determine if enlargement of the fourth ventricle represented a localized change or was associated with generalized enlargement of the ventricular system. Two of the seven studies included autistic subjects with associated neurologic disorders such as neurofibromatosis, asphyxia neonatorum, and intrauterine cytomegalovirus infection (Gaffney et al., 1987b; Garber et al., 1989). Six of the seven studies reported an absence of statistically significant differences in the size of the fourth ventricle (Jacobson et al., 1988; Rumsey et al., 1988; Garber et al., 1989; Piven et al., 1992; Kleiman, Neff, and Rosman, 1992; Holttum et al., 1992). One study (Gaffney et al., 1987a) reported an increase in fourth ventricular volume on midsagittal and coronal MR images, but not on axial images in samples of thirteen, six, and eight autistic individuals, respectively. Unfortunately, two of the autistic subjects studied had neurofibromatosis, and the history of other neurologic disorders or insults in the other subjects was not specified. Hence, it is not possible to determine if the findings were related to the autism or to the associated conditions.

In summary, preliminary research suggests that there may be a small subgroup of autistic individuals with a subtle increase in size of the third ventricle. It is not clear whether enlargement of the third ventricle occurs in isolation, suggesting abnormalities restricted to adjacent brain structures, or whether it occurs as part of a more generalized enlargement of the ventricular system. In addition, the relationship of ventricular enlargement to the mode of presentation, use of medication, seizures, and age have not been explored, so the contribution of brain deterioration and regressive events is unknown. In contrast, there is no evidence to support the presence of enlargement of the fourth ventricle in autistic populations that have been appropriately screened for associated neurologic conditions. Once again, the importance of studying only autistic subjects that have been screened for other conditions known to produce CNS abnormalities is paramount in determining the significance of brain abnormalities in autism. In unscreened autistic populations, it is not possible to determine if abnormalities are due to the autism or to the associated conditions.

STRUCTURAL BRAIN ABNORMALITIES IN AUTISM

Until the advent of MRI, the bulk of the neuroimaging literature in autism focused on measurements of the cerebral hemispheres, basal ganglia, and thalamus. However, notable for their absence from these studies are measurements of the cerebral cortex, hippocampus, and other structures in the limbic system that were not sufficiently defined by CT to allow measurement but figured prominently in neurobiologic theories. Studies of the cerebral hemispheres, other than area measurements of the subcortical nuclei, have been relatively crude, focusing on the presence or absence of gross structural abnormalities, radiodensity measurements, or brain volume. The introduction of MRI made the posterior fossa accessible for quantitative measurement for the first time.

As a newly emerging technology, MRI research is faced with a number of obstacles: the absence of normative data; the undefined but likely impact of age, gender, IQ, race, and socioeconomic status on normative values; and a lack of standardized methods of image acquisition and analysis. Such problems have characterized the developing stages of all new technologies. The absence in MRI of the radiation risk that posed a major obstacle for CT research in childhood disorders now makes it possible to enroll normal children as control subjects in MRI studies. Because of the expense of MRI studies, it is essential that standardized methods of image acquisition and analysis be developed and universally adopted so that data on disorders can be readily compared across research sites and a large normative data base accrued that considers the potential impact of all relevant subject variables.

GROSS STRUCTURAL ABNORMALITIES

Although early imaging studies emphasized the incidence of gross CT abnormalities in autism (Damasio et al., 1980; Gillberg and Svendsen, 1983), these abnormalities were ultimately traced to associated infectious, genetic, or neurologic conditions (Campbell et al., 1982; Prior et al., 1984; Harcherik et al., 1985; Creasey et al., 1986).

The screening of autistic subjects for infectious, metabolic, genetic, and neurologic disorders other than autism was implemented in imaging research by 1982, and the incidence of gross structural abnormalities in reports dropped substantially thereafter. The first imaging studies to employ rigorous screening procedures were those of Campbell et al. (1982) and Rosenbloom et al. (1984). With the exception of the low prevalence of enlargment of the lateral ventricles, the scans of these fifty-eight autistic children were normal. These studies were followed by the report of Prior et al. (1984) on nine screened autistic boys who were selected for their high functioning status to exclude the confound of mental retardation. According to Prior et al., because there was "no sign of abnormality of any kind on the CT scans or any asymmetry that might be related to lateralized cognitive functions" in this select group of autistic individuals, it was concluded that the abnormalities reported in previous studies were the result of the co-occurrence of various infectious, metabolic, genetic, and acquired neurologic conditions. This conclusion was supported by two subsequent negative studies (Harcherik et al., 1985; Creasey et al., 1986) of fourteen and twelve carefully selected autistic individuals spanning the range of IQs. As a result of this accumulated evidence, it was concluded that autistic individuals without other neurologic conditions were "very unlikely to have detectable CT abnormalities" (Harcherik et al., 1985) and that the "cerebral defect in autism was likely to be microscopic without major gross anatomic correlate" (Creasey et al., 1986). This conclusion was consistent with the neuropathologic findings of Bauman and Kemper (1985), who observed abnormalities at the cellular level in autism but no gross structural abnormalities other than a consistent increase in brain weight of about 100 g. It is important to note, however, that neuropathologic studies to date, although not observing gross structural abnormalities, have not included volume measurements.

Hence, two major issues at present for anatomic research are whether or not histologic abnormalities of the brain are detectable with quantitative measurements and whether or not there are changes in the volume of brain structures. The very limited availability of autopsy brain material in autism clearly makes imaging research the primary strategy at this time for investigating the neuroanatomy in a substantial age, gender, and IQ cross-section of the autistic population. Hence, the ultimate goal of imaging research is to achieve in vivo measurements that are highly correlated with measurements in fresh brain at autopsy, as exemplified by the preliminary work of Filipek et al. (1989). It is also important that future neuropathologic studies include measurements of brain volume analogous to the MRI measurements, particularly in view of the increase in brain weight of autopsy brain specimens and the increase in midsagittal brain area on MRI (Piven et al., 1992). Given the limits of imaging and neuropathologic resolution, a greater emphasis will also be needed on studies of in vivo functional anatomy and cellular chemistry using PET, functional MRI, and magnetic resonance spectroscopy (MRS).

CEREBRAL HEMISPHERES, BASAL GANGLIA, AND THALAMUS

Brain size. A number of studies have attempted to assess the size of the cerebral hemispheres using linear measurements of maximum transverse diameter of the hemispheres (Hoshino et al., 1984) or skull (Jacobson et al., 1988), brain area on single slices (Gaffney et al., 1987a, 1987b; Jacobson et al., 1988; Piven et al., 1992) or summed over a number of noncontiguous slices (Creasey et al., 1986), or skull area on single slices or summed over several noncontiguous slices (Rosenbloom et al., 1984; Gaffney et al., 1989). With one exception (Piven et al., 1992), there were no statistically significant differences between autistic and control groups and no increases in variance for any of these measurements. The study reporting a significant difference in brain size between autistic and control groups observed an increase in midsagittal brain area (excluding the brainstem and cerebellum) in the autistic group (12,773 ± 951 mm^2) as compared to age-and-IQ and socioeconomic status-and-IQ control groups (11,608 ± 1075 mm^2; 11,671 ± 956 mm^2) at the 0.002 level of significance (Piven et al., 1992). Although the biologic significance of this finding is unclear, it is consistent with the slight increase in brain weight that has been observed at autopsy (Piven et al., 1992).

Brain Density. CT brain densities have been examined in three studies (Prior et al., 1984; Harcherik et al., 1985; Jacobson et al., 1988). Prior et al. (1984) measured the density of white matter in the frontal lobes and gray matter in the lentiform nuclei. There was no control group for this study, and the findings were based on intragroup comparisons between left and right hemisphere structure size. Harcherik et al. (1985) measured the density of the right and left cerebral hemispheres. Jacobson et al. (1988) measured the densities of the right and left frontal lobes, caudate nuclei, and thalamic nuclei in autistic subjects compared to normal control subjects. No abnormalities were reported in the frontal lobes or the lentiform nuclei in two of the studies (Prior et al., 1984; Harcherik et al., 1985), but Jacobson et al. reported a statistically significant decrease in the densities of the right and left caudate nuclei in the autistic group as compared to the normal control group; the standard deviations for these measurements in the autistic group were also increased. The biologic significance of this finding is unclear, but medication status, seizure status, and movement disorders would be key factors to exclude before attaching etiologic significance to these findings. The subjects were not on psychotropic medication at the time of the study, but past history of medication use was not discussed. One subject was noted to have a history of seizures and anticonvulsant use, but no mention was made of the relationship of this case to the abnormal findings.

Cerebral Cortex. Quantitative measurements of the cerebral cortex were not provided by any of these studies. Jacobson et al. (1988) listed a measurement for the area of the "cortex," but this was actually a measurement of nonventricular brain on an axial slice. Qualitative abnormalities of the cortex were reported by Piven et al. (1990), who

described malformations of the cortical gyri consistent with development errors in neuronal migration, suggesting the need in future imaging and neuropathologic studies to look for heterotopias and gyral
abnormalities in addition to changes in volume.

A few recent studies published preliminary results of measurements
of the cerebral cortex in autism, using volumetric MRI data sets. These
findings are in abstract form at present but exemplify future developments and expectations for imaging research. Filipek et al. (1992)
reported an increase in the volume of cerebral cortex in autistic individuals compared to language-delayed and normal control children. In
contrast, Courchesne, Press, and Yeung-Courchesne (1992) reported a
decrease in parietal lobe volume in some autistic individuals. Much
larger samples, consistent methods of imaging and analysis, and normative data are needed to pursue both of these observations and to
investigate the potential role of cerebral cortical abnormalities in the
pathogenesis of autism.

The Size of Subcortical Nuclei.   Aside from the measurements of the
radiodensity of the basal ganglia and thalamus, two studies measured
the size of these structures (Creasey et al., 1986; Gaffney et al., 1988).
No abnormalities were found in the CT "volume" measurements of
Creasey et al. in twelve carefully selected high-functioning autistic subjects. The second study reported a decrease ($p < 0.02$) in the area of the
right lenticular nucleus in the autistic group without an increase in variance using univariate analysis; the analyses did not correct for multiple
comparisons, so the statistical strength of this finding is limited
(Gaffney et al., 1988). In addition, this sample included two autistic subjects with neurofibromatosis, one of whom also had a seizure disorder,
as well as an additional autistic subject with a seizure disorder. Again,
history of medication use was not discussed, also adding to the difficulty
of determining if such abnormalities are related to the autism or to acquired brain abnormalities.

Corpus Callosum.   Thus far, only two studies have reported measurements of the corpus callosum, although this structure provides an opportunity for assessing neuronal projections arising from the specific
areas of cortex. Gaffney et al. (1987a) reported no difference in the
midsagittal area of the corpus callosum in autistic subjects compared to
controls on MR images. Filipek et al. (1992) also reported no difference
in the volume of the corpus callosum in high-functioning autistic children compared to normal controls, but callosal volume in the autistic
subjects was disproportionately low relative to cerebral cortical and
white matter volume, both of which were significantly increased in the
autistic group. Because the corpus callosum provides an index of inter-

hemispheric connectivity, it is important that studies of the corpus callosum be pursued further with sample sizes sufficient to account for relevant demographic confounds.

Brainstem.   Many theories have postulated abnormalities of the brainstem as central to the pathophysiology of autism (Ornitz and Ritvo, 1968; Ornitz, 1985; Courchesne et al., 1988). However, much of the evidence of brainstem dysfunction that originally supported these theories was subsequently found to be related to the presence of associated neurologic and audiologic conditions (Rumsey et al., 1985) and to methodologic deficiencies (Ornitz, 1985). Neuropathologic studies have reported the persistence of a fetal pattern of circuitry in olivocerebellar pathways, which appears subject to later changes in the second to third decade of life (Bauman and Kemper, 1989). The brainstem was otherwise normal neuropathologically. Because of the inherent limitations of CT for the posterior fossa, imaging studies of brainstem structure had to await the development of MRI. Although MRI has greater resolution in the posterior fossa, studies of the brainstem have been few so far, and contradictory. Gaffney et al. (1988) measured the area of the pons, midbrain, medulla, and total brainstem area on midsagittal MR images in thirteen autistic and thirty-five nonmatched neurologic controls and reported a smaller pons and total brainstem area in the autistic group. The second study of brainstem size, however, reported an absence of pontine abnormalities in autism (Hsu et al., 1991). Piven et al. (1992), on the other hand, reported that the midsagittal area of the pons was significantly larger in their autistic group, but concluded that it was probably an IQ effect related to their control group that was not matched on IQ with the autistic group. Hence, the imaging anatomy of the brainstem in autism is relevant to a number of neurobiologic theories, but remains an unresolved issue.

Cerebellum.   The cerebellum in autism has attracted considerable interest in recent years due to reports by Courchesne and colleagues of selective hypoplasia of neocerebellar vermis on midsagittal MR images and the resulting theory hypothesizing cerebellar abnormalities as etiologic in autism (Courchesne et al., 1987, 1988; Murakami et al., 1989; Ciesielski et al., 1990). The findings in the original study (Courchesne et al., 1988) and the remeasurement study of the same cases (Murakami et al., 1989) had several significant methodologic limitations, including the lack of matching between autistic and control groups on age, gender, and IQ, the retrospective selection of controls chosen for the absence of neuroimaging abnormalities, and the lack of screening for fragile X syndrome, which is known to be associated with cerebellar hypoplasia.

Before the report of neuroradiologic abnormalities of the cerebellum, histologic abnormalities of the cerebellum had been reported in neuropathologic studies (Bauman and Kemper, 1985; Bauman, 1991). It was initially assumed that the imaging findings were a reflection of the neuropathologic changes, but it subsequently became clear that the histologic findings were not equivalent in either location or nature to the MRI findings. The neuropathologic abnormality was maximal in the posterior and inferior regions of the cerebellar hemispheres and involved cell loss, whereas the neuroimaging abnormalities were based on a decrease in tissue area and selectively involved the neocerebellar vermis. To address this disparity in findings, Purkinje cell counts were subsequently performed on the autopsy specimens, which confirmed the greatest cell loss in the posterior, inferior hemisphere regions; however, it also observed varying degrees of cell loss throughout the cerebellum (Arin, Bauman, and Kemper, 1991). Cell loss in the vermis involved 25–30 percent of cells but affected the vermis evenly; it was not confined to lobules vi and vii, as reported by the imaging studies.

Cerebellar abnormalities were reported in other imaging studies of autism, but were based on somewhat different parameters from those used by Courchesne and colleagues. Gaffney et al. (1987a, 1987b, 1987c) measured the cerebellum in the midsagittal, axial, and coronal planes and found no abnormalities in the cerebellar or vermal area in the midsagittal or axial planes, but did find a decrease in the cerebellum/posterior fossa and cerebellum/total brain area ratios and an increase in the fourth ventricle/posterior fossa ratio on the coronal scan. Area measurements were not provided for the coronal plane, and only the ratios were reported in support of an abnormality of the cerebellum.

In contrast, several recent imaging studies using the same imaging methods as the original study (Courchesne et al., 1988) failed to find evidence of vermal hypoplasia in autism (Ritvo and Garber, 1988; Holttum et al., 1992; Kleiman et al., 1992; Piven et al., 1992). These studies addressed the methodologic limitations of the prior positive studies (Courchesne et al., 1988; Murakami et al., 1989), including the retrospective selection and prescreening of controls, the lack of age, IQ, gender, and socioeconomic status matching between control and autistic subjects, and the failure to screen autistic subjects for fragile X syndrome. Each of these studies focused on a different age and IQ segment of the autistic population, but together they spanned the range of ages and severity. Ritvo and Garber (1988) studied cerebellar vermal size in fifteen autistic individuals (mean age 11.5 ± 4.1 years) of various IQs and fifteen normal controls matched for age, gender, and race using contiguous 5-mm midsagittal slices with negative findings. Piven et al. (1992) also found no difference in the midsagittal area of lobules vi and vii. An increase in the area of lobules i–v was observed in the autistic group when compared to an age-and-socioeconomic status matched control group, but not when compared to an age-and-IQ matched control group. This study suggests that socioeconomic status may have significance in its own right as a variable, although it may not be separate from intelligence, in that socioeconomic status may be a more accurate reflection of true intellect than IQ scores, particularly in small samples and in lower-functioning individuals.

Kleiman et al. (1992) studied seventeen young autistic children six to nine years of age with a mean IQ of 45 and age-, sex-, and gender-matched neurologic controls and found no differences in vermal size. This was followed by the study of Holttum et al. (1992) that focused on the opposite end of the age and IQ spectrum. The cohort consisted of eighteen non-mentally retarded (verbal and full scale IQ > 72) autistic individuals between the ages of twelve and forty years and eighteen normal controls individually matched for age, gender, race, and full-scale IQ. The findings with respect to the vermis and fourth ventricle size were again negative. In addition, Holttum et al. observed that the autistic subjects in Courchesne's study (1988) were on average four years younger than were their controls. Since normative data on the rate of growth of the vermal lobules has shown differential growth of lobules i–v relative to lobules vi–vii (Schaeffer et al., 1991), Holttum et al. suggested that the age differential between autistic and control groups in addition to the other factors already cited may have contributed to the abnormal findings of the Courchesne et al. study. Together these four studies suggest that the original findings of selective hypoplasia of vermal lobules vi–vii in autism were the result of the methods used for the selection of the controls and the lack of matching between autistic and control groups on age, IQ, and possibly gender and socioeconomic status. The absence of vermal abnormalities on these MRI studies is also consistent with the small magnitude and evenness of the Purkinje cell loss in the vermis on neuropathologic examination.

Recently, Courchesne et al. (in press) reported a bimodal distribution of the area of vermal lobules vi–vii in a larger sample of autistic individuals showing a subgroup with hypoplasia and a subgroup with hyperplasia but a large degree of overlap in between. They suggested that the negative results of recent MRI studies may have been the result of the inclusion in a small sample of autistic individuals with hypo- and hyperplasia of the vermis, resulting in an averaging of the values and failure to detect abnormalities. Although there was no evidence of an increase in variance in the measurements of the preceding negative studies, these samples included eighteen or fewer autistic individuals. This issue can be addressed only through further research substantially enlarging the collective autistic and normative database.

In summary, the cerebellum is neuropathologically abnormal in autism, but the involvement is at the cellular level and crosses all architectonic boundaries. The neuropathologic studies have not measured tissue volume and so are not directly comparable to the parameters measured in imaging studies. Although a few initial imaging studies reported abnormalities of the cerebellum, a number of studies with improved design have found no quantitative abnormalities of the vermis using the same imaging methods. These MRI studies in autism, in addition to the normative developmental data of Schaeffer et al. (1991), highlight the importance of carefully defined control groups, close matching with the autistic group on significant variables, and the need to develop adequate norms for MRI measurements.

SUMMARY

After nearly twenty-five years of imaging research in autism, it is now apparent that autism is infrequently associated with visible or gross radiologic abnormalities if cases are screened for associated infectious, genetic and metabolic causes of brain abnormalities. There may be a low incidence, on the order of 10–15 percent, of enlargement of the lateral ventricles that is not related to severity and is of unknown biologic significance. Quantitative morphometric technology is now under development, but little data are available so far, particularly on structures such as the cerebral cortex and limbic system, which are central to a number of neurobiologic theories. Further progress in imaging research depends on the continuing development of volumetric imaging and measurement methods that produce measurements with greater validity and make it possible to investigate structures such as the cerebral cortex and hippocampus. It is not yet clear if cell loss will be detectable on MRI with these improved methods, nor are neuropathological data available on volume changes. The lack of standardized methodology across sites is a reflection of this state of development, but will eventually be necessary if data are to be compared and pooled across sites. Over the past ten to fifteen years, neurobiologic research in autism has rather consistently provided evidence of functional abnormalities in frontal and parietal cortex and in neural connectivity (Minshew, 1991). In contrast, neuropathologic observations have emphasized abnormalities in the limbic system and failed to identify abnormality in cortex, with the initial methods of assessment. Volumetric imaging has the potential for providing valid structural measurements of cortex, hippocampus, white matter, and corpus callosum that may contribute to the resolution in the disparity between functional deficits and identified structural abnormalities in autism. In addition, the resolution limits of imaging and neuropathologic methods necessitates a greater emphasis on functional imaging methods such as functional MRI, MRS, and PET.

ACKNOWLEDGMENTS

The careful and dedicated technical assistance of Nancie E. Phillips, Susan R. Weldy, Kristin McCrory, and Evelyn Herbert is acknowledged and appreciated. This work was supported by NIMH grant MH40858 to Nancy Minshew.

REFERENCES

Arin, D. M., Bauman, M. L., and Kemper, T. L. 1991. The distribution of Purkinje cell loss in the cerebellum in autism. *Neurology* 41:307 (abstract).

Bauman, M. L. 1991. Microscopic neuroanatomic abnormalities in autism. *Pediatrics* 87(Suppl.):791–96.

Bauman, M. L., and Kemper, T. L. 1985. Histoanatomic observations of the brain in early infantile autism. *Neurology* 35:866–74.

Bauman, M. L., LeMay, M., Bauman, R. A., and Rosenberger P. B. 1985. Computerized tomographic (CT) observations of the posterior fossa in early infantile autism. *Neurology* 35:247 (abstract).

Campbell, M. S., Rosenbloom, S., Perry, R., George, A. E., Kricheff, I. I., Anderson, L., Small, A. M., and Jennings, S. J. 1982. Computerized axial tomography in young autistic children. *American Journal of Psychiatry* 139:510–12.

Chui, H. C., and Damasio, A. R. 1980. Human cerebral asymmetries evaluated by computed tomography. *Journal of Neurology, Neurosurgery, and Psychiatry* 43:873–78.

Ciesielski, K. T., Allen, P. S., Sinclair, B. D., Pabst, H. F., Yanossky, R., and Ludwig, R. 1990. Hypoplasia of cerebellar vermis in autism and childhood leukemia. In *Proceedings of the 5th International Child Neurology Congress.* Tokyo, Japan, pp. 650–(Abstract).

Courchesne, E., Townsend, J. P., Akshoomoff, N. A., Yeung-Courchesne, R., Press, G. A., Murakami, J. W., Lincoln, A. J., James, H. E., Saitoh, O., Egaas, B., Haas, R. H., Schreibman, L. In press. A new finding: Impairment in shifting attention in autistic and cerebellar patients. In S. H. Broman and J. Grafman, eds., *Atypical Deficits in Developmental Disorders: Implications for Brain Function.* Hillsdale, N.J.: Lawrence Erlbaum Associates.

Courchesne, E., Elmasian, R. O., and Yeung-Courchesne, R. 1987. Electrophysiologic correlates of cognitive processing: P3b and Nc, basic, clinical and developmental research. In A. M. Halliday, S. R. Butler, and R. Paul, eds., *A Textbook of Clinical Neurophysiology.* 645–76. Sussex, England: John Wiley and Sons.

Courchesne, E., Kilman, B. A., Galambos, R., and Lincoln, A. J. 1984. Autism: Processing of novel auditory information assessed by event-related brain potentials. *Electroencephalography and Clinical Neurophysiology* 59:238–48.

Courchesne, E., Press, G. A., and Yeung-Courchesne, R. 1992. Parietal lobe abnormalities detected by magnetic resonance in patients with infantile autism. *Society for Neuroscience Abstracts* 18:332.

Courchesne, E., Saitoh, O., Yeung-Courchesne, R., Press, G. A., Lincoln, A. J., Haas, R. H., and Schreibman, L. Two subtypes of cerebellar pathology detected with MR in patients with autism: hyperplasia and hypoplasia of vermal lobules VI and VII. *American Journal of Roentgenology.* In press.

Courchesne, E., Yeung-Courchesne, R., Press, G. A., Hesselink, J. R., and Jernigan, T. L. 1988. Hypoplasia of cerebellar vermal lobules VI and VII in autism. *New England Journal of Medicine* 318:1349–54.

Creasey, J., Rumsey, J. M., Schwartz, M., Duara, R., Rapoport, J. L., and Rapoport, S. I. 1986. Brain morphometry in autistic men as measured by volumetric computed tomography. *Archives of Neurology* 43:669–72.

Damasio, A. R. 1984. Autism (editorial). *Archives of Neurology* 41:481.

Damasio, H., Maurer, R. G., Damasio, A. R., and Chui, H. C. 1980. Computerized tomographic scan findings in patients with autistic behavior. *Archives of Neurology* 37:504–10.

Filipek, P. A., Kennedy, D. N., Caviness, V. S., Jr., Rossnick, S. L., Spraggins, T. A., and Starewicz, P. M. 1989. Magnetic resonance imaging-based brain morphometry: Development and application to normal subjects. *Annals of Neurology* 25:61–67.

Filipek, P. A., Richelme, C., Kennedy, D. N., Rademacher, J., Pitcher, D. A., Zidel, S., and Caviness, V. S. 1992. Morphometric analysis of the brain in developmental language disorders and autism. *Annals of Neurology* 32:475 (abstract).

Gaffney, G. R., Kuperman, S., Tsai, L. Y., and Minchin, S. 1988. Morphological evidence of brainstem involvement in infantile autism. *Biological Psychiatry* 24:578–86.

Gaffney, G. R., Kuperman, S., Tsai, L. Y., and Minchin, S. 1989. Forebrain structure in infantile autism. *Journal of the American Academy of Child and Adolescent Psychiatry* 28:534–37.

Gaffney, G. R., Kuperman, S., Tsai, L. Y., Minchin, S., and Hassanein, K. M. 1987a. Midsagittal magnetic resonance imaging of autism. *British Journal of Psychiatry* 151:831–33.

Gaffney, G. R., and Tsai, L. Y. 1987b. Brief report: Magnetic resonance imaging of high level autism. *Journal of Autism and Developmental Disorders* 17:433–38.

Gaffney, G. R., Tsai, L. Y., Kuperman, S., and Minchin, S. 1987c. Cerebellar structure in autism. *American Journal of Diseases of Children* 141:1330–32.

Garber, H. J., Ritvo, E. R., Chui, L. C., Griswold, V. J., Kashanian, A., and Oldendorf, W. H. 1989. A magnetic resonance imaging study of autism: Normal fourth ventricle size and absence of pathology. *American Journal of Psychiatry* 146:532–35.

Gillberg, C., and Svendsen, P. 1983. Childhood psychosis and computed tomographic brain scan findings. *Journal of Autism and Developmental Disorders* 13:19–33.

Harcherik, D. F., Cohen, D. J., Ort, S., Paul, R., Shaywitz, B. A., Volkmar, F. R., Rothman, S. L. G., and Leckman, J. F. 1985. Computed tomographic brain scanning in four neuropsychiatric disorders of childhood. *American Journal of Psychiatry* 142:731–34.

Hauser, S. L., DeLong, G. R., and Rosman, N. P. 1975. Pneumographic findings in the infantile autism syndrome: A correlation with temporal lobe disease. *Brain* 98:667–88.

Hier, D. B., LeMay, M., and Rosenberger, P. B. 1979. Autism and unfavorable left–right asymmetries of the brain. *Journal of Autism and Developmental Disorders* 9:153–59.

Holttum, J. R., Minshew, N. J., Sanders, R. S., and Phillips, N. E. 1992. Magnetic resonance imaging of the posterior fossa in autism. *Biological Psychiatry* 32:1091–1101.

Hoshino, Y., Manome, T., Kaneko, M., Yashima, Y., and Kumashiro, H. 1984. Computed tomography of the brain in children with early infantile autism. *Folia Psychiatrica et Neurologica Japonica* 38:33–44.

Hsu, M., Yeung-Courchesne, R., Courchesne, E., and Press, G. A. 1991. Absence of pontine abnormality in infantile autism. *Archives of Neurology* 48:1160–63.

Jacobson, R., LeCouteur, A., Howlin, P., and Rutter, M. 1988. Selective subcortical abnormalities in autism. *Psychological Medicine* 18:39–48.

Kleiman, M. D., Neff, S., and Rosman, N. P. 1992. The brain in infantile autism: Is the cerebellum really abnormal? *Annals of Neurology* 28:422 (abstract).

LeMay, M., and Kido, D. K. 1978. Asymmetries of the cerebral hemispheres on computed tomograms. *Journal of Computer Assisted Tomography* 2:471–76.

Murakami, J. W., Courchesne, E., Press, G. A., Yeung-Courchesne, R., and Hesselink, J. R. 1989. Reduced cerebellar hemisphere size and its relationship to vermal hypoplasia in autism. *Archives of Neurology* 46:689–94.

Ornitz, E. M. 1985. Neurophysiology of infantile autism. *Journal of the American Academy of Child Psychiatry* 24:251–62.

Ornitz, E. M., and Ritvo, E. R. 1968. Neurophysiologic mechanisms underlying perceptual inconstancy in autistic and schizophrenic children. *Archives of General Psychiatry* 19:22–27.

Piven, J., Berthier, M. L., Starkstein, S. E., Nehme, E., Pearlson, G., and Folstein, S. 1992. Magnetic resonance imaging evidence for a defect of cerebral cortical development in autism. *American Journal of Psychiatry* 14:734–39.

Piven, J., Nehme, E., Simon, J., Barta, P., Pearlson, G., and Folstein, S. E. 1992. Magnetic resonance imaging in autism: Measurement of the cerebellum, pons, and fourth ventricle. *Biological Psychiatry* 31:491–504.

Prior, M. R., Tress, B., Hoffman, W. L., and Boldt, D. 1984. Computed tomographic study of children with classic autism. *Archives of Neurology* 41:482–84.

Ritvo, E., and Garber, J. H. 1988. Cerebellar hypoplasia and autism. *New England Journal of Medicine* 319:1152 (abstract).

Rosenbloom, S., Campbell, M., and George, A. E. 1984. High resolution CT scanning in infantile autism: A quantitative approach. *Journal of the American Academy of Child Psychiatry* 23:72–77.

Rumsey, J. M., Creasey, H., Stepanek, J. S., Dorwart, R., Patronas, N., Hamburger, S. D., and Duara, R. 1988. Hemispheric asymmetries, fourth ventricular size, and cerebellar morphology in autism. *Journal of Autism and Developmental Disorders* 18:127–37.

Rumsey, J. M., Duara, R., Grady, C., Rapoport, J. L., Margolin, R. A., Rapoport, S. I., and Cutler, N. R. 1985. Brain metabolism in autism: Resting cerebral glucose utilization as measured with positron emission tomography (PET). *Archives of General Psychiatry* 15:448–57.

Rutter, M. 1988. Biological basis of autism: Implications for intervention. In F.J. Menolascino and J.A. Stark, eds., *Preventive and Curative Intervention in Mental Retardation.* 265–94. Baltimore: Brookes Publishing.

Schaeffer, G. B., Thompson, J. N., Jr., Bodensteiner, J. B., Gingold, M., Wilson, M., and Wilson, D. 1991. Age-related changes in the relative growth of the posterior fossa. *Journal of Child Neurology* 6:15–19.

Tsai, L. Y., Jacoby, O. G., and Stewart, M. A. 1983. Morphological cerebral asymmetries in autistic children. *Biological Psychiatry* 18:317–27.

5

IN VIVO BRAIN CHEMISTRY OF AUTISM
³¹P MAGNETIC RESONANCE
SPECTROSCOPY STUDIES

Nancy J. Minshew, M.D.

Magnetic resonance spectroscopy (MRS) is a powerful tool for studying the in vivo chemistry of the brain. It is likely to join positron emission tomography (PET) and single-photon emission tomography (SPECT) over the next decade as a method for the direct analysis of brain chemistry. Although spectroscopy was the original scientific application of the nuclear magnetic resonance phenomenon, in vivo MRS has lagged considerably behind magnetic resonance imaging (MRI) in the development of clinical applications. The reasons for this difference have been several. MRI was largely able to follow in the mold established by computerized axial tomography (CT) and was supported by its immediate clinical acceptance and the attendant financial reimbursement. The development of in vivo spectroscopy, on the other hand, did not have these advantages. It was further limited by a greater dependence on specialized expertise in biophysics and by competition for instrument time and institutional resources with clinical interests. In addition, the development of in vivo spectroscopy required a high-field magnet with good field homogeneity, whereas most of the clinical magnets purchased for imaging were low-field models, thus eliminating the option for spectroscopy.

The major advantages of MRS over PET and SPECT are the capacity to directly assay tissue metabolites and to do so noninvasively and without the use of radiation. The primary limitations of MRS are the low signal-to-noise ratio, necessitating recording periods on the order of five to ten minutes, the potential limitations of spatial localization methods for measurements of phospholipid metabolism, and the need to validate the localization and quantification aspects of these procedures. However, ongoing development of MRS methodology are progressively reducing these limitations as evidenced by the recent evolution in spatial localization methodology and fast magnetic resonance technology.

THE PHYSICOCHEMICAL BASIS OF MRI AND MRS

Both MRI and MRS rely on the same basic physical chemical properties of atoms, but exploited in slightly different ways. Specifically, the resonance frequency of a nucleus is modified by neighboring atoms, resulting in a resonance shift along the frequency spectrum that is characteristic of each chemical environment; this phenomenon is referred to as *chemical shift*. In addition, the relaxation time of an excited atom is dependent on its rotational and longitudinal motion freedom, which is in turn determined by its environment; these processes are referred to as T_1 or T_2 *relaxation*, depending on the mechanisms involved in the dissipation of energy as the nucleus goes from its excited state to the ground state. In the case of imaging, the differences in the relaxation time of the water proton in three different environments (cerebrospinal fluid, gray matter, and white matter) are used to define neuroanatomic structure. The progressive decrement in the mobility of water protons in these three environments produces the tissue contrast used to generate the image format. In MRS, the modification of nuclear resonance frequency by the chemical environment is used to identify and quantify the different chemical species containing the paramagnetic atom under study, resulting in a spectrum in which the different molecules containing the atom are displayed as peaks dispersed over the observed frequency range. The resonance frequency or location of the peak identifies the chemical species, whereas the area under the peak indicates its quantity.

BIOLOGICALLY RELEVANT NUCLEI

MRS is dependent on the presence of atomic nuclei with magnetic moments. For biologic studies, the relevant nuclei include hydrogen (^{1}H), carbon (^{13}C), sodium (^{23}Na), and phosphorus (^{31}P). In addition, lithium (^{7}Li) and fluoride (^{19}F) are of value for pharmacologic studies. These nuclei enable the study of cellular energy metabolism, membrane lipid metabolism, glycogen, some amino acids and neurotransmitters, as well as lithium and fluorinated pharmacologic agents.

^{31}P MAGNETIC RESONANCE SPECTROSCOPY

For technical and scientific reasons, the phosphorus nucleus has significant advantages over the other biologically relevant nuclei for the study of neuropsychiatric disorders, particularly those with a developmental or degenerative origin (i.e., disorders in which abnormalities of brain membrane metabolism with or without alterations in bioenergetics are likely to be part of the pathophysiology). With ^{31}P MRS, it is possible to investigate both high-energy phosphate metabolism and membrane phospholipid metabolism, two major aspects of brain function and structure.

^{31}P MRS AND BIOENERGETICS

The energy status of the brain is assayed through the resonances for phosphocreatine (PCr), adenosine triphosphate (ATP), adenosine diphosphate (ADP), and inorganic phosphate (P_i), as well as the determination of intracellular pH. In the in vivo spectrum (Figure 5.1), ATP and ADP are represented in three resonance regions, reflecting the γ, α, and β phosphoruses of ATP and the α and β phosphoruses of ADP. These three regions of the spectrum also contain contributions other than ATP and ADP and so are also referred to as the *ionized ends, esterified ends,* and *middles regions.* The ionized ends region is composed of the resonances from γ ATP and β ADP. The esterified ends region is comprised of the α phosphoruses of ATP and ADP, the dinucleotides (such as nicotinamide adenine dinucleotide, cytidine diphosphocholine, and cytidine diphosphoethanolamine), and the uridine diphosphosugars. The middles region consists of the β phosphorus of ATP. Intracellular pH can be calculated by the chemical shift difference between the PCr

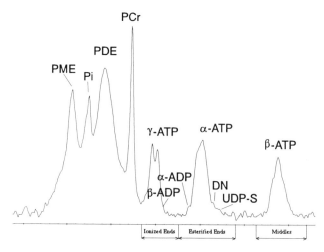

Figure 5.1. *In Vivo* [31]P Nuclear Magnetic Resonance Spectroscopy of the Dorsal Prefrontal Cortex.

and P_i peaks or between the γ and α peaks of ATP (Petroff et al., 1985; Pettegrew et al., 1988).

^{31}P MRS AND MEMBRANE PHOSPHOLIPID METABOLISM

Brain phospholipid metabolism is assessed through the phosphomonoester (PME) and phosphodiester (PDE) resonances. In brain extracts, the PME resonance is shown to consist predominantly of contributions from α-glycerol phosphate, phosphoethanolamine, and phosphocholine. In the mammalian brain, these three metabolites are found predominantly in the anabolic pathway for membrane phospholipids. Similarly, the PDE resonance has been shown to contain primarily glycerol 3-phosphoethanolamine and glycerol 3-phosphocholine, the catabolic products of phospholipid metabolism in mammalian brain. These metabolites are involved in the metabolism of the two phospholipids phosphatidylcholine and phosphatidylethanolamine, which are major components of all membranes, including those in the brain. Phosphatidylethanolamine is unusually abundant in brain membranes.

THE VALIDATION OF IN VIVO MRS FINDINGS

The characterization of the various contributors to the in vivo phosphorus spectrum of the human brain relies heavily on in vitro studies. In vitro studies provide chemical conditions more favorable to ^{31}P MRS and utilize higher-field magnets, resulting in significant enhancement of sensitivity and resolution (Figure 5.2). Peak identity is further verified by other biochemical and spectroscopic procedures. In vitro MRS studies of autopsy human brain or mammalian brain also provide an opportunity for confirming and further characterizing the findings observed on the lower-resolution in vivo spectra. Additionally, in vitro MRS data on brain chemistry can be compared with the results of classic biochemical assays performed on the same tissue sample. The in vitro investigations are therefore a significant and essential component of MRS research.

VARIOUS IN VIVO MRS TECHNIQUES

In vivo spectroscopy of the human brain can be accomplished with varying degrees of spatial localization using one of three techniques: a surface coil, pulse sequences with spatial localization to a designated slice of brain, and region-specific localization sequences. The surface coil technique was the initial method developed for in vivo MRS and, hence, the most MRS data are available with this technique.

As the name suggests, the surface coil technique for MRS involves the positioning of a receiver-transmitter coil on the external surface of the

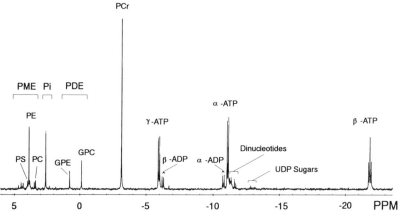

Figure 5.2. High-resolution phosphorus-31 nuclear magnetic resonance spectrum of a perchioric acid extract of freeze-clamped brain from a 3-month-old Fischer 344 rat.
Source: Pettegrew, Keshavan & Minshew, 1993

Note: Easily identifiable resonances and their chemical shifts (δ) include the phosphomonoesters (PME); α-glyc-erol phosphate (α-GP, 4.298), L-phosphoserine (PS, 3.898), phosphoethanolamine (PE, 3.848), and phosphocholine (PC, 3.338); inorganic orthophosphate (PI, 2.638); the phosphodiesters (PDE): glycerol 3-phosphoethanolamine (GPE, 0.818) and glycerol 3-phosphocholine (GPC, –0.138); phosphocreatine (PCr. –3.128); the nucleotide triphos-phates (especially adenosine triphosphate [ATP]; γ –5.808, α –10.928, β –21.48); the nucleotide diphosphates (es-pecially adenosine diphosphate [ADP]; β –6.118, α –10.618); dinucleotides such as nicotinamide adenine dinucleotide (NAD, –11.378); and a complex resonance band centered around –12.898, which is composed of nucle-oside diphospho-derivatives such as uridine diphospho (UDP) sugars and cytidine diphospho-derivatives such as cy-tidine diphosphocholine and cytidine diphosphoethanotamine. PPM = parts per million.

body over the organ or tissue to be studied. The sampling profile under the surface coil is that of a truncated cone in which the depth of tissue penetration is equal to the radius of the coil. For studies of the brain, the pulse sequence can be designed so as to neutralize contributions from scalp, whereas the phosphorus-containing molecules in bone are highly immobile and, hence, do not contribute to the spectrum. Similarly, the phosphorus-containing molecules of myelin are highly immobilized and are also unlikely to contribute significantly to brain spectra obtained with a surface coil. The actual brain tissue contributing signal to a spectrum can be defined with a "coil image." Although the boundaries of the sam-pled brain are not precisely defined, the location and size of the coil re-strict the origin of the signal to immediately subjacent brain. The primary limitation of the surface coil method is that it is restricted to the study of structures located at the surface of the body. For some tissues or regions such as muscle or frontal cortex, this restriction does not constitute a lim-itation. However, in vivo studies of the brain are limited with a surface coil to the cortex of the frontal lobes, due to the interference from mus-cle and blood sinuses overlying the temporal, parietal, and occipital cor-tex and the distance of subcortical structures from the scalp surface.

Pulsed-gradient spatial localization methods have been developed re-cently to address these limitations, but do so at the potential expense of the initial portion of the MRS signal due to the time required to turn off the gradients before signal can be recorded. The initial part of the signal contains contributions to the phospholipid resonances and, hence, the localization methods may sacrifice the accuracy or validity of the phospholipid data. These spectroscopy methods and issues are described in detail in recent publications (Pettegrew, 1991; Pettegrew et al., 1991; Minshew et al., 1993).

Two different localization techniques are currently available for in vivo MRS. The least sophisticated of these identifies a cross-sectional slice and sums all of the MRS signal over the entire slice. This approach is the least desirable of the three MRS methods because it averages data across two parameters that are often of pathophysiologic significance in disorders of the central nervous system—distinctions between gray and white matter, and distinctions between the left and right hemispheres and anterior and posterior regions within the hemispheres. The most advanced MAS methods and equipment allow for localization of the signal to small preselected regions of the brain, although the actual boundaries of the tissue sampled may be less precise. Because the spatial localization methods are relatively recent and require the purchase of new MRI–MRS equipment, the majority of the ^{31}P in vivo MRS studies of the brain thus far have relied on the surface coil method.

THE QUANTITATION OF MRS RESULTS

The methods for quantitating MRS data are also subject to variation, each with its strengths and limitations. The derivation of accurate quantitation from MRS data requires the presence of an external phosphorus-containing standard in the imaging field at the time of the study and an accurate determination of tissue volume. The accuracy or validity of the quantitation depends on the accuracy of the brain volume determination and the comparability of the molecular environment in the external standard solution to the tissue environment. Because of the requirement for spatial localization, absolute quantitation is restricted to the spatial localization MRS methods. Lacking an accurate determination of tissue volume, the data from in vivo surface coil studies are often expressed in terms of relative percentages of the total phosphorus signal. However, this quantification method has been demonstrated to be equivalent to results expressed in μmole/g[klunk, submitted], in in vitro experiments with an internal standard. The advantage of this data format is that the data are independent of variations in tissue volume, which has been an important confound in PET studies of CNS disorders.

^{31}P MRS STUDIES OF NORMAL BRAIN DEVELOPMENT

The study of normal brain development from birth through senescence with ^{31}P MRS is a prerequisite for understanding pathophysiologic processes. To investigate the normal developmental and aging changes in brain chemistry as detected by ^{31}P MRS, in vitro MRS studies of brain extracts were studied in Fischer 344 rats ranging in age from newborn through senescence, which is about 2 years in the rat (Pettegrew et al., 1985, 1987, 1990). These studies revealed high levels of PMEs (membrane building blocks) beginning in the newborn period, which declined rapidly thereafter to the low levels maintained throughout adult life. The PDE levels (membrane breakdown products) demonstrated the reverse phenomenon, with low levels in the newborn period that rose rapidly to stabilize at adult levels. These developmental changes in phospholipid metabolism reflected in the developmental changes in PME and PDE levels coincide with neuronal organizational events. The early high levels of PMEs or membrane building blocks coincide with the development of the dendritic tree and synaptogenesis. The rise in PDE levels and drop in PME levels coincides with the end of dendritic proliferation. The developmental data for bioenergetics revealed low PCr and ATP levels initially and a rise to adult levels coincident with the development of brain electrical activity.

Normative data for humans has been derived from in vivo MRS studies of normal controls involved in studies of various neuropsychiatric disorders. These data are limited and are mostly from older adults, although data on individuals between twelve and thirty years of age has been accrued more recently (Minshew et al., 1992b). With normal brain aging in humans, the PME levels were observed to decline slightly and the PDEs to rise slightly, without changes in PCr or ATP (Panchalingam et al., 1990, 1991a, 1991b). These small changes in phospholipid metabolism with normal aging are suggestive of decreased synthesis and increased breakdown of brain membranes and are consistent with neuropathologic observations of a reduction in dendritic spines with normal aging. In contrast, adolescence and early adulthood are considered times of synaptic pruning in the human dorsal prefrontal cortex. The ^{31}P MRS studies of normal subjects between twelve and thirty years of age have revealed a significant decrease in the levels of PME, an increase in PDE levels, and no significant changes in the levels of PCr, ATP, or P$_i$ as a function of increasing age in adolescents and young adults (Minshew et al., 1992b). These MRS results are consistent with decreased synthesis and increased catabolism of phospholipids, which is in keeping with synaptic pruning. Studies such as these suggest that ^{31}P MRS will provide additional insight into important developmentally regulated processes in the brain.

^{31}P MRS FINDINGS IN AUTISM

MRS remains a relatively new method of clinical research, and consequently few studies of neuropsychiatric disorders, other than hypoxia or stroke, have been reported. Only one study has appeared on autism so far (Minshew et al., 1993) and is described here. Due to the limited sample size and lack of replication to date of this study, the findings described are preliminary, but are particularly interesting in the context of what is known about brain development and the neurobiology of autism from neurophysiologic, neuropathologic, neuropsychologic, and PET studies. This study and the others described also demonstrate the potential contributions of MRS to clinical neuroscience research.

The first MRS study in autism was undertaken to investigate the in vivo brain chemistry of the cerebral cortex in autism and its relationship to the pathophysiology of this disorder (Minshew et al., 1993). The cerebral cortex had been implicated in the pathophysiology of autism by a number of studies, beginning with the reports of diminution of auditory and, to a lesser extent, visual P300s. Because the subjects were able to perform the cognitive task correctly, the neurophysiologic abnormality was initially hypothesized to be the consequence of reliance on less-efficient, alternative pathways for the processing of information by parietal cortex (Novick, Kurtzberg, and Vaughan, 1979; Novick et al., 1980).

These observations were subsequently confirmed by other laboratories and were followed by reports of the absence of the frontally distributed negative component Nc during selective attention paradigms (Courchesne, Elmasian, and Yeung-Courchesne, 1987; Courchesne et al., 1989; Grillon, Courchesne, and Akshoomoff, 1989; Ciesielski, Courchesne, and Elmasian, 1990), suggesting the presence in the frontal lobes of a similar neurophysiologic abnormality. This neurophysiologic evidence of abnormal neural connectivity coincided with a 2-fluoro-3-deoxy-D-glucose PET study reporting decreased functional connectivity with the frontal and parietal cortex. These data revealed fewer interhemispheric functional correlations between homologous regions in the frontal and parietal cortices and decreased intrahemispheric correlations between the frontal and parietal cortices and the striatum and thalamus (Horwitz et al., 1987). These findings suggested dysfunction at the neural network level of brain organization with widespread involvement of cortex and functionally related subcortical areas.

The third area of evidence suggesting abnormalities in the cortex and in neural connectivity came from neuropsychologic studies of high-functioning autistic individuals (Rumsey and Hamburger, 1988; Minshew et al., 1992a; Minshew and Goldstein, 1993a). These studies reported a pattern of cognitive abnormalities in autism that was characterized by deficits in complex cognitive functions such as complex memory, complex language comprehension, concept formation, and problem solving, and by intact function in more elementary cognitive functions such as basic attention, sensory perception, rote memory, and formal language abilities. This pattern has been interpreted as consistent with either frontal-systems dysfunction or more widespread dysfunction (Rumsey and Hamburger, 1988) or dysfunction in a distributed neural network of cortical origin responsible for complex information processing (Minshew and Goldstein, 1993a, 1993b).

In this ^{31}P MRS study of autism, high-energy phosphate and membrane phospholipid metabolism was investigated in dorsal prefrontal cortex under resting conditions in eleven nonsedated nonmentally retarded autistic adolescents and young adults who met research diagnostic criteria for Autistic Disorder and eleven closely matched normal controls (Minshew et al., 1993). Emphasis was placed on the study of nonmentally retarded autistic individuals, the accuracy of the diagnosis of autism using research diagnostic instruments and outside verification of diagnosis, and close matching between the autistic and control groups on variables most likely to have an impact on the structure and function of the central nervous system (e.g., age, full-scale and verbal IQ, gender, and possibly socioeconomic status). Neuropsychologic and language parameters reflecting the overall severity of autism and of the cognitive and language deficits in high-functioning autistic individuals (Minshew et al., 1992b; Rumsey and Hamburger, 1988; Venter, Lord, and Schopler, 1992) were chosen a priori for comparison with the MRS metabolite levels to investigate the relationship between measures of brain chemistry and the clinical disorder.

INTERGROUP METABOLITE DIFFERENCES

The significant metabolic alterations observed in the dorsal prefrontal cortex of the autistic subjects relative to the controls were decreased levels of PCr and decreased levels of esterified ends or αATP. The levels of PME, P^i, PDE, ionized ends (αATP and βADP), middles (βATP), and intracellular pH were not significantly different between autistic and control subjects.

A decrease in PCR levels, in the absence of changes in intracellular pH, suggested increased utilization of PCr to maintain ATP levels (e.g., a hypermetabolic state). The biologic import of this finding is unknown, but neurophysiologic studies have suggested that alterations in bioenergetics may be the consequence of neurophysiologic alterations. As previously mentioned, Novick and co-workers (1979, 1980) suggested that the P300 abnormalities in autism may be the consequence of reliance on less-efficient, alternative pathways for information processing. In neurophysiologic studies of normal individuals, Gevins and co-workers observed that incorrect responses during cognitive evoked potential paradigms resulted in greater activation of frontal cortex and related pathways than correct answers (Gevins et al., 1983, 1987, 1989). Similarly, PET studies in normal individuals have suggested that brain function was more efficient (e.g., fewer neural circuits are activated) in individuals with higher IQ and once a new task has been learned (Haier et al., 1992; Squire et al., 1992). Additional MRS, PET, and functional MRI studies using cortical activation techniques are needed to further investigate brain connectivity and function in autism.

The decrease in esterified ends observed in the autistic group could be of multiple origins. Contributors to this resonance include the α-phosphate of ATP and ADP, dinucleotides such as nicotinamide adenine dinucleotide, cytidine diphosphocholine, cytidine diphosphoethanolamine, and uridine diphosphosugars. Hence, a decrease in this resonance could reflect diminished levels of one or more of these constituents. In addition to ATP and the dinucleotides, the contributors to this resonance are found predominantly in the pathways of membrane biosynthesis and lipid and protein glycosylation. The absence of alterations in β-ATP levels, the only peak whose sole contribution is from ATP, suggested that the decrease in esterified ends in autism may be related to alterations in these membrane- and glycosylation-related biosynthetic activities. The significance of this finding for the pathophysiology of autism is unknown. However, alterations in protein glycosylation could theoretically be related to the alterations reported in immune status in autism (Warren et al., 1986, 1990a, 1990b) because highly glycosylated proteins are involved in normal immune function (Gennis, 1989).

INTRAGROUP CLINICAL–METABOLIC CORRELATIONS

When the ^{31}P MRS metabolite levels were compared with IQ scores (Wechsler, 1974, 1981) and selected scores from tests of reasoning ability (Wisconsin Card Sorting Test—Grant and Berg, 1948; Making Inferences subtest from the Test of Language Competence—Wiig and Secord, 1989), secondary memory (delayed recall scores from the California Verbal Learning Test—Delis et al., 1987) and semantic language comprehension (Wiig and Secord, 1989; Token Test—Benton and Hamsher, 1978), a number of significant clinical–metabolic correlations were observed in the autistic group that were not present in the control group. The correlations were generally quite robust and demonstrated a consistent pattern across the different clinical parameters. As test performance declined, the levels of the most labile high-energy phosphate compound (PCr) and of the membrane building blocks (PME) decreased, and the levels of the membrane breakdown products (PDE) increased (Figure 5.3). These findings are consistent with a hypermetabolic energy state and with undersynthesis and enhanced degradation of brain membranes. The clinical–metabolic correlations with PCr provide additional support for the biologic significance of an altered energy state, probably secondary to the neurophysiologic abnormalities in autism. The phospholipid correlations are more intriguing, in view of the histoanatomic observations of a truncation in the development of the dendritic tree in autism (Bauman and Kemper, 1985; Raymond, Bauman, and Kemper, 1989). The metabolic evidence of undersynthesis and enhanced degradation of brain phospholipids may provide a possible molecular metabolic basis for the observed histoanatomic findings, as the presence of this metabolic pattern during fetal brain development could be expected to result in undersynthesis of brain membranes in affected neural systems. In addition, this metabolic pattern also has the potential for membrane degradation. It may, therefore, provide a potential molecular metabolic basis for the clinical regression that occurs at presentation in nearly one-third of autistic children and the deterioration that occurs in a small minority in adolescence.

The clinical–metabolic correlations observed in the autistic subjects were not present in the control subjects. This suggests that the correlations in the autistic subjects were not merely an exaggerated form of normal biologic variability, but instead may represent a true qualitative alteration in brain metabolism.

In summary, this preliminary study reported alterations in high-energy phosphate and membrane phospholipid metabolism in the brain in autism, which correlated with the clinical deficits and severity of this disorder. As with the PET findings in autism (Chapter 6), the clinical–metabolic correlations were scientifically and statistically the most sig-

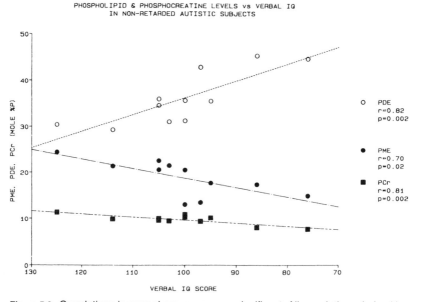

Figure 5.3. Correlations in normal group were nonsignificant. All correlations derived by linear regression analysis.

nificant, and provided the greatest insights into the pathophysiology of autism. This would suggest that future MRS studies should incorporate such correlations as a central element of their design.

^{31}P MRS FINDINGS IN SCHIZOPHRENIA

The overlap in clinical symptomatology between autism and schizophrenia has long been recognized. This overlap was formally investigated in the study by Rumsey, Andreasen, and Rapoport (1986), who noted significant clinical overlap in the area of "negative symptoms" but not in the "positive symptom" area. Neurobiologic studies in autism and schizophrenia have also provided evidence of significant areas of overlap, as shown by the high degree of similarity between findings for these two disorders on neuropsychologic functioning, oculomotor physiology, and cognitive evoked potentials. This pattern of similarities and dissimilarities makes these two clinical disorders excellent comparison groups for neurobiologic research studies.

A ^{31}P MRS study of first-episode, nonmedicated schizophrenic individuals similar to the study described above has reported findings similar to those in autism, with the significant exception of the abnormalities involving energy metabolism (Pettegrew et al., 1991). In schizophrenia, the ^{31}P MRS high energy phosphate findings were indicative of frontal lobe hypometabolism, consistent with previous PET findings in schizophrenia. The phospholipid findings in schizophrenia were similar to those in autism, providing evidence of decreased synthesis and enhanced membrane degradation. Because schizophrenia develops in the second or third decade of life rather than during prenatal or early childhood years, the pathophysiologic ramifications of this molecular metabolic abnormality would differ somewhat from autism. Given the stage of brain development at the time of onset of schizophrenia, the ^{31}P MRS findings would support an exaggeration or loss of control of the synaptic pruning that is normally occurring at this time. The clinical, neurobiologic, and MRS similarities between autism and schizophrenia suggest that these two disorders may involve the same neural systems but differ primarily as a result of the timing of the neuropathologic process relative to the stage of brain development and the differing mode of progression (static congenital with regression in a subgroup versus episodic with or without complete reconstitution after each episode).

SUMMARY

Magnetic resonance spectroscopy has significant potential for increasing the understanding of the neurobiology of the brain in health and in various disorders. This technology is in its infancy as a clinical research tool, but NMR technology itself is in an advanced state, providing the opportunity for the rapid development of this technology for clinical research.

At this juncture in the development of clinical research applications of MRS, it is important that significant consideration be given early on to the development of adequate normative data by age, gender, IQ, and possibly also race and socioeconomic status. It is equally important that the early research efforts give careful consideration to the definition of subject groups, particularly the matching criteria for control subjects. Finally, MRS and PET studies so far have both suggested that functional correlations are likely to be more valuable than intergroup differences and should be a central part of the study design of future research.

ACKNOWLEDGMENTS

The careful and dedicated technical assistance of Melissa Nicholson, Stephen M. Dombrowski, Nancie E. Phillips, Susan R. Weldy, and Kristin C. McCrory are acknowledged and appreciated. This work was supported by NIMH grant MH40858 to Nancy J. Minshew.

REFERENCES

Bauman, M. L., and Kemper, T. L. 1985. Histoanatomic observations of the brain in early infantile autism. *Neurology* 35:866–74.

Benton, A. L., and Hamsher, K. deS. 1978. *Multilingual Aphasia Examination*. Iowa City: University of Iowa.

Ciesielski, K. T., Courchesne, E., and Elmasian, R. 1990. Effects of focused selective attention tasks on event-related potentials in autistic and normal individuals. *Electroencephalography and Clinical Neurophysiology* 75:207–20.

Courchesne, E., Elmasian, R. O., and Yeung-Courchesne, R. 1987. Electrophysiologic correlates of cognitive processing: P3b and Nc, basic, clinical and developmental research. In A. M. Halliday, S. R. Butler, and R. Paul, eds., *A Textbook of Clinical Neurophysiology*. 645–76. Sussex, England: John Wiley and Sons.

Courchesne, E., Lincoln, A. J., Yeung-Courchesne, R., Elmasian, R., and Grillon, C. 1989. Pathophysiologic findings in non-retarded autism and receptive developmental language disorders. *Journal of Autism and Developmental Disorders* 19:1–17.

Delis, D.C., Kramer, J. H., Kaplan, E., and Ober, B. A. 1987. *California Verbal Learning Test*. New York: Psychological Corporation.

Gennis, R. B. 1989. *Biomembranes: Molecular Structure and Function*. New York: Springer-Verlag.

Gevins, A. S., Cutillo, B. A., Bressler, S. L., Morgan, N. H., White, R. M., Illes, J., and Greer, D. S. 1989. Event-related covariances during a bimanual visuomotor task. II. Preparation and feedback. *Electroencephalography and Clinical Neurophysiology* 74: 147–60.

Gevins A. S., Morgan, N. H., Bressler, S. L., Cutillo, B. A., White, R. M., Illes, J., Greer, D. S., Doyle, J. C., and Zeitlin, G. M. 1987. Human neuroelectric patterns predict performance accuracy. *Science* 235:580–85.

Gevins, A. S., Schaffer, R. E., Doyle J. C., Cutillo, B. A., Tannehill, R. S., and Bressler, S. L. 1983. Shadows of thought: Shifting lateralization of human brain electrical patterns during brief visuomotor task. *Science* 220:97–99.

Grant, D. A., and Berg, E. A. 1948. *Wisconsin Card Sorting Test.* Odessa, FL: Psychological Assessment Resources.

Grillon, C., Courchesne, E., and Akshoomoff, N. 1989. Brainstem and middle latency auditory evoked potentials in autism and developmental language disorder. *Journal of Autism and Developmental Disorders* 19:255–69.

Haier, R. J., Siegel, B. V., MacLachlan, A., Soderling, E., Lottenberg, S., and Buchsbaum, M. S. 1992. Regional glucose metabolic changes after learning a complex visuospatial/motor task: A positron emission tomographic study. *Brain Research* 570:134–43.

Horwitz, B., Rumsey, J. M., Grady, C., and Rapoport, S. I. 1987. Interregional correlations of glucose utilization among brain regions in autistic adults. *Annals of Neurology* 22:118 (abstract).

Maurer, R. G., and Damasio, A. R. 1982. Childhood autism from the point of view of behavioral neurology. *Journal of Autism and Developmental Disorders* 12:195–205.

Minshew, N. J., and Goldstein, G. 1993a. Autism: A distributed neural network defect? *Archives of Clinical Neuropsychology* 8:252 (abstract).

Minshew, N. J., and Goldstein, G. 1993b. Is autism an amnesic disorder? Evidence from the California Verbal Learning Test. *Neuropsychology* 7:209–16.

Minshew, N. J., Goldstein, G., Muenz, L. R., and Payton, J. B. 1992a. Neuropsychological functioning in nonmentally retarded autistic individuals. *Journal of Clinical and Experimental Neuropsychology* 14:749–61.

Minshew, N. J., Panchalingam, K., Dombrowski, S. M., and Pettegrew, J. W. 1992b. Developmentally regulated changes in brain membrane metabolism. *Biological Psychiatry* 31:62A (abstract).

Minshew et al. 1993 publication.

Novick, B., Kurtzberg, D., and Vaughan, H. G., Jr. 1979. An electrophysiologic indication of defective information storage in childhood autism. *Psychiatry Research* 1:101–8.

Novick, B., Vaughan, H. G., Jr., Kurtzberg, D., and Simson, R. 1980. An electrophysiologic indication of auditory processing defects in autism. *Psychiatry Research* 3:107–14.

Panchalingam, K., Pettegrew, J. W., Branthoover, G., and Tretta, M. 1991a. ATP utilization in dorsal prefrontal cortex of Alzheimer's disease brain is correlated with severity of dementia. *Society for Neuroscience Abstracts* 17:1258 (abstract).

Panchalingam, K., Pettegrew, J. W., Strychor, S., and Tretta, M. 1990. Effect of normal aging on membrane phospholipid metabolism by ^{31}P *in vivo* NMR spectroscopy. *Society for Neuroscience Abstracts* 16:843 (abstract).

Panchalingam, K., Strychor, S., Tretta, M., Newton, A., and Pettegrew, J.W. 1991b. *In vivo* ^{31}P NMR shows decreased brain ATP utilization is correlated with severity of dementia in Alzheimer's disease. *Neurology* 41:269 (abstract).

Petroff, O. A. C., Prichard, J. W., Behar, K. L., Alger, J. R., den Hollander, J. A., and Shulman, R. G. 1985. Cerebral intracellular pH by ^{31}P nuclear magnetic resonance spectroscopy. *Neurology* 35:781–88.

Pettegrew, J. W. 1991. Nuclear magnetic resonance: Principles and applications to neuroscience research. In F. Boller and J. Grafman, eds., *Handbook of Neuropsychology, Vol. 5.* 39–56. Amsterdam: Elsevier Science Publishers.

Pettegrew, J. W., Keshavan, M. S., Panchalingam, K., Strychor, S., Kaplan, D. B., Tretta, M. G., and Allen, M. 1991. Alterations in brain high-energy phosphate and membrane phospholipid metabolism in first-episode, drug-naive schizophrenics. *Archives of General Psychiatry* 48:563–68.

Pettegrew, J. W., Kopp, S. J., Minshew, N. J., Glonek, T., Feliksik, J. M., Tow, J. P., and Cohen, M. M. 1985. ^{31}P NMR studies of phospholipid metabolism in developing and degenerating brain. *Neurology* 35:257.

Pettegrew, J. W., Kopp, S. J., Minshew, N. J., Glonek, T., Feliksik, J. M., Tow, J. P., and Cohen, M. M. 1987. ^{31}P nuclear magnetic resonance studies of phosphoglyceride metabolism in developing and degenerating brain: Preliminary observations. *Journal of Neuropathology and Experimental Neurology* 46:419–30.

Pettegrew, J. W., Panchalingam, K., Withers, G., McKeag, D., and Strychor, S. 1990. Changes in brain energy and phospholipid metabolism during development and aging in the Fischer 344 rat. *Journal of Neuropathology and Experimental Neurology* 49:237–49.

Pettegrew, J. W., Withers, G., Panchalingam, K., and Post, J. F. M. 1988. Considerations for brain pH assessment by ^{31}P NMR. *Magnetic Resonance Imaging* 6:135–42.

Pettegrew, J. W., Keshavan, M. S., and Minshew, N. J. 1993 ^{31}P Nuclear Magnetic Resonance Spectroscopy: Neurodevelopment and Schizophrenia. *Scizophrenia Bulletin* 19(1): 35–53.

Raymond, G., Bauman, M., and Kemper, T. 1989. The hippocampus in autism: Golgi analysis. *Annals of Neurology* 26:483–84 (abstract).

Rumsey, J. M., Andreasen, N. C., and Rapoport, J. L. 1986. Thought, language, communication, and affective flattening in autistic adults. *Archives of General Psychiatry* 43:771–77.

Rumsey, J. M., Duara, R., Grady, C., Rapoport, J. L., Margolin, R. A., Rapoport, S. I., and Cutler, N. R. 1985. Brain metabolism in autism: Resting cerebral glucose utilization as measured with positron emission tomography (PET). *Archives of General Psychiatry* 15:448–57.

Rumsey, J. M., and Hamburger, S. D. 1988. Neuropsychological findings in high-functioning men with infantile autism, residual state. *Journal of Clinical and Experimental Neuropsychology* 10:201–21.

Squire, L. R., Ojemann, J. G., Miezin, F. M., Petersen, S. E., Videen, T. O., and Raichle, M. E. 1992. Activation of the hippocampus in normal humans: A functional anatomical study of memory. *Proceedings of the National Academy of Science, U.S.A.* 89:1837–41.

Venter, A., Lord, C., and Schopler, E. 1992. A follow-up study of high functioning autistic children. *Journal of Child Psychology and Psychiatry* 33:489–507.

Warren, R. P., Cole, P., Odell, J. D., Pingree, C. B., Warren, W. L., White, E., Yonk, J., and Singh, V. K. 1990a. Detection of maternal antibodies in infantile autism. *Journal of the American Academy of Child and Adolescent Psychiatry* 29:873–77.

Warren, R. P., Yonk, L. J., Burger, R. A., Cole, P., Odell, J. D., Warren, W. L., White, E., and Singh, V. K. 1990b. Deficiency of suppressor-inducer (CD4+CD45RA+) T cells in autism. *Immunology Investigations* 19:245–51.

Warren, R. P., Margaretten, N. C., Pace, N. C., and Foster, A. 1986. Immune abnormalities in patients with autism. *Journal of Autism and Developmental Disorders* 16:189–97.

Wechsler, D. 1974. *Wechsler Intelligence Scale for Children—Revised Manual.* New York: Psychological Corporation.

Wechsler, D. 1981. *Wechsler Adult Intelligence Scale—Revised Manual.* New York: Psychological Corporation.

Wiig, E. H., and Secord, W. 1989. *Test of Language Competence—Expanded Edition.* New York: Psychological Corporation.

6

POSITRON EMISSION TOMOGRAPHY: IMPLICATIONS FOR CEREBRAL DYSFUNCTION IN AUTISM

Barry Horwitz, Ph.D.
Judith M. Rumsey, Ph.D.

Developmental disorders, such as autism, have generally presented formidable problems for scientific investigation. Often, no discernable gross anatomic abnormalities suggest which brain regions are particularly affected by the disorder. On the other hand, neuro-chemical and cellular abnormalities can sometimes be seen, suggesting that the disorder may involve abnormal functional organization rather than region-specific impairments. For these reasons, the investigation of developmental disorders using functional neuroimaging techniques may shed light on the neurobiologic bases for the symptoms.

PET and other functional neuroimaging techniques offer the possibility of studying numerous biochemical brain processes in patient groups and control subjects. In particular, the oxidative metabolism and blood flow of the brain are of great interest because of their relation to neural activity. In this chapter, we review studies of autism using PET and other functional neuroimaging modalities that measure the regional cerebral metabolic rate for glucose (rCMRglc), regional cerebral metabolic rate for oxygen (rCMRO2), or regional cerebral blood flow (rCBF).

AN OVERVIEW OF METABOLIC FUNCTIONAL NEUROIMAGING

The central hypothesis underlying metabolic imaging is that regions participating in a cognitive operation become more active and increase their rates of oxidative metabolism. This increased metabolic demand is thought to be due to an increased pumping of ions across nerve cell membranes to restore ionic gradients to the steady-state levels that were disrupted by neuronal activity (Mata et al., 1980). Because glucose is the primary substrate for brain oxidative metabolism, the most direct metabolic measures are rCMRO2 or rCMRglc. The rCBF also increases to supply the needed oxygen and glucose, and the coupling between rCBF and rCMRglc appears to be linear under most conditions (Raichle et al., 1976; Baron et al., 1985). Subsequent work, however, suggests that rCMRO$_2$ may sometimes be uncoupled from rCBF and rCMRglc, with rCMRO$_2$ being less responsive to increases in activity (Fox and Raichle, 1986; Raichle et al., 1987).

A large number of radiotracers have been developed to measure rCBF, rCMRO$_2$, and rCMRglc. The isotopes incorporated in radiopharmaceuticals fall into two classes: those that emit single gamma rays (e.g., ^{133}Xe, ^{123}I, ^{99}Tc) and those that emit positrons (e.g., ^{15}O, ^{11}C, ^{18}F). Isotopes that emit single gamma rays allow nontomographic surface imaging and relatively low resolution tomographic imaging with SPECT. Positron-emitting isotopes allow high-resolution tomographic imaging with PET.

PET makes use of the fact that when a positron (positive electron), after ejection from the nucleus of a positron-emitting nucleus of an atom, encounters an electron, mutual annihilation occurs in which two high-energy gamma rays are produced and move away at nearly 180 degrees relative to each other. Detecting these two gamma rays in coincidence determines the line along which the decay occurred. An image of the distribution of radioactivity in the imaged organ is generated by using the principles of computed tomography on the detected coincidence events. The distribution of radioactivity in the organ is converted into a quantitative image of a specific physiologic process by using a kinetic model for tracer distribution.

The measurement of rCMRglc in humans involves the application of the deoxyglucose method, developed by Sokoloff and colleagues (1977), to PET by labeling the molecule with ^{18}F or ^{11}C (Phelps et al., 1979; Reivich et al., 1979, 1985). This method integrates activity over a period of thirty to forty-five minutes. Reviews of the application of PET/deoxyglucose to studies of normal human subjects and patient populations can be found in Reivich and Alavi (1985), Phelps, Mazziotta, and Schelbert (1986), and Pawlik and Heiss (1989).

The principal methods of measuring rCBF using positron-emitting isotopes involve bolus injections of H$_2$^{15}O (Herscovitch, Markham, and Raichle, 1983; Raichle et al., 1983) or the inhalation of C^{15}O$_2$ (Lammertsma et al., 1990). Because the half life of ^{15}O is only 123 seconds, these methods also allow repeated scans spaced twelve to fifteen minutes apart, with the added advantage of high-resolution PET imaging.

Since the time interval over which rCBF is integrated is forty seconds to four minutes, these methods also provide a time frame conducive to cognitive studies. The measurement of rCMRO2 with PET is possible with a complicated procedure involving the measurement of rCBF, regional cerebral blood volume, and regional oxygen extraction ratio (e.g., Frackowiak et al., 1980) with separate scans. For reviews of the use of rCBF to investigate human brain function, see Friston and Frackowiak (1991) and Haxby et al. (1991).

Most of the early studies using PET, especially those examining rCMRglc, were performed with the subject in the resting state: awake, but with no specific cognitive demands. The goal was to see if specific abnormalities in cerebral metabolism could be detected and related to the neuropsychologic impairments or psychiatric symptoms in the population under study. For example, Haxby et al. (1985) found that many patients with dementia of the Alzheimer type showed asymmetries in posterior cortical glucose metabolism. Patients with a relative left-sided hypometabolism had greater language impairment compared to their visuospatial skills than did patients with a relatively greater right-sided hypometabolism, who showed the opposite pattern of cognitive abnormalities. Recently, cognitive studies performed while the subject is undergoing PET have become more frequent, especially when rCBF is the quantity being measured. For example, Grady et al. (1993) found frontal as well as posterior cortical activation during a face discrimination task in patients with dementia of the Alzheimer type. In contrast, age-matched normal subjects showed only posterior activation. Thus, to perform the same cognitive task, Alzheimer patients may need to recruit greater cerebral resources than healthy subjects.

An important methodologic point associated with functional neuroimaging studies concerns the use of normalized data. One advantage PET has over SPECT is that rCBF can be determined absolutely (that is, in units of milliliters per 100g per minute) in the former. The reason for this is that an accurate correction for photon attenuation can be obtained in PET because both photons have to be detected to have a coincidence. This results in the sensitivity for detection of activity being independent of depth within the tissue being imaged (see Horwitz, 1990a, for a discussion of this technical issue). Because of this, measurements of rCBF in SPECT usually are relative to the value in some other brain region, or relative to the value in the whole brain. However, even in PET studies of rCBF, most groups present their values in normalized form (i.e., relative to whole brain CBF), since differences in pCO2 and other physiologic variables can affect global CBF.

A number of other methodologic issues involving metabolic imaging will be discussed after we review the metabolic imaging studies of autism. These points will clarify possible interpretations of the autism results. However, it is worth mentioning at the beginning why there have been so few metabolic imaging studies of autistic patients. Because the primary interest is focused on autistic children, the problem of giving radioactive isotopes to minors becomes a major obstacle. Because children are more sensitive to the effects of radiation, dosages must be lowered in children, which reduces the imaging sensitivity of the scanning method. Moreover, the use of radiation makes it difficult to scan healthy age-matched control subjects. Patient cooperation with the demands of the scanning procedure (e.g., not moving in the scanner for a specified time interval) likewise restricts the number of autistic patients who can be studied. Finally, the need to minimize the effects of medication, possible health complications (e.g., seizures), and emotional reactions to the scanning procedure also serves to confound the results obtained by metabolic imaging.

METABOLIC IMAGING STUDIES OF AUTISM

Rumsey et al. (1985) published the first PET study of patients with autism. Ten healthy autistic men (eighteen to thirty-six years of age) and fifteen healthy age-matched control men were examined using [^{18}F]fluorodeoxyglucose (^{18}FDG) and an ECAT II positron tomograph (spatial resolution: 1.7 cm in the image plane). Most of the autistic men were high functioning. All were selected on the basis of childhood symptoms and diagnoses, documented in childhood medical records. Both patients and controls were screened to exclude diseases that may affect brain function, including infectious, metabolic, and neurologic diseases; only idiopathic cases of autism were studied. Patients with seizures likewise were excluded. All autistic patients were medication-free for a minimum of thirty days before scanning, and most had little or no history of neuroleptic treatment. All patients had CT scans that were clinically read as normal. A quantitative CT volumetric study of autistic men that included many of these subjects showed no volumetric differences between patients and controls (Creasey et al., 1986).

During the forty-five-minute uptake period for ^{18}FDG and PET, subjects were at rest, with eyes covered and ears plugged. Data were obtained from seven slices parallel to the inferior orbitomeatal (IOM) line. rCMRglc was determined in fifty-nine regions of interest (ROIs).

Although the global mean metabolic rate for the autistic group relative to controls was elevated by about 20 percent (mean ± SD: 5.84 ± 0.99 mg/100g/min versus 4.87 ± 0.95 mg/100g/min; $p < .05$), there was considerable overlap in the values of global mean metabolic rate between the two groups. Horwitz et al. (1988), combining data from four additional autistic men with that from the ten of Rumsey et al. (1985), likewise found a significant global elevation for the autistic group relative to controls (fourteen healthy age-matched males, including seven from the Rumsey et al. study), although the increased global mean was just 12 percent higher (5.84 ± 0.84 versus 5.22 ± 0.61 mg/100g/min). As in the first study, the regional rates were generally higher in the autistic group, but there were few localized foci of increased rCMRglc. Indeed, when ratios of regional-to-global CMRglc were compared, only one of fifty-nine ROIs differed between the two groups, a result consistent with chance.

Even though the mean relative metabolic rates did not differ between the two groups, there was more heterogeneity in the autistic group than in the control group. Significantly more autistic patients showed extreme relative metabolic rates and asymmetries than did control subjects in one or more brain regions.

Autistic children were studied with PET and ^{18}FDG by De Volder et al. (1987). Eighteen patients between the ages of two and eighteen years were examined and compared to fifteen adults (mean age: twenty-two years) and six children. All autistic subjects had normal or nearly normal CT scans and EEGs; in particular, no epileptic activity was present. Some of the autistic children were affected by low to moderate levels of mental retardation. Patients were medication-free for several weeks before scanning. However, to maintain cooperation during the PET procedure, many of the patients were sedated with intramuscular droperidol, and some with etybenzatropine added to prevent extrapyramidal symptoms. Because normal children could not be scanned, three of the control children were evaluated as nearly normal at the time of the scan. The remaining three displayed unilateral brain damage, and only PET data from the intact side was used. Scanning was performed on an ECAT III tomograph with 9-mm spatial resolution in the image plane. Data were obtained from six to ten slices, and both absolute and relative rCMRglc were determined in twenty ROIs.

The mean values of rCMRglc did not differ between control children and patients, although the autistic subjects showed more variable rates. Rates were slightly elevated in the autistic group compared to the normal, adult subjects, but the differences were not statistically significant. The pattern of metabolic rates appeared normal in the autistic group, although there seemed to be more heterogeneity in neocortical association areas.

A PET study by Herold et al. (1988) investigated cerebral glucose and oxygen metabolism and blood flow in six young (twenty-one to twenty-five years of age) men with autism. Except for one patient with a history of epilepsy, none had any other neurologic illness, and none was taking medication at the time of the PET study nor for several years before the study. Intelligence in the patients ranged from mildly retarded to average. A control group consisting of six men and two women was used for all three measures (rCMRglc, rCMRO2, and rCBF); they were significantly older than the patients (twenty-two to fifty-three years of age). For data on oxygen and blood flow, an age-matched control group of four males and two females also was used.

Scanning was performed on an ECAT II scanner (in-plane resolution of 1.7 cm). Subjects were examined while listening to music of their choice, but without task demands. Because of the time constraints needed to measure rCBF, rCMRO2, and rCMRglc, only one PET slice through the basal ganglia and temporal gray matter was obtained. Blood flow and metabolic rates were determined in twenty-four to twenty-seven cortical regions per hemisphere and in twelve regions in the territory of the middle cerebral artery. There were no significant differences in rCMRO2, rCMRglc, and rCBF between autistic subjects and either control group, either globally or regionally.

One other PET study has been reported in the literature (Heh et al., 1989). After the report of hypoplasia in the cerebellar lobules in autistic patients (Courchesne et al., 1987, 1988), Heh et al. (1989) investigated glucose metabolism in the cerebellum of seven autistic adults (nineteen to thirty-six years of age) and eight age-matched control subjects. Using a NeuroECAT IV scanner (resolution 7.6 mm) and [18]FDG, they determined rCMRglc in a single slice through the cerebellum, superior posterior cerebellar vermis (lobules VI and VII), and pons parallel to the canthomeatal line. During the uptake period, subjects performed a visual vigilance task. There were no significant differences in normalized rCMRglc in ten ROIs between patients and control subjects.

Two non-PET rCBF studies of autism also have been performed. Using the nontomographic ^{133}Xe inhalation method, Sherman et al. (1984) examined seven retarded autistic males (eighteen to thirty-three years of age) and thirteen age-matched male volunteers. Four of the seven autistic subjects were on medication (anticonvulsants, neuroleptics) at the time of the study. pCO_2 values, which can significantly affect rCBF, were not reported. Their results suggested depressed left- and right-hemisphere gray matter rCBF in the autistic patients, with a pattern of hyperfrontal flow different from that in control subjects (in their control group, hyperfrontality was greater in the right than in the left hemispheres; in the autistic patients, the hyperfrontal pattern was more symmetric, with the pattern in the right hemisphere attenuated from that in control subjects). Zilbovicius et al. (1991) used SPECT with ^{133}Xe to measure rCBF in twenty-one autistic children (five to eleven years of age) and fourteen age-matched children with developmental language disorder. All examinations were performed during sleep after the administration of droperidol and phenobarbital. No differences in rCBF between the two groups were found.

All these studies indicate that focal reductions or increases in brain metabolism do not occur in either autistic children or adults in the relatively nondemanding conditions studied to date. The lack of focal reductions differs from findings in patients with acquired lesions, suggesting that resting energy metabolism and blood flow may not be decreased in developmental disorders such as autism. The reason for the overall global elevation reported by Rumsey et al. (1985) and Horwitz et al. (1988) is not clear. Anxiety induced by the procedure may have been a factor, although ratings of the subjects' anxiety levels by the neurologist performing the scans did not differ between patients and controls, and failed to correlate with global metabolic rate within the autistic group (Rumsey et al., 1985).

Therefore, autism, which is frequently accompanied by normal macroscopic brain anatomy, is characterized by normal regional resting brain metabolism and blood flow, without focal reductions or elevations in rCMRglc, rCMRO2, and rCBF. It is possible that the lack of focal abnormalities may have resulted from the use of relatively low resolution scanners. This is an especially prominent problem when examining metabolism in temporal lobe and limbic structures, where bone and the absence of easily identifiable (in the metabolic image) landmarks result in unreliable metabolic values. Perhaps differences between autistic patients and control subjects will be found when scanning is performed on high-resolution scanners, and when metabolic and anatomic data, obtained from MRI, are registered so that precise region identification can be made (e.g., Pelizzari et al., 1989).

METHODOLOGIC INTERLUDE: THE BRAIN AS AN INTEGRATED SYSTEM

Bauman and Kemper (1985, 1987) showed in autopsied brain tissue from autistic patients that there is increased cell packing densities and reduced neuronal size in limbic structures, and reduction in the number of Purkinje cells in the cerebellum. In addition, the persistence of a clear zone, or lamina dessicans, deep to the superficial cell layer in the entorhinal cortex, which normally disappears by fifteen months of age, was noted. Findings of this sort suggest that the neuropathology of autism may involve anomalous structural and functional organization, rather than the cell death and tissue loss as seen in disorders acquired later in life. Such abnormalities may lead to abnormal functional associations among brain regions, rather than large local changes in energy metabolism and blood flow. The performance of complex behaviors depends on the interaction of particular brain regions with one another

(Luria, 1973; Horwitz, 1990a; Mesulam, 1990), and therefore alterations in these relations may result in pathologic disruptions in integrated cerebral activity.

To determine whether or not functional relations between brain areas are disrupted, neural data must be obtained simultaneously from multiple brain regions and the covariance of such data assessed. If, in a given group of subjects under specific experimental conditions, two brain regions are functionally associated, then their activity will be highly correlated. That is, a change or difference in activity in one region would be expected to systematically affect other regions to which it was functionally associated. Numerous efforts to implement this approach have been undertaken, using multielectrode-obtained electrical data in experimental animals (Gerstein, Perkel, and Subramanian, 1978; Ts'o, Gilbert, and Wiesel, 1986), scalp-recorded electrical activity in humans (Gevins et al., 1985), and cerebral metabolic measures of functional activity (Clark et al., 1984; Horwitz, Duara, and Rapoport, 1984, 1986; Horwitz et al., 1990, 1992; Friston and Frackowiak, 1991).

Correlational analysis of PET/FDG data have been employed to investigate differences between control subjects and a number of patient groups. By correlating rCMRglc or rCBF between pairs of regions (and across subjects), an interregional correlation matrix is obtained that displays the pattern of functional associations for the entire brain (Horwitz, Duara, and Rapoport, 1984, 1986; Horwitz et al., 1990). Comparisons between matrices obtained from patients and control subjects can then be made. Correlations are usually performed on normalized PET data (the ratio of regional to global CMRglc) because intraindividual differences in rCMRglc are generally smaller than are interindividual differences, and this global scaling effect must be removed (Horwitz, Duara, and Rapoport, 1984; Horwitz and Rapoport, 1988). Partial validation for the use of correlational analysis on PET data to investigate brain functional relations has been provided both by simulation studies (Horwitz, 1990b) and by correlational analysis of data on rCBF activation during two kinds of visual processing paradigm (Horwitz et al., 1992).

ALTERED FUNCTIONAL RELATIONS IN AUTISM

The correlation method was applied to PET/FDG data obtained from adults with autism and control subjects (Horwitz et al., 1988). ECAT II PET data from fourteen autistic men (eighteen to thirty-nine years of age) and fourteen age-matched healthy male control subjects were used in the analysis. As mentioned earlier, ten of the fourteen were in the Rumsey et al. (1985) study. The autistic patients were primarily a high-

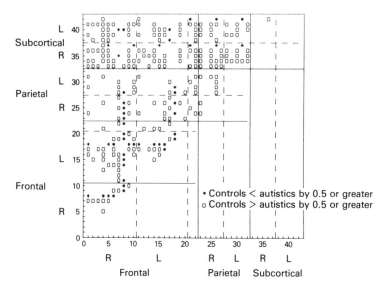

Figure 6.1. The correlations of normalized rCMRglc that differed between patients with autism and control subjects. The correlation coefficients that were numerically larger by at least 0.5 in the control group relative to the autistic group are indicated by "O"; those that were numerically smaller in control subjects by at least 0.5 are denoted by "*." *Source:* Modified from Horwitz et al., 1988.

functioning group. Scanning was performed with subjects at rest (i.e., eyes closed, ears plugged).

Figure 6.1 shows the interregional difference correlation matrix for the autistic patients and control subjects. The major subdivisions of the matrix are the frontal lobe (ten bilateral and two midline regions), the parietal lobe (five bilateral regions), and subcortical and other gray matter structures (bilateral caudate nucleus, thalamus, lenticular nucleus, insula, and cerebellum). The numbers along the axes correspond to the region numbers listed in Table 2 of Horwitz et al. (1988). Correlations involving temporal and occipital regions did not show dramatic differences between patients and controls, and thus are not displayed.

As illustrated in Figure 6.1, more correlations between normalized rCMRglc were lower in the autistic group than were higher. These reductions included both lower positive correlations and more negative correlations in the autistic group where controls showed positive correlations. Reduced correlations in the autistic group involved region pairs within the frontal lobe, frontal–parietal region pairs, and, perhaps most dramatically, region pairs involving subcortical structures (including the thalamus and basal ganglia) and frontal and parietal neocortex. Correlations involving the cerebellum did not show many large differences between autistic patients and control subjects. [Note that the slice including the cerebellum in this study did not include the cerebellar structures that Courchesne et al. (1988) found to be abnormal in autism.]

It was hypothesized (Horwitz et al., 1988) that the reduction in frontal–parietal intercorrelations in the autistic group relative to the control group represented an imbalance in mutually inhibitory neural circuits associated with attention, as mutual inhibition would result in positive correlations. According to Mesulam (1986), mutually inhibitory frontal–parietal interactions mediate an approach–avoidance equilibrium with the external environment, with the frontal lobe mediating an inward-looking avoidance of the environment and the parietal lobe directing an outward-looking approach to the environment. Given that the major neocortical regions that integrate the sensory and motor components of directed attention are in posterior parietal and frontal association cortex (Mesulam, 1981), this approach–avoidance equilibrium may be related to a balance between shifting and directed attention. In this view, damage to the frontal lobe releases the inhibition of parietal structures, resulting in a reduced ability to sustain the focus of attention and leading to such symptoms as distractibility and disinhibition of behavior. On the other hand, by releasing the frontal lobe from inhibition, damage to parietal structures would result in neglect and a reduced ability to shift the focus of attention.

The imbalance in the mutually inhibitory frontal–parietal interactions in autism, reflected in the decreased frontal–parietal correlations, was hypothesized (Horwitz et al., 1988) to indicate a dominance of the outward-directed parietal lobe by the inward-directed frontal lobe, accounting, in part, for the deficient ability to shift the focus of attention that is characteristic of autism. Other studies have demonstrated attentional deficits in autism involving frontal lobe regions (Ciesielski, Courchesne, and Elmasian, 1990). This is not to say that the primary deficit in autism resides in either the frontal or the parietal lobes. Rather, the idea is that in autism the approach–avoidance relationship between the frontal and parietal lobes is abnormal. Damasio and Maurer (1978) proposed a similar notion, hypothesizing that inappropriate control of parietal command function may be one of the causes of the attentional deficits in autism. It is interesting that a similar reduction in frontal—parietal correlations was found in young adults with Down syndrome (Horwitz et al., 1990), where it was suggested that the imbalance in the mutually inhibitory frontal–parietal attentional interactions indicated a dominance of frontal regions by parietal structures. Patients with Down syndrome show greater distractibility, and less behavioral inhibition, than do normal subjects. Moreover, the frontal lobes in Down syndrome relative to the rest of the brain are smaller than in controls (Crome and Stern, 1972).

In addition the reduction in the size of frontal–parietal correlations between normalized rCMRglc values, the autistic group also had reduced values for correlations between frontal and parietal regions and subcortical structures. These subcortical structures included the basal ganglia and the thalamus. There also were reductions in correlations between frontal and parietal regions and the insula, a paralimbic region. Damasio and Maurer (1978) suggested that autistic patients often demonstrate disturbances in motility that are similar to classic neurologic signs indicative of dysfunction in the basal ganglia and related frontal lobe structures.

CONCLUSIONS AND FUTURE DIRECTIONS FOR PET STUDIES OF AUTISM

Despite the marked, but selective, behavioral abnormalities seen in autism, the PET studies published to data have failed to document focal reductions or elevations in brain metabolism. Thus, resting brain metabolism may not be altered in autism, which is frequently accompanied by normal macroscopic brain anatomy and lack of gross neurologic abnormality. Yet, the limited neuropathologic data available to date (Bauman and Kemper, 1985, 1987) suggest anomalous prenatal development and microscopic organization of brain structure with major implications for functional reorganization. The correlational analysis reviewed above supports the view that the functional associations among brain regions in autism, especially those involving frontal and parietal cortex and subcortical regions including the basal ganglia, differ from normal subjects.

What kind of neuroimaging studies of autistic subjects can yield insight into the neurobiology of this disorder? Biochemically based abnormalities might be explored in autism with receptor labeling studies using PET or SPECT. However, the lack of consistent biochemical findings and drug efficacy in autism fail to provide clear hypotheses for such studies at present. A more fruitful avenue may be the pursuit of sensory, motor, and cognitive activation studies.

Functional neuroimaging activation studies involve imaging the brain while the subject is actively engaged in some specific behavior. These techniques may be used to examine residual activity of dysfunctional brain regions or circuits (e.g., the ability to activate a brain region), compensatory activity (i.e., the use of anomalous brain circuits to perform a task) or increased reliance on normal alternative neural pathways. Converging evidence across a variety of tasks that normally activate a structure, and convergent data from correlational analyses implicating dysfunction of a structure, might provide compelling data for localizing dysfunction. Because prenatal lesions can alter brain anatomy and connectivity far from the lesion site (Goldman-Rakic and Galkin, 1978; Galaburda et al., 1985), PET and other functional neuroimaging techniques may prove uniquely capable of determining the functional implications of prenatal pathology. Unlike acquired disorders where structural abnormalities are easily imaged, subtle developmental disorders may require the added sensitivity of activation studies for localizing abnormalities.

Such studies of autistic subjects raise issues concerning the heterogeneity of the population and selection of tasks. Homogeneous subgroups selected for particular levels of functioning, neurocognitive profiles, or neuropsychiatric symptomatology may provide for stronger study design, given the extreme heterogeneity in each of these areas associated with autism. Increased homogeneity would have the added practical advantage for designing tasks or conditions that all patients may perform with a reasonable degree of cooperation and competence in order for brain activity to be examined under well-controlled conditions. Tasks may be selected as probes for specific brain regions hypothesized to be dysfunctional or because they engage cognitive processes thought to be abnormal and to constitute key features of the syndrome.

While neuropathologic studies suggest the involvement of limbic and cerebellar circuitry in autism, limbic structures and the cerebellum, as studied thus far with PET, appear normal. Behavioral symptoms involving emotion, memory, and unusual gait (clinically observed in older patients though as yet poorly documented) may reflect dysfunction of these neural circuits. Thus, PET or SPECT might be used in conjunction with tasks that increase metabolic demands on these regions and that normally activate these structures. A failure to activate normally a region might then be interpreted as evidence of dysfunction, whereas excessive activation of other related structures might be interpreted as compensatory.

Although functional deficits in autism remain poorly understood, considerable progress has been made over the past twenty years in defining cognitive deficits in autism. Uneven Wechsler Intelligence Scale profiles, consistent across studies (Rumsey, 1992), suggest that cognitive deficits may provide a key to localizing brain dysfunction in autism. A review of studies in high-functioning patients, where the usual confounds of mental retardation and developmental language disorders are minimized or avoided, suggests several domains as reasonable candidates for activation studies with PET (Rumsey, 1992): pragmatic deficits (i.e., deficits in the social use of speech) and dysprosodies (disordered rhythm and intonation) are specifically impaired in autism and are not attributable to general delays in the development of language (Tager-Flusberg, 1981; Macdonald et al., 1989). Deficits in executive problem solving (Rumsey and Hamburger, 1988; Prior and Hoffman, 1990) and abnormalities in the ability to direct, maintain, and shift attention also appear characteristic and worthy of study (Courchesne, Akshoomoff, and Townsend, 1990).

Rote memory skills are frequently intact, but limited processing and difficulty extracting rules have been noted (Frith, 1970; Hermelin and O'Connor, 1970; Prior and Chen, 1976). Whereas specific aspects of memory function, as defined by current nosologies, have yet to be examined in depth, relationships between memory and clinical symptoms and reported limbic pathology make it a particularly suitable candidate for future studies.

PET activation studies of another equally subtle disorder—developmental dyslexia—have demonstrated a failure to activate the left temporoparietal cortex (Rumsey et al., 1992). This experience with cognitive activation during PET suggests that the use of activation tasks during functional neuroimaging will indeed provide a more sensitive method for examining brain function in developmental disorders.

REFERENCES

Baron, J. C., Rougemont, D., Collard, P., Bustany, P., Bousser, M. G., and Comar, D. 1985. Coupling between cerebral blood flow, oxygen consumption, and glucose utilization: Its study with positron tomography. In *Positron Emission Tomography*, M. Reivich and A. Alavi, eds. New York: Alan R. Liss, pp. 203–18.

Bauman, M., and Kemper, T. L. 1985. Histoanatomic observations of the brain in early infantile autism. *Neurology* 35:866–74.

Bauman, M., and Kemper, T. L. 1987. Limbic involvement in a second case of early infantile autism. *Neurology* 37 (Suppl. 1):147.

Ciesielski, K. T., Courchesne E., and Elmasian, R. 1990. Effects of focused selective attention tasks on event-related potentials in autistic and normal individuals. *Electroencephalography and Clinical Neurophysiology* 75:207–20.

Clark, C. M., Kessler, R., Buschsbaum, M. S., Margolin, R. A., and Holcomb, H. H. 1984. Correlational methods for determining regional coupling of cerebral glucose metabolism: A pilot study. *Biological Psychiatry* 19:663–78.

Courchesne, E., Akshoomoff, N. A., and Townsend, J. 1990. Recent advances in autism. *Current Opinion in Pediatrics* 2:685–93.

Courchesne, E., Hesselink, J. R., Jernigan, T. L., and Yeung-Courchesne, R. 1987. Abnormal neuroanatomy in a nonretarded person with autism: Unusual findings with magnetic resonance imaging. *Archives of Neurology* 44:335–41.

Courchesne, E., Yeung-Courchesne, R., Press, G. A., Hesselink, J. R., and Jernigan, T. L. 1988. Hypoplasia of cerebellar vermal lobules VI and VII in infantile autism. *New England Journal of Medicine* 318:1349–54.

Creasey, H., Rumsey, J. M., Schwartz, M., Duara, R., Rapoport, J. L., and Rapoport, S. I. 1986. Brain morphometry in autistic men as measured by volumetric computed tomography. *Archives of Neurology* 43:669–72.

Crome, L., and Stern, J. 1972. *Pathology of Mental Retardation*. Baltimore: Williams and Wilkins.

Damasio, A. R., and Maurer, R. G. 1978. A neurological model for childhood autism. *Archives of Neurology* 35:777–86.

De Volder, A., Bol, A., Michel, C., Congneau, M., and Goffinet, A. M. 1987. Brain glucose metabolism in children with the autistic syndrome: Positron tomography analysis. *Brain and Development* 9:581–87.

Fox, P. T., and Raichle, M. E. 1986. Focal physiological uncoupling of cerebral blood flow and oxidative metabolism during somatosensory stimulation in human subjects. *Proceedings of the National Academy of Science* 83:1140–44.

Frackowiak, R. S. J., Lenzi, G. L., Jones, T., and Heather, J. D. 1980. Quantitative measurement of regional cerebral blood flow and oxygen metabolism in man using ^{15}O and positron emission tomography: Theory, procedure, and normal values. *Journal of Computer Assisted Tomography* 4:727–36.

Friston, K. J., and Frackowiak, R. S. J. 1991. Imaging functional anatomy. In *Brain Work and Mental Activity (Alfred Benzon Symposium 31)*, N. A. Lassen, D. H. Ingvar, M. E. Raichle, and L. Friberg, eds. Copenhagen: Munksgaard, pp. 267–77.

Frith, U. 1970. Studies in pattern detection in normal and autistic children. II. Reproduction and production of color sequence. *Journal of Experimental Child Psychology* 10:120–35.

Galaburda, A. M., Sherman, G. F., Rosen, G. D., Aboitiz, F., and Geschwind, N. 1985. Developmental dyslexia: Four consecutive cortical anomalies. *Annals of Neurology* 18:222–33.

Gerstein, G. L., Perkel, D. H., and Subramanian, K. N. 1978. Identification of functionally related neural assemblies. *Brain Research* 140:43–62.

Gevins, A. S., Doyle, J. C., Cutillo, B. A., Schaffer, R. E., Tannehill, R. S., and Bressler, S. L. 1985. Neurocognitive pattern analysis of a visuospatial task: Rapidly-shifting foci of evoked correlations between electrodes. *Psychophysiology* 22:32–43.

Goldman-Rakic, P. S., and Galkin, T. W. 1978. Prenatal removal of frontal association cortex in the fetal rhesus monkey: Anatomical and functional consequence in postnatal life. *Brain Research* 152:451–85.

Grady, C. L., Haxby, J. V., Horwitz, B., Gillette, J., Salerno, J. A., Gonzalez-Aviles, A., Carson, R. E., Herscovitch, P., Schapiro, M. B., and Rapoport, S. I. 1993. Activation of cerebral blood flow during a face perception task in patients with dementia of the Alzheimer type. *Neurobiology of Aging* 14:35–44.

Haxby, J. V., Duara, R., Grady, C. L., Rapoport, S. I., and Cutler, N. R. 1985. Relations between neuropsychological and cerebral metabolic asymmetries in early Alzheimer's disease. *Journal of Cerebral Blood Flow and Metabolism* 5:193–200.

Haxby, J. V., Grady, C. L., Ungerleider, L. G., and Horwitz, B. 1991. Mapping human functional neuroanatomy with brain work imaging. *Neuropsychologia* 29:539–55.

Heh, C. W. C., Smith, R., Wu, J., Hazlett, E., Russel, A., Asarnow, R., Tanguay, P., and Buschsbaum, M. S. 1989. Positron emission tomography of the cerebellum in autism. *American Journal of Psychiatry* 146:242–45.

Hermelin, B., and O'Connor, N. 1970. *Psychological Experiments with Autistic Children*. Oxford: Pergamon Press.

Herold, S., Frackowiak, R. S. J., Le Couteur, A., Rutter, M., and Howlin, P. 1988. Cerebral blood flow and metabolism of oxygen and glucose in young autistic adults. *Psychological Medicine* 18:823–31.

Herscovitch, P., Markham, J., and Raichle, M. E. 1983. Brain blood flow measured with intravenous O-15 water: I. Theory and error analysis. *Journal of Nuclear Medicine* 24:782–89.

Horwitz, B. 1990a. Quantification and analysis of PET metabolic data. In *Positron Emission Tomography in Dementia*, R. Duara, ed. New York: Wiley-Liss, pp. 13–70.

Horwitz, B. 1990b. Simulating functional interactions in the brain: A model for examining correlations between regional cerebral metabolic rates. *International Journal of Biomedical Computing* 26:149–70.

Horwitz, B., Duara, R., and Rapoport, S. I. 1984. Intercorrelations of glucose metabolic rates between brain regions: Application to healthy males in a state of reduced sensory input. *Journal of Cerebral Blood Flow and Metabolism* 4:484–99.

Horwitz, B., Duara, R., and Rapoport, S. I. 1986. Age differences in intercorrelations between regional cerebral metabolic rates for glucose. *Annals of Neurology* 19:60–67.

Horwitz, B., Grady, C. L., Haxby, J. V., Ungerleider, L. G., Schapiro, M. B., Mishkin, M., and Rapoport, S. I. 1992. Functional associations among human posterior extrastriate brain regions during object and spatial vision. *Journal of Cognitive Neuroscience* 4:311–22.

Horwitz, B., and Rapoport, S. I. 1988. Partial correlation coefficients approximate the real intrasubject correlation pattern in the analysis of interregional relations of cerebral metabolic activity. *Journal of Nuclear Medicine* 29:392–99.

Horwitz, B., Rumsey, J., Grady, C., and Rapoport, S. I. 1988. The cerebral metabolic landscape in autism: Intercorrelations of regional glucose utilization. *Archives of Neurology* 45:749–55.

Horwitz, B., Schapiro, M. B., Grady, C. L., and Rapoport, S. I. 1990. Cerebral metabolic pattern in young adult Down's syndrome subjects: Altered intercorrelations between regional rates of cerebral glucose utilization. *Journal of Mental Deficiency Research* 34:237–52.

Lammertsma, A. A., Cunningham, V. J., Deiber, M. P., Heather, J. D., Bloomfield, P. M., Nutt, J., Frackowiak, R. S .J., and Jones, T. 1990. Combination of dynamic and integral methods for generating reproducible functional CBF images. *Journal of Cerebral Blood Flow and Metabolism* 10:675–86.

Luria, A. R. 1973. *The Working Brain*. New York: Basic Books.

Macdonald, H., Rutter, M., Howlin, P., Rios, P., LeCouteau, A., Evered, C., and Folstein, S. 1989. Recognition and expression of emotional cues by autistic and normal adults. *Journal of Child Psychology and Psychiatry* 30:865–77.

Mata, M., Fink, D. J., Gainer, H., Smith, C. B., Davidsen, L., Savaki, H., Schwartz, W. J., and Sokoloff, L. 1980. Activity-dependent energy metabolism in rat posterior pituitary primarily reflects sodium pump activity. *Journal of Neurochemistry* 34:213–15.

Mesulam, M.-M. 1981. A cortical network for directed attention and unilateral neglect. *Annals of Neurology* 10:309–25.

Mesulam, M.-M. 1986. Frontal cortex and behavior. *Annals of Neurology* 19:320–25.

Mesulam, M.-M. 1990. Large-scale neurocognitive networks and distributed processing for attention, language, and memory. *Annals of Neurology* 28:597–613.

Pawlik, G., and Heiss, W.-D. 1989. Positron emission tomography and neuropsychological function. In *Neuropsychological Function and Brain Imaging*, E. D. Bigler, R. A. Yeo, and E. Turkheimer, eds. New York: Plenum Press, pp. 65–137.

Pelizzari, C. A., Chen, G. T. Y., Spelbring, D. R., Weichselbaum, R. R., and Chen, C.-T. 1989. Accurate three-dimensional registration of CT, PET, and/or MR images of the brain. *Journal of Computer Assisted Tomography* 13:20–26.

Phelps, M., Mazziotta, J., and Schelbert, H. 1986. *Positron Emission Tomography and Autoradiography*. New York: Raven Press.

Phelps, M. E., Huang, S. C., Hoffman, E. J., Selin, M. S., Sokoloff, L. and Kuhl, D. E. 1979. Tomographic measurement of local glucose metabolic rate in humans with (F-18)2-fluoro-2-deoxy-D-glucose: Validation of method. *Annals of Neurology* 6:371–88.

Prior, M., and Chen, C. 1976. Short-term and serial memory in autistic, retarded, and normal children. *Journal of Autism and Childhood Schizophrenia* 6:121–31.

Prior, M. R., and Hoffman, W. 1990. Neuropsychological testing of autistic children through an exploration with frontal lobe tests. *Journal of Autism and Developmental Disorders* 20:581–90.

Raichle, M. E., Fox, P. T., Mintun, M. A., and Dense, C. 1987. Cerebral blood flow and oxidative glycolysis are uncoupled by neuronal activity. *Journal of Cerebral Blood Flow and Metabolism* 7 (Suppl. 1):S300.

Raichle, M. E., Grubb, R. L., Gado, M. H., Eichling, J. O., and Ter-Pogossian, M. H. 1976. Correlation between regional cerebral blood flow and oxidative metabolism. *Archives of Neurology* 33:523–26.

Raichle, M. E., Martin, W. R. W., Herscovitch, P., Mintun, M. A., and Markham, J. 1983. Brain blood flow measured with intravenous O-15 water: II. Implementation and validation. *Journal of Nuclear Medicine* 24:790–98.

Reivich, M., and Alavi, A. 1985. *Positron Emission Tomography*. New York: Alan R. Liss.

Reivich, M., Alavi, A., Wolf, A., Fowler, J., Russell, J., Arnett, C., MacGregor, R. R., Shiue, C. Y., Atkins, H., Anand, A., Dann, R., and Greenberg, J. H. 1985. Glucose metabolic rate kinetic model parameter determination in humans: The lumped constants and rate constants for [18-F]fluorodeoxyglucose and [11-C]deoxyglucose. *Journal of Cerebral Blood Flow and Metabolism* 5:179–92.

Reivich, M., Kuhl, D., Wolf, A., Greenberg, J., Phelps, M., Ido, T., Casella, V., Hoffman, E., Alavi, A., and Sokoloff, L. 1979. The [18F] fluorodeoxyglucose method for the measurement of local cerebral glucose utilization in man. *Circulation Research* 44:127–37.

Rumsey, J. M., Andreason, P., Zametkin, A. J., Aquino, T., King, C., Hamburger, S. D., Pikus, A., Rapoport, J. L., and Cohen, R. 1992. Failure to activate the left temporoparietal cortex in dyslexia. *Archives of Neurology* 49:527–34.

Rumsey, J. M. 1992. Neuropsychological studies of high-level autism. In *High-Functioning Individuals with Autism*, E. Schopler and G. Mesibov, eds. New York: Plenum Press, pp. 41–64.

Rumsey, J. M., Duara, R., Grady, C., Rapoport, J. L., Margolin, R. A., Rapoport, S. I., and Cutler, N. R. 1985. Brain metabolism in autism. *Archives of General Psychiatry* 42:448–55.

Rumsey, J. M., and Hamburger, S. D. 1988. Neuropsychological findings in high-functioning men with infantile autism, residual state. *Journal of Clinical and Experimental Neuropsychology* 10:201–21.

Sherman, M., Nass, R., and Shapiro, T. 1984. Regional blood flow in autism. *Journal of Autism and Developmental Disorders* 14:439–46.

Sokoloff, L., Reivich, M., Kennedy, C., Des Rosiers, M. H., Patlak, C. S., Pettigrew, K. D., Sakurada, O., and Shinohara, M. 1977. The [14-C]deoxyglucose method for the measurement of local cerebral glucose utilization: Theory, procedure and normal values in the conscious and anesthetized albino rat. *Journal of Neurochemistry* 28:897–916.

Tager-Flusberg, H. B. 1981. On the nature of linguistic functioning in early infantile autism. *Journal of Autism and Developmental Disorders* 11:45–56.

Ts'o, D. Y., Gilbert, C. D., and Wiesel, T. N. 1986. Relationships between horizontal interactions and functional architecture in cat striate cortex as revealed by cross-correlation analysis. *Journal of Neuroscience* 6:1160–70.

Zilbovicius, M., Garreau, B., Tzourio, N., Mazoyer, B. M., Bruck, B., Raynaud, C., Syrota, A., and Lelord, G. 1991. SPECT rCBF study in childhood autism. *Journal of Cerebral Blood Flow and Metabolism* 11 (Suppl. 2):S825.

7

NEUROANATOMIC OBSERVATIONS
OF THE BRAIN IN AUTISM

Margaret L. Bauman, M.D.
Thomas L. Kemper, M.D.

Early infantile autism is a behaviorally defined disorder, initially described by Kanner in 1943. Symptoms typically become evident before three years of age and are generally associated with varying degrees of developmental delay. Clinical features may include abnormal social responses and behavior, disordered speech, language, and cognitive skills, repetitive and stereotypic behavior, poor eye contact, and an obsessive insistence on sameness. Many affected individuals appear to have islands of rote memory, and some show exceptional isolated talents in the face of otherwise general functional disability. Although normal in physical appearance, a significant number demonstrate hypotonia, dyspraxia, and disordered modulation of sensory input (Rapin, 1991). Some aspects of the syndrome have been observed in conditions such as phenylketonuria, tuberous sclerosis, and fragile X syndrome, but the majority of cases are without identified etiology. Twin and sibling studies have suggested evidence for a genetic liability, the mechanism of which remains unknown (Folstein and Piven, 1991).

Autism was historically believed to be caused by parental and social influences. However, with more detailed clinical observation and with advances in medical technology, evidence for an underlying neurologic basis for autism has become increasingly compelling. Many anatomic sites within the brain have been suggested as potential regions of abnormality, most commonly the medial temporal lobe (Delong, 1978; Damasio and Maurer, 1978; Maurer and Damasio, 1982). Although early pneumoencephalographic findings seemed to support this view (Hauser et al., 1975), CT studies have not shown consistent findings (Hier et al., 1979; Caparulo et al., 1981; Tsai et al., 1982; Gillberg and

Svendsen, 1983; Bauman et al., 1985; Rumsey et al., 1988). Other areas of suspected pathology have included the thalamic nuclei (Coleman, 1979), the basal ganglia (Vilensky et al., 1981), and the vestibular system (Ornitz and Ritvo, 1968). In more recent years, some MRI have suggested that the cerebellum may also play a role in this disorder (Courchesne et al., 1988; Gaffney et al., 1988; Murakami et al., 1989; Courchesne, 1991).

There have been few neuropathologic studies of infantile autism. A brief report by Aarkrog (1968) noted "slight thickening of the arterioles, slight connective tissue increase in the leptomeninges, and some cell increase" in a right frontal lobe brain biopsy. In a review of thirty-three cases of childhood psychosis, Darby (1976) suggested a relationship between limbic system lesions and the affective component of autism, but no specific pathology was delineated. Williams et al. (1980) examined autopsy material obtained from four individuals with autistic features, looking primarily for evidence of cell loss or gliosis. No consistent abnormalities were noted. Coleman et al. (1985) performed glial and neuronal cell counts in multiple areas of the cerebral cortex in an autistic patient and two age and sex-matched controls. No differences were found. The authors concluded that abnormalities during the early stages of nervous system development and migration were unlikely in autism and that the probable pathologic process was more likely to occur later during the elaboration of neuronal processes and synapses. In 1986, Ritvo et al. observed decreased numbers of Purkinje cells in the vermis and cerebellar hemispheres of four autistic patients in comparison with subjects having no known pathology of the central nervous system. These authors raised a number of interesting questions in regard to their findings and the possible implications for some of the clinical features of autism.

NEUROANATOMIC OBSERVATIONS

In 1985, we reported the results of a systematic study of the brain of a twenty-nine-year-old well-documented man with autism using the technique of whole brain serial section (Bauman and Kemper, 1985). This brain was studied in comparison with an identically processed age and sex-matched control. Since that initial report, five additional clinically well-documented cases have been studied using the same methodology (Table 7.1).

All six brains have shown no gross abnormalities. Myelination has been found to be comparable to the controls in all cases. Microscopic study of multiple areas of the cerebral cortex showed mild cytoarchitectonic abnormalities, which were confined to the cortex of the anterior cingulate gyrus in five of the six patients. Systematic examination of the

Table 7.1 The Clinical Features of Six Autistic Patients

Feature	Age (Years)/Sex					
	9/male	10/female	12/male	22/male	28/male	29/male
IQ	severe MR	severe MR	105	moderate MR	moderate MR	severe MR
Seizures	++	–	–	+	+	+
Cause of death	dead in bed	sepsis	Ewing sarcoma	drown	sepsis	drown

Note: Two children had no seizures. Most of the autistic individuals were cognitively impaired, except for the twelve-year-old boy, who was documented as being of average intelligence.

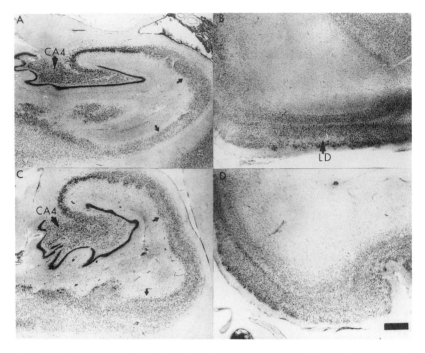

Figure 7.1. Nissl-stained sections from the hippocampal complex (A) and the entorhinal cortex (B) in the brain of a twenty-nine-year-old autistic male, with comparable sections from an age- and sex-matched control subject (C and D). Neuronal cell packing density is increased throughout these areas in the autistic brain. This can best be seen by comparing area CA4 in the hilum of the fascia dentata in A and C, and in the deep layer of the entorhinal cortex in B and D. In the entorhinal cortex of this autistic man (B), there is a clear zone deep to the superficial cell layer (LD), which is not present in the control (D). This clear zone is referred to as a lamina dessicans and normally disappears in early childhood.
Source: Bauman and Kemper, 1985

basal forebrain, thalamus, hypothalamus, and basal ganglia showed no differences from controls.

Areas of the forebrain that were found to be abnormal were confined to the hippocampus (Figures 7.1 and 7.2), subiculum, entorhinal cortex, amygdala, mammillary body, anterior cingulate cortex, and septum. In comparison with the controls, these areas showed reduced neuronal cell size and increased cell-packing density (increased numbers of neurons per unit volume) bilaterally. Further analysis of the CA1 and CA4 pyramidal neurons of the hippocampus, using the rapid Golgi technique (Figure 7.3), showed decreased complexity and extent of the dendritic arbors in these cells (Raymond et al., 1989). In the amygdala, the medial, corti-

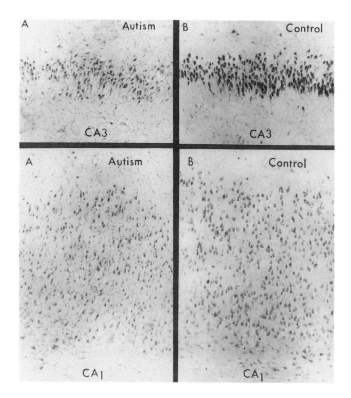

Figure 7.2. Photomicrograph of a Nissl-stained section of the hippocampus at higher power. Note the abnormally small, tightly packed cells in the CA3 and CA1 hippocampal subfields in the autistic brain as compared with the control.
Source: Kemper and Bauman, 1992

cal, and central nuclei consistently demonstrated the most significant increase in cell-packing density. With the exception of the child of normal intelligence, the lateral nucleus was uninvolved. All areas found to be abnormal in these autistic patients are known to be connected by closely interrelated circuits and comprise a major portion of the limbic system of the forebrain. These findings are summarized in Table 7.2.

In the septal region, additional abnormalities were found in the vertical limb of the nucleus of the diagonal band of Broca (NDB) and in the medial septal nucleus (MSN). In the latter, cell-packing density was found to be significantly and consistently increased, and the neuronal cell size strikingly reduced, a pattern similar to that observed elsewhere in the limbic system. However, a different pattern of abnormality was noted in the NDB. In the younger autistic brains, ages nine, ten, and twelve years, the neurons of the NDB were unusually large and were

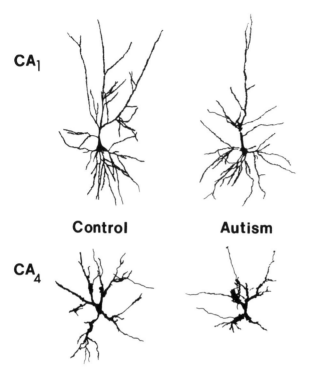

Figure 7.3. Camera lucida drawings of Golgi-stained neurons from the CA4 and CA1 subfields of the hippocampus. Note the stunting of some of the dendritic arbors in the cells from the autistic brain, and the limited amount of secondary and tertiary branching in these neurons.
Source: Kemper and Bauman, 1992

present in adequate numbers. In contrast, in the older autistic cerebra, ages twenty-two, twenty-eight, and twenty-nine years, the neurons of this same nucleus were small in size and were markedly reduced in number (Figure 7.4).

Except for the findings in the limbic system, the only other abnormalities in the autistic brain have been confined to the cerebellum and related inferior olive. All six brains have shown a significant decrease in the number of Purkinje cells and a variable decrease in granule cells throughout the cerebellar hemispheres (Figures 7.5 and 7.6), with the most marked decrease being found in the posterolateral neocerebellar cortex and adjacent archicerebellar cortex (Arin et al., 1991). In addition, abnormalities have been observed in the fastigeal, emboliform, and globose nuclei in the roof of the cerebellum that appear to differ with the age of the patient. Small pale neurons, which are decreased in number, characterize these nuclei in the three older

Table 7.2. A Summary of the Distribution of Pathologic Abnormalities
in Six Autistic Patients

Site	Age (Years)/Sex					
	9/male	10/female	12/male	22/male	28/male	29/male
Hippocampus						
CA4	+++	+	+	++	++	+++
CA3	+++	++	+	++	++	+++
CA2	+++	++	++	++	+++	+++
CA1	+++	+++	+++	++	+++	+++
Subiculum	++	+++	+++	+++	+++	+++
Entorhinal cortex	++	++	++	++	++	+++
Mammilary body	++	+	++	++	+	+++
Medial septal nuclei	++	?	++	++	++	++
Amygdala						
Cortical n.	+++	+++	+++	+++	+++	+++
Medial n.	++	+++	++	+++	++	+++
Central n.	+++	+++	++	++	++	+++
Medial basal n.	+	+++	++	++	++	0
Lateral basal n.	++	++	++	++	++	0
Lateral n.	0	0	++	0	0	0
Anterior cingulate gyrus	++	++	++	++	++	0

Note: For simplicity, significant abnormalities are shown with +++, lesser abnormalities with + or ++, and the absence of abnormality with 0. Although there is some variation in the degree of abnormality in various portions of the limbic system in each case, the pattern of involvement is generally consistent between cases.

autistic brains (Figure 7.7). In the younger cases, however, these same nerve cells, as well as those of the dentate nucleus, are enlarged in size and are present in adequate numbers (Figure 7.8) (Kemper and Bauman, 1992).

Areas of the principal inferior olivary nucleus of the brainstem in the autistic brains, which are known to be related to the abnormal cerebellar cortex (Holmes and Stewart 1908), failed to show retrograde cell loss and atrophy, which is invariably seen following perinatal or postnatal Purkinje cell loss in human pathology (Norman, 1940; Greenfield, 1954). The olivary neurons in the three older autistic brains were present in adequate numbers, but they were small and pale (Figure 7.9). In the three younger cases, however, these same neurons were significantly enlarged, but were otherwise normal in appearance and number (Figure 7.10). In all of the autistic cerebra, some of the olivary neurons tended to cluster at the periphery of the nuclear convolutions, a pattern that has been reported in some syndromes of prenatal origin associated with mental retardation (Sumi, 1980; DeBassio et al., 1985).

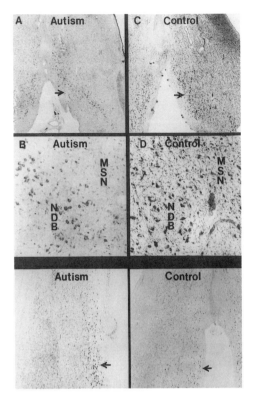

Figure 7.4. Nissl-stained photomicrographs of the septal nuclei from a twenty-nine-year-old autistic male (A, B, C, D) and a ten-year-old autistic child (lower two photographs). Neurons of the nucleus of the diagonal band of Broca (NDB) are small and reduced in number in the older patient, but are enlarged and plentiful in the child (NDB indicated by arrows).
Source: Kemper and Bauman, 1992

IMPLICATIONS OF LIMBIC SYSTEM OBSERVATIONS

Based on the neuroanatomic investigations to date, abnormalities in the autistic brain have been confined to portions of the limbic system, and to the cerebellum and related inferior olive. Decreased neuronal cell size and increased cell-packing density characterize the hippocampal complex and the amygdala as well as areas related to them. This pattern of small, closely packed neurons resembles that typically seen during an earlier stage of brain maturation and may, therefore, represent a curtailment of normal development. Consistent with this notion is the decreased complexity and extent of the dendritic arbors observed in some pyramidal cells of the hippocampus.

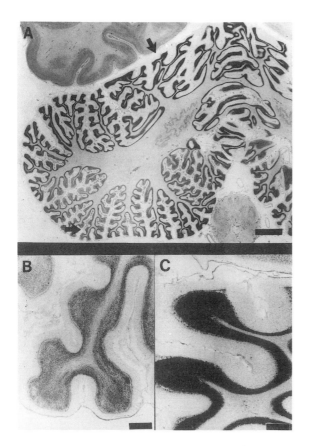

Figure 7.5. Nissl-stained section of the cerebellum from the brain of an adult autistic male. Note the atrophy of the cerebellar cortex in the lateral and inferior portions of the hemispheres, and the relatively normal appearing anterior lobe and vermis. In B, the markedly reduced number of Purkinje cells and, to a lesser extent, granule cells can be appreciated as compared with more normal appearing anterior cerebellum (C). Systematic counting of the Purkinje cells, however, indicates a decreased number in the anterior lobe as well, but this reduction is less pronounced than in the posterior and inferior portions of the hemispheres.
Source: Bauman and Kemper, 1985

The hippocampal complex is related by sequential projections from the dentate gyrus through the ammonic subfields and into the subiculum (Rosene and Van Hoesen, 1987). The entorhinal cortex projects to all areas of the hippocampus and has reciprocal projections with the subiculum (Van Hoesen and Pandya, 1975a and 1975b; Rosene and Van Hoesen, 1977). The entorhinal and perirhinal cortices and, to a lesser extent, the subiculum, are the site of afferent projections from multiple limbic neocortical areas, auditory and visual association cortex, and a polysen-

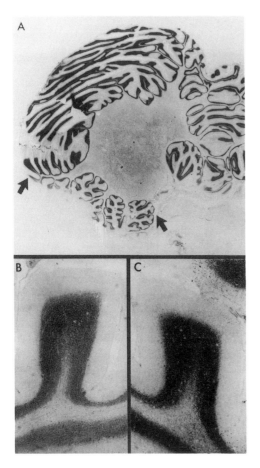

Figure 7.6. Nissl-stained low-power photograph of the cerebellum from an autistic child. Note the atrophy of the folia in the posterior lateral hemispheres. At higher power (B and C), the reduction in Purkinje cells can be seen, in association with some slight pallor of the granule cells.
Source: Kemper and Bauman, 1992

sory cortical area on the bank of the superior temporal sulcus (Van Hoesen and Pandya, 1975a; Van Hoesen et al., 1972; Van Hoesen et al., 1975; Van Hoesen et al., 1979; Amaral et al., 1983; Rosene and Van Hoesen, 1987). Additionally, nearly all efferent projections from the hippocampal complex are from the subiculum and/or the prosubiculum, and, to a lesser extent, the adjacent CA1 subfields and include projections back to the limbic neocortical areas and limbic nuclei of the thalamus (Rosene and Van Hoesen, 1977; Rosene and Van Hoesen, 1987). The mammillary body receives a dense projection from the subiculum, and both septal nuclei (NDB and MSN) are related to the hippocampal–subiculum complex

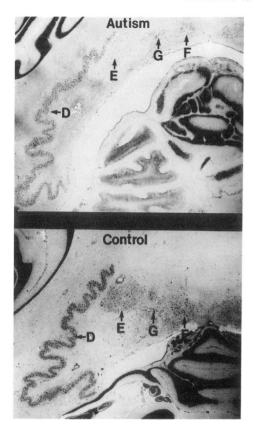

Figure 7.7. Photomicrograph of the deep cerebellar nuclei from the brain of an adult autistic male. The neurons of the fastigeal (F), globose (G), and emboliform (E) nuclei are small and pale and reduced in number. The dentate nucleus (D) appears distorted and the nerve cells are small but present in adequate numbers.
Source: Bauman and Kemper, 1985

by reciprocal projections (Rosene and Van Hoesen, 1977; Rosene and Van Hoesen, 1987). The cingulate cortex has complex interrelationships with many of these areas (Papez, 1937; Pandya et al. 1981). Thus, the central focus of these anatomically related circuits is the hippo-campal–subiculum complex, with many of the abnormal areas in the forebrain related to it by direct projections.

Similar histoanatomic abnormalities were also found in the amygdala, with the most marked increased cell-packing density found in the corti-cal, medial, and central nuclei. Of these, the cortical nucleus directly ter-minates in the molecular layer of the CA3 and CA2 subfields of the hippocampus as well as in the subiculum and prosubiculum (Rosene and Van Hoesen, 1987). The medial and central nuclei represent the

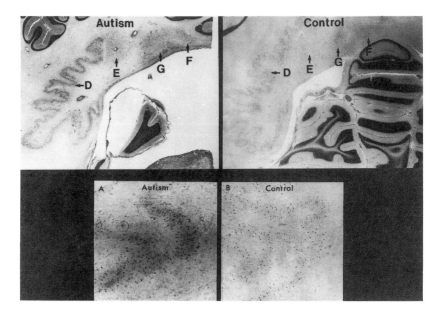

Figure 7.8. Nissl-stained photomicrograph of the deep cerebellar nuclei from the brain of an autistic child. Note the prominent cerebellar nuclei with neuronal enlargement which characterizes this autistic brain. Similar findings are noted in the dentate nucleus in the lower panels.
Source: Kemper and Bauman, 1992

most lateral extension of the rostral part of the reticulate core of the brain; they are directly related to it by reciprocal connections from the hypothalamus to the medulla oblongata (Leontovich and Zhukova, 1963; Price and Amaral, 1981; Amaral et al., 1982). Afferent projections to the medial and central amygdaloid nuclei are also received from the basolateral complex of the amygdala (Price and Amaral, 1981; Krettek and Price, 1978), which is in turn directly related to many of the limbic, visual, and auditory association cortices that are directly and reciprocally related to the hippocampal–subicular complex of circuits. In addition, more recent studies indicate that the amygdala projects massively to the perirhinal and entorhinal cortices (Saunders and Rosene, 1988). Thus, the abnormalities in the forebrain of the autistic brain could disrupt the function of the circuitry of the hippocampal complex, and the amygdala, as well as that of the limbic and sensory association neocortical areas and the reticulate core of the brain.

The only brain to show involvement of all nuclei of the amygdala was that of the normally intelligent twelve-year-old boy. His most significant clinical deficits were in pragmatic language and behavior. This observation raises the possibility that variation in symptoms may be re-

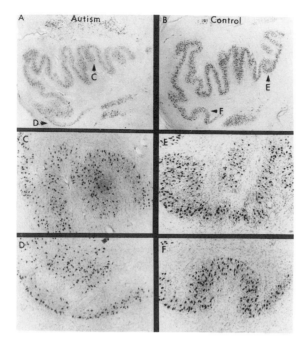

Figure 7.9. High- and low-power photomicrographs of the neurons of the inferior olive from the brain of an adult autistic male. Note that the neurons are small in size but present in adequate numbers. Note also the presence of a peripheral distribution of neurons along the edge of the inferior loop of this nucleus (D).
Source: Kemper and Bauman, 1992

flected in the extent to which parts of the limbic system are involved. In this regard, Bachevalier (1992) bilaterally lesioned the amygdala in infant monkeys. With maturation, these animals appeared to be behaviorally similar to high-functioning autistic children. These observations are in contrast to the significant autisticlike behavior exhibited by infant monkeys subjected to bilateral lesions of both the hippocampus and the amygdala (Bachevalier, 1991), which seems to give credance to this hypothesis.

The findings in the NDB of the septum are somewhat difficult to interpret. In the younger autistic individuals, the neurons of the NDB are unusually large, while these same cells are small and decreased in number in the older patients. This variable pattern with the age of the patient may represent an unstable circuitry. In the adult monkey, this nucleus provides a strong highly focused cholinergic projection to the amygdala and hippocampus (Rosene and Van Hoesen, 1987). The extent of its projection during fetal life is unknown. We suggest that the abnormally small neurons observed in the hippocampal complex and

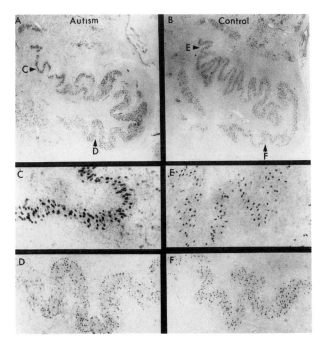

Figure 7.10. High- and low-power Nissl-stained photomicrographs of the inferior olivary nucleus from an autistic child and a control subject. In contrast to the findings in the adult autistic patient, the neurons in this brain are significantly larger than are those in the control; otherwise, they are normal in appearance. Note the peripheral distribution of neurons along the edges of the inferior loop of this nucleus (D).
Source: Kemper and Bauman, 1992

the amygdala in the autistic brains may fall within the fetal distribution pattern of this septal projection.

The behavioral significance of this medial temporal lobe circuitry has been experimentally demonstrated in animals whereby lesions in these regions have produced effects on emotion, motivation, memory, and learning, many of which resemble some of the clinical features of childhood autism. Atypical behaviors similar to those seen in autism were described in monkeys by Kluver and Bucy in 1939 following bilateral surgical ablation of the medial temporal lobe. Purposeless hyperactivity, hyperexploratory behavior, severe impairment of social interaction, and the inability to recognize or remember the significance of visually or manually examined objects were observed. Similar behaviors have also been reported in humans following comparable neurosurgical lesions (Terzian and Delle-Ore, 1955). When bilateral ablations in animals were confined to the hippocampus, stereotypic motor behavior, hyperactivity, and a disordered response to novel stimuli resulted (Roberts et al., 1962; Kimble, 1963). Bilateral lesions in adult monkeys that have been confined to the amygdala have led to a loss of fear of normally adversive stimuli, withdrawal from previously rewarding social interactions, compulsive indescriminate examination of objects, and the reduced ability to attach meaning to a specific situation based on past experience, resulting in the inability to adapt behavior to new environmental situations (Mishkin and Aggleton, 1981). Furthermore, ablations of the central, medial, and cortical nuclei of the amygdala were more effective in repressing the influence of familiarization than laterally placed amygdalar lesions (Vergnes, 1981). In a later study, Murray and Mishkin (1985) demonstrated that monkeys with bilateral ablations of the amygdala experienced severely impaired long-term cross-modal, associative memory. These lesioned monkeys failed to recognize an object by vision that they had examined by touch or taste. These results suggest that cross-modal association may be one of the major functions of the amygdala and that an abnormality in this circuitry could lead to difficulty in generalizing information from one experience to another, a characteristic seen in many autistic individuals.

It is important to recognize that the majority of these lesion studies have been performed in adult animals. In 1981, Thompson reported the results of bilateral amygdaloidectomies in infant monkeys. The surgically treated animals initially appeared to be behaviorally similar to controls. However, by eight months of age, the treated animals were noted to have poor social skills; hyperactivity was evident by three years of age. Thus, the lesioned monkeys appeared to have "grown into" their symptoms, a series of events not unlike the early clinical picture seen in some autistic children. Bilateral surgical resection of both the hippocampus and the amygdala in neonatal monkeys resulted in gross motor stereotypies, tantrums in novel situations, blank and unexpressive faces, little eye contact, poor body expression, and deficits in cognitive memory (Bachevalier 1991). As in the Thompson study, these behaviors became more apparent with increasing age. However, considerable variability in these autisticlike behaviors were noted in the lesioned animals. This suggests that subtypes of autistic symptoms may not necessarily result from differing pathologies; rather, they may derive from a common locus of pathology that may produce variable phenotypic features.

In addition to altered behavior, limbic system structures found to be abnormal in the autistic brain have been implicated in disturbances of memory and learning. Severe loss of recognition and associative visual memory have been reported by Mishkin (1978) following ablations of both the hippocampus and the amygdala in adult monkeys, and by Mahut et al. (1982) following bilateral hippocampal lesions. Profound loss of tactile memory has also been noted in adult monkeys following bilateral combined lesions of the amygdala and hippocampus (Murray and Mishkin, 1983). These observations suggest that damage to these structures results in a severe memory deficit that is at least bimodal and is comparable to the global retrograde amnesia seen following medial temporal lobe surgery or pathology in humans. Furthermore, it has been suggested that the hippocampus and the amygdala participate equally in object-recognition memory. The amygdala appears to be important for memory related to object–reward, object–punishment, and object–object associations across modalities (Parkinson et al., 1988). In contrast, the hippocampus has been found to be critical to object–place associations. Monkeys subjected to bilateral hippocampal ablations are incapable of associating objects with their spatial locations.

Since then, Squire and Zola-Morgan (1991) re-examined the relationship of medial temporal lobe structures to memory. They found that the severe memory loss previously attributed to bilateral ablations of both the hippocampus and the amygdala was the result of inadvertent injury to the cortical regions adjacent to the amygdala during surgery, and not to the inclusion of the amygdala as had been previously thought (Mishkin, 1978). Additional studies determined that the medial temporal lobe memory system consisted of the hippocampal formation, including the entorhinal cortex and the anatomically related perirhinal and parahippocampal cortices. The amygdala did not appear to be a component of this memory system, nor did it contribute to the kind of memory related to this system.

Studies in the forebrain of human and nonhuman primates have suggested the presence of at least two memory systems, representational or declarative memory, and procedural or habit memory (Mishkin and Appenzeller, 1987; Murray, 1990; Squire and Zola-Morgan, 1991). Representational memory involves all sensory modalities and mediates the processing of facts, experience and events, and the integration and generalization of information that leads to higher-order cognition and learning. Habit memory is involved in skill learning and automatic connections between a stimulus and a response. In contrast to declarative memory, habit learning is not accessible to conscious recollection and is acquired by repeated presentation of the same stimulus until the task has reached criteria. These two systems are believed to be anatomically separate, representational memory depending on the hippocampus, amygdala, and areas related to them, while the substrate for habit memory is thought to reside in the striatum and neocortex of the cerebral hemispheres.

In our studies of the neuropathology of infantile autism, the striatum has shown no abnormalities. With the exception of a mild cytoarchitectonic irregularity in the cingulate cortex, the neocortex also appears to be uninvolved. In contrast, the hippocampal complex, amygdala, entorhinal cortex, septum, and medial mammillary body have all shown significant abnormalities. Thus, the substrate for representational memory appears to be selectively abnormal in the autistic brain, while that for habit memory appears to be spared.

Limbic system abnormalities in relationship to memory in humans have been described following surgical resection of the hippocampus, amygdala, and immediate adjacent areas. The most famous of these patients, H. M., had essentially no recall of facts or events that occurred after bilateral medial temporal lobe resection (Milner, 1972). Thus, failure to recall daily experiences and acquire new information following surgery have been characteristic of these patients. The effect of a congenital disturbance to this memory system is unknown. However, it is likely that the clinical picture resulting from the surgical removal of specific areas of the limbic system in adult human and nonhuman primates may be substantially different from that resulting from prenatal abnormalities in these same areas. Early lesions and curtailments of development within these structures could be in a position to disrupt or distort the acquisition and meaning of information derived from continually occurring novel stimuli that are characteristic of daily life. Such a disturbance in the processing of information could potentially lead to the disordered cognition, social interaction, and language characteristic of the autistic child.

Consistent with the probable preservation of the rigidly specific habit memory system in autism is the presence and preoccupation with repetitive and stereotypic behavior and the seemingly obsessive need for sameness. The autistic individual may become comfortable in specific well-memorized environments, but may become upset with small changes in that environment, possibly because even minor alterations may render that setting unrecognizable. The preservation of the habit memory system could also account for the outstanding memory for rote information seen in some autistic individuals.

Memory and learning have also been examined in normal monkeys from infancy to adulthood. During the first months of life, infant monkeys have been able to demonstrate the presence of a well-developed noncognitive habit memory system. When evaluated for the presence of representational memory however, these same monkeys did not begin to acquire that ability until late infancy, failing to reach adult-level mastery until two years of age. Thus, the ability to make cognitive associations (representational memory) appears to develop gradually in the normal animal, presumably because the neuronal circuitry upon which it depends matures slowly over time (Bachevalier and Mishkin, 1991). Similar findings have recently been reported in normal human infants by Overman (1990). In this study, infants as young as twelve months of age were able to handle object discrimination tasks as well as adults, a skill dependent on the presence of rote memory. However, when presented with a delayed nonmatching to sample task (DNMS) that required the learning of the rules of the task in order to be successful, the young children did not begin to solve this task until nineteen months of age, plus or minus three months. Although children ages forty-five to eighty-one months performed the DNMS task at increasingly higher levels with increasing age, their scores remained significantly below that seen in adults. Based on these studies, there is the suggestion that, in both human and nonhuman primates, these different cognitive processes are mediated by two independent neural systems that mature at different times (Overman et al., 1992).

Thus, the limbic system, which is believed to be responsible for representational memory, appears to be a later-developing system in both human and nonhuman primates, while the habit memory system seems to be fully functional in early life. Given this pattern of cognitive maturation, it is possible that a developmentally dysfunctional neuronal circuitry involving the limbic system would have little developmental impact during the first one to two years of life. However, as the substrate for normal representational memory and higher cognitive function gradually increases in functional importance, the effects of this dysfunctional circuitry may become evident, leading to what appears to be social, language, and cognitive deterioration, features reported in some cases of childhood autism.

CEREBELLUM AND CEREBELLAR CIRCUITS

Areas of abnormality outside of the forebrain have been confined to the cerebellum and the related inferior olive in all cases studied to date. The relationship of these lesions to those in the forebrain is unclear. In the cerebellar cortex there was a bilaterally symmetrical decrease in number of Purkinje cells and, to a lesser extent, granule cells without significant gliosis involving primarily the hemispheres, and appearing most prominently in the posterior inferior neocerebellar cortex and adjacent archicerebellar cortex. The absence of glial cell hyperplasia suggests that the lesion was acquired early in development. In animals, Brodal (1940) noted a progressively decreasing glial response following cerebellar lesions at increasingly early ages. Further support for the early acquisition of the cerebellar abnormalities relates to the preservation of the neurons in the principal inferior olive. Retrograde loss of olivary neurons regularly occurs following cerebellar lesions in the immature postnatal and adult animal (Brodal 1940) and in neonatal and adult humans (Holmes and Stewart, 1908; Norman, 1940; Greenfield,

1940). According to the topographic map of Holmes and Stewart (1908), a lesion of the neocerebellum corresponding in distribution to that seen these six autistic brains, would result in neuronal loss in the lateral part of the principal inferior olive. In all cases, these neurons, although enlarged in the three youngest brains, but smaller in the three older cerebra, are present in adequate numbers bilaterally.

The occurrence of retrograde loss of olivary neurons after cerebellar lesions is presumably due to the close relationship of the olivary climbing fiber axons to the Purkinje cell dendrites (Eccles et al., 1967). It has been shown in the fetal monkey that the olivary climbing fibers, prior to establishing their definitive relationship with the Purkinje cell dendrites, synapse in a transitory zone beneath the Purkinje cells called the *lamina dissecans* (Rakic, 1971). Since this zone is no longer evident in the human fetus after thirty weeks of gestation (Rakic and Sidman, 1970), it is likely that the cerebellar cortical lesion occurred at or before this time. Further support for this concept is provided by the study of Goldman and Galkin (1978), where, in an analogous situation, the expected retrograde loss of neurons of the medial dorsal nucleus of the thalamus failed to occur following prefrontal lesions in the rhesus monkey, prior to but not after, 106 days of gestation.

The abnormalities of the deep cerebellar nuclei show an inconsistent relationship to the abnormalities noted in the cerebellar cortex and to those noted in the inferior olivary complex. The least involved cerebellar nucleus, the dentate, normally receives direct projections from the most involved cerebellar area, the neocerebellum. Additionally, one of the most involved nuclei, the fastigeal, receives direct projections from the histologically least involved areas, the cerebellar vermal cortex (Brodal, 1981). Similarly, the principal inferior olivary nucleus, which has abnormally small neurons in three young adult patients and abnormally enlarged neurons in three young individuals, is reciprocally related to the dentate nucleus, which appears to be histologically normal in the brains from the older individuals, but which shows neuronal enlargement in the three younger cases. However, the apparently uninvolved medial and dorsal accessory olivary nuclei are reciprocally related to the globose and emboliform nuclei which are abnormal in all cases. With few exceptions, since the efferent projections from the cerebellum are provided by the deep cerebellar nuclei, the combination of lesions in these nuclei and those in the cerebellar cortex are in a position to broadly disrupt these efferent projections (Brodal, 1981).

The fact that the neurons of the deep cerebellar nuclei and those of the inferior olive are enlarged in young autistic brains and are small and decreased in number in these same areas in young adult patients is intriguing. According to Flechsig (1920) and Yakovlev and Lecours

(1967), the olivocerebellar tracts in the inferior cerebellar peduncle show advanced myelination at twenty-eight weeks of gestation, suggesting the existence of a functional circuit between the olivary nucleus and the cerebellum at this stage of development. As noted previously, since the intimate relationship of the inferior olive to the Purkinje cells has not yet been established at this time, this prenatal olivary projection is presumed to be to the cerebellar nuclei. This evidence suggests that this pathway may be the dominant cerebellar circuit prior to thirty weeks gestation. In the infant and adult human brain, the presence of retrograde cell loss of olivary neurons following cerebellar cortical lesions indicates that the predominant inferior olivary projection in the postnatal period of development is to the Purkinje cells, with the more primitive circuitry remaining as a collateral projection to the cerebellar nuclei. Therefore, based on these observations, we have hypothesized that, in the autistic brain, the early lack of availability of adequate numbers of Purkinje cells, the target cells for the mature inferior olivary projections, leads to the postnatal persistence of the prenatal projection to the cerebellar nuclei. Assuming that this hypothesis is correct, the abnormal persistence of this primitive fetal circuit may account for the neuronal enlargement characteristic of the cells of the cerebellar nuclei and inferior olive seen in the young autistic brains. We further suggest that, since this fetal circuit was probably not "designed" to function as a dominant postnatal pathway, it is likely that it is unable to sustain itself over time. This may then account for the reduced size and eventual loss of neurons in older autistic patients.

The relationship of the cerebellar abnormalities to the clinical features of autism remain unclear. In general, cerebellar dysfunction beginning in early life, including congenital absence of the cerebellum, has been associated with few neurologic symptoms (Norman, 1940; Adams et al., 1984). Animal studies have shown the existence of a direct pathway between the fastigeal nucleus and the septal nuclei and the amygdala, and a reciprocal relationship with the hippocampal cortex, suggesting that the cerebellum may play a role in the modulation of emotion and higher cortical function (Heath & Harper, 1974; Heath et al., 1978). Furthermore, animal and human studies have suggested a role for the cerebellum in the control of affective behavior (Berman et al., 1974) and functional psychiatric disorders (Heath et al., 1979). Experiments in rabbits have implicated the dentate and the interpositus nuclei in the elaboration of classic conditioned reflex responses (McCormick and Thompson 1984). Studies in patients with cerebellar lesions have suggested a role for the cerebellum in mental imagery, anticipatory planning (Leiner et al., 1987), and some aspects of language processing (Petersen et al., 1989). The cerebellum has also been implicated in autistic patients in the control of attention, possibly due to its relationship with the parietal association cortices through connections in the pons (Courchesne et al., 1992). Grafman et al. (1992) also suggested that the cerebellum may be involved in cognitive planning that is independent of memory and which is most significant in novel situations. In an extensive overview of the potential role of the cerebellum in higher cortical function, Schmahmann (1991) hypothesized that the cerebellum may regulate the speed, consistency, and appropriateness of mental and cognitive processes. Thus, there is growing evidence from both experimental and clinical studies suggesting that cerebellar lesions in adult animals and humans may result in disturbances of emotion, behavior, learning, and possibly language. Future studies will need to address the effect of cerebellar lesions occuring early in prenatal and postnatal life and their relationship to the later development of cognition.

CONCLUSIONS

Consistent pathologic abnormalities have been found in the brains of autistic individuals that have been confined to the limbic system and cerebellar circuits. Anatomic evidence suggests that the limbic system abnormalities may represent a developmental maturational curtailment involving this circuitry. The findings in the cerebellum and related olivary nucleus further suggest that the process that results in these abnormalities has its onset prior to birth. Lesion studies in animals, humans, and nonhuman primates support the role of the medial temporal lobe structures, most especially the hippocampus and the amygdala, in cognition, memory, emotion and behavior. In addition, there is growing evidence from studies in animals and adult humans that the cerebellum may also be involved in some aspects of learning. Although the effect of prenatal abnormalities within the limbic system and cerebellum are not known, it is likely that dysfunction in these circuits may be in a position to disrupt the aquisition and understanding of information throughout life and could lead to many of the clinical features characteristic of autism.

The etiology of the brain abnormalities seen in autism is unknown. Four of the six patients studied to date had seizures and were treated with anticonvulsant medications; two patients did not. The anatomic findings in the cerebellum in all cases, while showing some differences that appeared to be age-related, were similar, suggesting that neither the presence of seizures nor medication were factors. Furthermore, although most the patients studied to date have had significant cognitive impairments, one child was of normal intelligence. This child's major disability was pragmatic language and behavior. Anatomic findings in this case were similar in distribution to the other five patients, suggesting that the findings in the limbic system and cerebellum in autism are not related to mental retardation. Furthermore, the variation in clinical presentation among the patients studied, despite similar anatomic findings in all brains, lends support to the hypothesis that subsets of phenotypic expression may be derived from the same or similar patterns of pathologic abnormality.

Future anatomic studies in autism will need to address the question of variation in neuronal size and the number of neurons present that, in the cerebellar circuits and the nucleus of the diagonal band of Broca in the septum, differ with the age of the patient. Since there is no animal model for autism at this time, continued heavy reliance on human tissue will be necessary. While we have hypothesized that these changes may represent retained fetal circuitry, this will need to be further analyzed in patients at ages younger than those already studied. In addition, the question of variable phenotypic expression in autism will need closer scrutiny, with continued systematic analysis of anatomic abnormalities in autistic patients who have been carefully studied and documented during life. The mechanisms by which autistic individuals acquire and process information remain to be elucidated. However, some clues appear to be forthcoming as more information is learned about behavioral development and how and when infant and young human and nonhuman primates achieve cognition. Continued clinical studies combined with anatomic observations will be crucial to our future understanding of autism.

ACKNOWLEDGMENTS

We would like to thank the many parents and families who, by their gift to brain research, have made this work possible. We would also like express our appreciation to the late Dr. Paul I. Yakovlev, our teacher and friend, whose process of whole brain serial section as a method for the study of neurodevelopmental anatomy has provided the basis for this research.

This work was supported in part by the Nancy Lurie Marks Charitable Foundation, the Natalie Z. Haar Foundation, and the June Rockwell Levy Foundation.

REFERENCES

Aarkrog, T. 1968. Organic factors in infantile psychoses and borderline psychoses: Retrospective study of 45 cases subjected to pneumoencephalography. *Danish Medical Bulletin* 15: 283–88.

Adams, J. H., Corsellis, J. A. N., and Duchen, L. W. 1984. *Greenfield's Neuropathology*. New York: John Wiley.

Amaral, D. G., Veazey, R. B., and Cowan, W. M. 1982. Some observations on the hypothalamoamygdaloid axonal connections. *Brain Resaerch* 252: 13–27.

Amaral, D. G., Inshusti, R., and Cowan, W. M. 1983. Evidence for direct projection from the superior temporal gyrus to the entorhinal cortex in the monkey. *Brain Research* 275: 263–77.

Arin, D. M., Bauman, M. L., and Kemper, T. L. 1991. The distribution of Purkinje cell loss in the cerebellum in autism. *Neurology* 41(Suppl): 307.

Bachevalier, J. 1991. An animal model for childhood autism. In C. A. Tamminga and S. C. Schultz, eds., *Advances in Neuropsychiatry and Psychopharmacology*. 129–40. New York: Raven Press.

Bachevalier, J. 1992. Personal communication.

Bauman, M. L. and Kemper, T. L. 1985. Histoanatomic observations of the brain in early infantile autism. *Neurology* 35: 866–74.

Bauman, M. L., LeMay, M., Bauman, R. A., and Rosenberger, P. B. 1985. Computerized Tomographic (CT) observations of the posterior fossa in early infantile autism. *Neurology* 35(Suppl.): 347.

Berman, A. J., Berman, D., and Prescott, J. W. 1974. The effect of cerebellar lesions on emotional behavior in the rhesus monkey. In I. S. Cooper, M. Riklan, and R. S. Snider, eds., *The Cerebellum, Epilepsy and Behavior*. 277–84. New York: Plenum Press.

Brodal, A. 1940. Modification of Gudden method for study of cerebral localization. *Archives of Neurology and Psychiatry* 43: 46–58.

Brodal, A. 1981. *Neurological Anatomy in Relation to Clinical Medicine*. New York: Oxford University Press.

Caparulo, B. K., Cohen, D. J., Rothman, S. L., Young, J. G., Katz, J. D., Shaywitz, S. E., and Shaywitz, B. A. 1981. Computed tomographic brain scanning in children with developmental neuropsychiatric disorders. *Journal of the American Academy of Child Psychiatry* 20: 338–57.

Coleman, M. 1979. Studies of the autistic syndromes. In R. Katzman, ed., *Congenital and Acquired Cognitive Disorders*. 265–303. New York: Raven Press.

Coleman, P. D., Romano, J., Lapham, L., and Simon, W. 1985. Cell counts in cerebral cortex in an autistic patient. *Journal of Autism and Developmental Disorders* 15: 245–55.

Courchesne, E., Yeung-Courchesne, R., Press, G. A. C., Hesselink, J. R., and Jernigan, T. L. 1988. Hypoplasia of cerebellar lobules VI and VII in autism. *New England Journal of Medicine* 318: 1349–54.

Courchesne, E. 1991. Neuroanatomic imaging in autism. *Pediatrics* (Suppl.) 87: 781–790.

Courchesne, E., Akshoomoff, N. A., and Townsend, J. 1992. Recent advances in autism. In H. Naruse and E. M. Ornitz, eds., *Neurobiology of Infantile Autism*. Amsterdam: Elsevier Science Publishers, pp. 111–128.

Darby, J. H. 1976. Neuropathologic aspects of psychosis in childhood. *Journal of Autism and Childhood Schizophrenia* 6: 339–52.

DeBassio, W. A., Kemper, T. L., and Knoefel, J. E. 1985. Coffin-Siris syndrome: Neuropathologic findings. *Archives of Neurology* 42: 350–53.

Delong, G. R. 1978. A neuropsychological interpretation of infantile autism. In M. Rutter and E. Schopler, eds., *Autism*. 207–18. New York: Plenum Press.

Damasio, A. R. and Maurer, R. G. 1978. A neurologic model for childhood autism. *Archives of Neurology* 35: 777–86.

Eccles, J. C., Ito, M., and Szentagothai, J. 1967. *The Cerebellum as a Neuronal Machine*. New York: Springer.

Flechsig, P. 1920. *Anatomie des Menchlichen Gehim und Ruchenmachs auf Myelogenetischer Grundlage*. Leipzig: George Theime.

Folstein, S. E., and Piven, J. 1991. Etiology of autism: Genetic factors. *Pediatrics* (Suppl.) 87: 767–73.

Gaffney, G. R., Kuperman, S., Tsai, L. Y., and Minchin, S. 1988. Morphologic evidence of brainstem involvement in infantile autism. *Biological Psychiatry* 24: 578–86.

Gillberg, C., and Svendsen, P. 1983. Childhood psychosis and computed tomographic brain scan findings. *Journal of Autism and Developmental Disorders* 13: 19–32.

Goldman, P. S., and Galkin, T. W. 1978. Prenatal removal of frontal association cortex in the fetal rhesus monkey: Anatomic and functional consequence in postnatal life. *Brain Research* 152: 451–85.

Grafman, J., Litvan, I., Massaquoi, S., Stewart, M., Sivigu, A., and Hallet, M. 1992. Cognitive planning deficit in patients with cerebellar atrophy. *Neurology* 42: 1493–96.

Greenfield, J.G. 1954. *The Spino-Cerebellar Degenerations*. Springfield, IL: C. C. Thomas.

Hauser, S. L., Delong, G. R., and Rosman, N. P. 1975. Pneumographic findings in the infantile autism syndrome. *Brain* 98: 667–88.

Heath, R. G., and Harper, J. W. 1974. Ascending projections of the cerebellar fastigeal nucleus to the hippocampus, amygdala, and other temporal lobe sites: Evoked potential and histological studies in monkeys and cats. *Experimental Neurology* 45: 268–87.

Heath, R. G., Dempsey, C. W., Fontana, C. J., and Myers, W. A. 1978. Cerebellar stimulation: Effects on septal region, hippocampus and amygdala of cats and rats. *Biological Psychiatry* 113: 501–29.

Heath, R. G., Franklin, D. E., and Shraberg, D. 1979. Gross pathology of the cerebellum in patients diagnosed and treated as functional psychiatric disorders. *Journal of Nervous and Mental Disorders* 167: 585–92.

Hier, D. B., LeMay, M., and Rosenberger, P. B. 1979. Autism and unfavorable left-right asymmetries of the brain. Journal of Autism and Developmental Disorders 9: 153–59.

Holmes, G., and Stewart, T. G. 1908. On the connection of the inferior olives with the cerebellum in man. *Brain* 31: 125–37.

Kanner, L. 1943. Autistic disturbances of affective contact. *Nervous Child* 2: 217–50.

Kemper, T. L., and Bauman, M. L. 1992. Neuropathology of infantile autism. In H. Naruse and E. M. Ornitz, eds., *Neurobiology of Infantile Autism*. 43–57. Amsterdam: Elsevier Science Publishers.

Kimble, D. P. 1963. The effects of bilateral hippocampal lesions in rats. *Journal of Physical Psychology* 56: 273–83.

Kluver, H., and Bucy, P. 1939. Preliminary analysis of functions of the temporal lobe in monkeys. *Archives of Neurology and Psychiatry* 42:979–1000.

Krettek, J. E., and Price, J. L. 1977. Projections from the amygdaloid and adjacent olefactory structures of the entorhinal cortex and to the subiculum in the rat and cat. *Journal of Comparative Neurology* 172: 723–52.

Krettek, J. E., and Price, J. L. 1978. A description of the amygdaloid complex in the rat and cat with observations on the intra-amygdaloid axonal connections. *Journal of Comparative Neurology* 178: 255–80.

Leiner, H. C., Leiner, A. L., and Dow, R. S. 1987. Cerebrocerebellar learning loops in apes and humans. *Italian Journal of Neurological Science* 8: 425–36.

Leontovich, T. A., and Zhukova, G. P. 1963. The specificity of the neuronal structure and topography of the reticular formation of the brain and spinal cord of carnivora. *Journal of Comparative Neurology* 121: 347–79.

Mahut, H., Zola-Morgan, S., and Moss, M. 1982. Hippocampal resections impair associative learning and recognition memory in the monkey. *Journal of Neuroscience* 2: 1214–29.

Maurer, R. G., and Damasio, A. R. 1982. Childhood autism from the point of view of behavioral neurology. *Journal of Autism and Developmental Disorders* 12: 195–205.

McCormick, D. A., and Thompson, R. F. 1984. Cerebellum: Essential involvement in the classically conditioned eyelid response. *Science* 223: 296–99.

Milner, B. 1972. Disorders of learning and memory after temporal lobe lesions in man. *Clinical Neurosurgery* 19: 421–46.

Mishkin, M. 1978. Memory in monkey severely impaired by combined but not separate removal of amygdala and hippocampus. *Nature* 273: 297–98.

Mishkin, M., and Aggleton, J. P. 1981. Multiple functional contributors of the amygdala in the monkey from the amygdaloid complex. In Y. Ben-Ari, ed., *INSERM Symposium, No. 20.* 409–19. Amsterdam: Elsevier/North Holland Biomedical Press.

Mishkin, M., and Appenzeller, T. 1987. The anatomy of memory. *Scientific American* 256: 80–89.

Murakami, J. W., Courchesne, E., Press, G. A., Yeung-Courchesne, R., and Hesselink, J. R. 1989. Reduced cerebellar hemisphere size and its relationship to vermal hypoplasia in autism. *Archives of Neurology* 46: 689–94.

Murray, E. A., and Mishkin, M. 1983. Severe tactile memory deficits in monkeys after combined removal of the amygdala and hippocampus. *Brain Research* 270: 340–44.

Murray, E. A., and Mishkin, M. 1985. Amygdaloidectomy impairs crossmodal association in monkeys. *Science* 228: 604–6.

Murray, E. A. 1990. Representational memory in non-human primates. In R. P. Kesner and D. S. Olton, eds., *Neurobiology of Comparative Cognition.* 127–55. Hillsdale, NJ: Lawrence Erlbaum Associates.

Norman, R. M. 1940. Cerebellar atrophy associated with etat marbre of the basal ganglia. *Journal of Neurology and Psychiatry* 3: 311–18.

Ornitz, E. M., and Ritvo, E. R. 1968. Neurophysiologic mechanisms underlying perceptual inconstancy in autistic and schizophrenic children. *Archives of General Psychiatry* 19: 22–27.

Overman, W. H. 1990. Performance on traditional match-to-sample and non-match-to-sample, and object descrimination tasks by 12 and 32 month old children: A developmental progression. In A. Diamond, ed., *Developmental and Neural Basis of Higher Cognitive Function.* 365–93. New York: Academic Press.

Overman, W., Bachevalier, J., Turner, M., and Peuster, A. 1992. Object recognition versus object descrimination: Comparison between human infants and infant monkeys. *Behavioral Neuroscience* 106: 15–29.

Pandya, D. N., Van Hoesen, G. W., and Mesulam, M. M. 1981. Efferent connections of the cingulate gyrus in the rhesus monkey. *Brain Research* 42: 319–30.

Papez, J. W. 1937. A proposed mechanism for emotion. *Archives of Neurology and Psychiatry* 38: 725–43.

Parkinson, J. K., Murray, E. A., and Mishkin, M. 1988. A selective mnemonic role for the hippocampus in monkeys: Memory for the location of objects. *Journal of Neuroscience* 8: 4159–67.

Petersen, S. E., Fox, P. T., Posner, M. I., Mintum, M. A., and Raichle, M. E. 1989. Positron emission tomographic studies of the processing of single words. *Journal of Cognitive Neuroscience* 1: 153–70.

Rakic, P., and Sidman, R. L. 1970. Histogenesis of the cortical layers in human cerebellum particularly the lamina dissecans. *Journal of Comparative Neurology* 139: 473–500.

Rakic, P. 1971. Neuron–glia relationship during granule cell migration in developing cerebellar cortex. A Golgi and electron microscopic study in macacus rhesus. *Journal of Comparative Neurology* 141: 282–312.

Rapin, I. 1991. Autistic children: Diagnostic and clinical features. *Pediatrics* (Suppl). 87: 751–60.

Raymond, G., Bauman, M. L., and Kemper, T. L. 1989. The hippocampus in autism: Golgi analysis. *Annals of Neurology* 26: 483–84.

Ritvo, E. R., Freeman, B. J., Scheibel, A. B., Duong, T., Robinson, H., Guthrie, D., and Ritvo, A. 1986. Lower Purkinje cell counts in the cerebella of four autistic subjects: Initial findings of the UCLA–NSAC autopsy research report. *American Journal of Psychiatry* 146: 862–66.

Roberts, W. W., Dember, W. N., and Brodwick, H. 1962. Alteration and exploration in rats with hippocampal lesions. *Journal of Comparative Psychiatry.* 55:695–700.

Rosene, D. L., and Van Hoesen, G. W. 1977. Hippocampal efferents reach widespread areas of cerebral cortex and amygdala in rhesus monkey. *Science* 198: 315–17.

Rosene, D. L., and Van Hoesen, G. W. 1987. The hippocampal formation of the primate brain. In E. G. Jones and A. Peters, eds., *Cerebral Cortex, Volume 6.* 345–450. New York: Plenum Press.

Rumsey, J. H., Creasey, J., Stepanik, J. S., Dorwart, R., Patronas, N., Hamburger, S. D., and Duara, R. 1988. Hemispheric asymmetries, fourth ventricular size, and cerebellar morphology in autism. *Journal of Autism and Developmental Disorders* 18: 127–37.

Saunders, R. C., and Rosene, D. L. 1988a. A comparison of the efferents of the amygdala and the hippocampal formation in the rhesus monkey. I. Convergence in the entorhinal, prorhinal and perirhinal cortices. *Journal of Comparative Neurology* 271: 153–84

Saunders, R. C., and Rosene, D. L. 1988b. A comparison of the amygdala and the hippocampal formation in the rhesus monkey. II. reciprocal and non-reciprocal connections. *Journal of Comparative Neurology* 271: 185–207.

Schmahmann, J. D. 1991. An emerging concept. The cerebellar contribution to higher function. *Archives of Neurology* 48: 1178–87.

Squire, L. R., and Zola-Morgan, S. 1991. The medial temporal lobe memory system. *Science* 253: 1380–86.

Sumi, S. M. 1980. Brain malformation in the trisomy 18 syndrome. *Brain* 93: 821–30.

Terzian, H., and Delle-Ore, G. 1955. Syndrome of Kluver and Bucy reproduced in man by bilateral removal of the the temporal lobes. *Neurology* 3: 373–80.

Thompson, E. I. 1981. Long-term behavioral development of rhesus monkeys after amygdaloidectomy in infancy. In Y. Ben-Ari, ed., *The Amydaloid Complex. INSERM Symposium, No. 20.* 259–70. Amsterdam: Elsevier/North Holland Biomedical Press.

Tsai, L., Jacoby, C. G., Stewart, M. A., and Beisler, J. M. 1982. Unfavorable left-right asymmetries of the brain in autism: a question of methodology. *British Journal of Psychiatry* 140: 312–19.

Van Hoesen, G. W., Pandya, D. N., and Butters, N. 1972. Cortical afferents to the entorhinal cortex of the rhesus monkey. *Science* 175: 1471–73.

Van Hoesen, G. W., and Pandya, D. N. 1975a. Some connections of the entorhinal (area 28) and the perirhinal (area 35) cortices in the rhesus monkey. I. Temporal lobe afferents. *Brain Research.* 95: 1–24.

Van Hoesen, G. W., and Pandya, D. N. 1975b. Some connections of the entorhinal (area 28) and perirhinal (area 35) cortices of the rhesus monkey. III. Efferent connections. *Brain Research* 95: 39–59.

Van Hoesen, G. W., Pandya, D. N., and Butters, N. 1975. Some connections of the entorhinal (area 28) and perirhinal (area 35) cortices of the rhesus monkey. II. Frontal lobe afferents. *Brain Research* 95: 25–38.

Van Hoesen, G. W., Rosene, D. L., and Mesulam, M. M. 1979. Subicular input from temporal cortex in the rhesus monkey. *Science* 205: 608–10.

Vergnes, M. 1981. Effect of prior familiarization with mice on elicitation of mouse killing in rats: Role of the amygdala. In Y. Ben-Ari, ed. T*he Amygdaloid Complex. INSERM Symposium, No. 20.* 293–304. Amsterdam: Elsevier/North Holland Biomedical Press.

Vilensky, J. A., Demasio, A. R., and Maurer, R. G. 1981. Gait disturbances in patients with autistic behavior. *Archives of Neurology* 38: 646–49.

Williams, R. S., Hauser, S. L., Purpura, D. P., Delong, G. R., and Swisher, C. W. 1980. Autism and mental retardation. *Archives of Neurology.* 37: 749–53.

Yakovlev, P. I., and Lecours, A. R. 1967. Myelogenetic cycles of regional maturation of the brain. In A. Minkowski, ed., *Regional Development of the Brain in Early Life.* 3–70. Oxford: Blackwell Scientific Publications.

8

THE CONTRIBUTION OF MEDIAL TEMPORAL LOBE STRUCTURES IN INFANTILE AUTISM: A NEUROBEHAVIORAL STUDY IN PRIMATES

Jocelyne Bachevalier, Ph.D.
Patricia M. Merjanian, Ph.D.

Early infantile autism is a descriptive term identifying a distinctive disorder of behavioral development in a young child. The syndrome was first recognized by Kanner in 1943 and was demonstrated to have an early onset, usually before the age of thirty months, and a prevalence in male subjects. The distinctive characteristics are impairment in reciprocal social interactions, verbal and nonverbal communication, and restricted repertoire of activities and interests (often including ritualistic and self-stimulatory behaviors). Associated features are unusual fears and anxiety, hyperorality, pica, and inability to adequately modulate sensory input.

Despite considerable research efforts over the last decade, the causes of infantile autism remain unknown. Although the causes are likely to be diverse (Rutter, 1978; Ornitz, 1983), it has become accepted that a primary defect in brain function is present in autistic children. During the last two decades, it has been proposed that the behavioral disturbances seen in autistic children could follow dysfunction in different brain regions, ranging from subcortical structures, such as the brainstem, thalamus, and striatum (Ornitz, 1983), cerebellum (Courchesne et al., 1988), mesolimbic dopaminergic system (Damasio and Maurer, 1978), and medial temporal lobe (DeLong, 1978, 1993), to association areas of the cortex, including the prefrontal cortex (Rumsey and Hamburger, 1988; Prior and Hoffman, 1990; Minshew, 1991; Bishop, 1993). There is growing evidence to support the hypothesis that infantile autism results from early neuropathology of the medial temporal lobe (for review, see DeLong and

Bauman, 1987; Fein et al., 1987; Merjanian and Nadel, 1993). For example, there are similarities between the disturbed behaviors noted in autism and those found in the Klüver–Bucy syndrome; this syndrome results from bilateral damage to the temporal lobes in both adult monkeys (Kluüver and Bucy, 1938, 1939) and humans (Marlowe et al., 1975; Lilly et al., 1983). In addition, autistic children have been shown to have memory defects similar in some respects to those of both amnesic adult humans with temporal lobe pathology (Boucher and Warrington, 1976; Boucher, 1981; but see also Ameli et al., 1988; Minshew and Goldstein, 1993) and adult monkeys with medial temporal lobe lesions (Chapter 9; Merjanian et al., 1984; Merjanian, 1985). Finally, strong implications of medial temporal pathology, and even direct evidence of it, have been found in some cases of autism (Hetzler and Griffin, 1981; Bauman and Kemper, 1988, Chapter 7; Hof et al., 1991; Hoon and Reiss, 1992; Deonna et al., 1992). Accumulating evidence from our ongoing neurobehavioral study in infant monkeys provides additional support for this hypothesis. Indeed, neonatal damage to the medial temporal lobe structures in primates yields behavioral disturbances strikingly similar to those seen in autistic children (Merjanian et al., 1986, 1988; Bachevalier, 1991).

This chapter begins with a summary of clinical and experimental evidence of the involvement of the medial temporal lobe structures in memory and emotion. The major behavioral disturbances seen in infant monkeys that had received lesions of the amygdalohippocampal complex are then described. It can be seen from this survey that neonatal damage to the amygdalohippocampal complex yields severe memory loss associated with profound socioemotional abnormalities. Furthermore, separate neonatal lesions of the amygdaloid complex and the hippocampal formation produce distinct patterns of memory and socioemotional disturbances. The potential value of these experimental findings for an understanding of infantile autism is discussed in the final section of the chapter.

THE MEDIAL TEMPORAL LOBE STRUCTURES AND INFANTILE AUTISM

It is now well established that medial temporal structures (i.e., the amygdala, the hippocampus, and the surrounding cortical areas) are involved in the regulation of memory functions and emotional reactions. Evidence for this regulation has come principally from experiments in primates in which damage to these regions resulted in prominent effects on learning, memory, motivation, emotion, and social interaction.

Much of our knowledge concerning the role of the medial temporal lobe in memory functions is derived from well-studied clinical patients who either underwent selective medial temporal lobe operations for relief of epilepsy or demonstrated neuropathology in this brain region secondary to anoxia or ischemia. Among these patients are the famous cases H. M. (Scoville and Milner, 1957) and, later, D. R. B. (Damasio et al., 1985) and R. B. (Zola-Morgan et al., 1986). All three patients have a profound inability to remember recent events and to learn many types of new information. They can, however, recollect old events and their intelligence, perception, and language are either unaffected or only minimally impaired.

Paradoxically, despite their profound memory defects, amnesic patients have demonstrated normal performance in certain kinds of learning tasks (Milner, 1962; Corkin, 1968; Warrington and Weiskrantz, 1968; Brooks and Baddeley, 1976; Cohen and Squire, 1980; Squire at al., 1984). For example, amnesic subjects demonstrate steady learning of mirror-drawing, tactile mazes, or rotary pursuit, and they can improve on other cognitive tasks such as completing jigsaw puzzles or solving the Tower-of-Hanoi problem. Subsequent studies conducted with nonhuman primates have converged upon a similar dichotomy of spared learning abilities in the presence of profound amnesia (Mishkin and Petri, 1984; Mishkin et al., 1984; Zola-Morgan and Squire, 1985). Monkeys with bilateral damage to medial temporal lobe structures are unable to recognize an object they had seen just a minute or two earlier (Mishkin, 1982; Saunders et al., 1984; Zola-Morgan and Squire, 1985) or to remember whether or not the object had been associated with a food reward for even a few seconds (Spiegler and Mishkin, 1979). Nevertheless, the same monkeys have no difficulty mastering a multiple-trial concurrent-object discrimination task in which successive trials on a given pair are separated by twenty-four-hour intertrial intervals (Malamut et al., 1984).

These clinical and experimental findings have led to the proposal that retaining the effects of experience depends on two fundamentally different neural systems (Hirsh, 1974; Mishkin and Petri, 1984; Mishkin et al., 1984; Zola-Morgan and Squire, 1985; Mishkin and Appenzeller, 1987). One is a *memory* or representational system that serves both recognition and recall and utilizes a *corticolimbic* circuit. This system is presumed to be *impaired* in subjects rendered amnesic by damage to the medial temporal lobe structures. The other is a *habit* system that mediates the formation of stimulus-response connections and is thought to depend in large part on a *corticostriatal* circuit (Mishkin et al., 1984; Wang et al., 1990). This system is presumed to be *preserved* in amnesic subjects. Complementary evidence from our developmental behavioral studies in infant monkeys suggests that the two retention systems are developmentally dissociable; that is, the corticolimbic memory system appears to mature considerably later than does the corticostriatal habit system (Bachevalier and Mishkin, 1984; Bachevalier, 1990). A similar delay in the maturation of the limbic memory system was demonstrated in rat pups (Freeman and Stanton, 1991) and human infants (Overman, 1990; Overman et al., 1992).

Other behavioral and emotional changes after bilateral damage to the medial temporal lobe region in adult monkeys were first described by Brown and Schafer (1888). These changes included hypoemotionality as reflected by a tendency to become unnaturally fearless and tame (hyperexploratory behavior), excessive examination of objects (often with the mouth), purposeless hyperactivity, and impairment in social interaction (Klüver and Bucy, 1938, 1939). Later studies have shown that many similar behavioral changes can be observed after restricted bilateral damage to either the amygdala (Rosvold et al., 1954; Weiskrantz, 1956; Kling, 1972; Aggleton and Passingham, 1981; Aggleton and Mishkin, 1986; Zola-Morgan et al., 1991) or the inferior temporal cortex (Horel et al., 1975; Iwai et al., 1986). It is interesting that emotional changes also follow selective lesions of the ento- and perirhinal cortical areas (the most mediorostral portion of the inferior temporal cortex); monkeys with such lesions exhibit an increased amount of freezing behavior and an absence of facial expressions in the presence of fear-inducing stimuli (Meunier et al., 1991).

The role of the medial temporal lobe structures in emotional behavior has also received support from clinical cases. Hypoemotionality has been described both in patients suffering from viral encephalitis, a disease that can produce extensive damage to the limbic structures and the neocortex in the temporal lobe (Friedman and Allen, 1969; Gascon and Gilles, 1973; Marlowe et al., 1975), and in patients who received bilateral temporal lobectomy as a treatment either for psychosis (Obrador, 1947; Pool, 1952; Terzian and Delle Ore, 1955) or for otherwise untreatable epileptic seizures, such as case H. M. (Scoville and Milner, 1957; Hebben et al., 1981). In addition to the hypoemotionality, some of these patients have exhibited the complete pattern of behavioral disturbances seen in Klüver–Bucy syndrome.

The severe memory loss and accompanying disturbances in emotional behavior produced by damage to the medial temporal structures in adult primates are in some respect similar to the behavioral abnormalities observed in autistic children. These similarities have led to the proposal that infantile autism may also result from damage to the medial temporal structures (DeLong and Bauman, 1987; Fein et al., 1987; DeLong, 1992). Yet, the clinical picture of an autistic child is considerably different from that of an amnesic adult. For example, the impairment in normal social interactions is more dramatic in the autistic children than it is in the amnesic adults. Autistic children suffer disturbances of verbal and nonverbal communication and stereotypies not seen in amnesic adults. Thus, if the neural dysfunction in autism resides in the medial temporal lobe, then the question of why autistic children differ so greatly in their cognitive, emotional, and social behaviors from amnesic adults arises. A possible answer is that while the medial temporal lobe is damaged in both populations of patients, the damage has occurred during different time periods of development and thus has yielded different patterns of cognitive impairment and behavioral disturbances. According to this hypothesis, one would expect that the memory loss of a young individual would have a greater impact on the development of cognitive abilities than that of an individual acquiring the same neural damage in adulthood. While amnesic adults might be able to retrieve old memories, amnesic infants might never have been able to form and store memories in the first place; consequently, they would develop additional intellectual deficits and behavioral abnormalities (see also DeLong, 1992). Furthermore, because the medial temporal structures also play an important role in the early expression of emotion and the subsequent establishment of normal social relationships, it is probable that differences comparable to those seen in memory would occur. Early damage might significantly impair the acquisition of appropriate socioemotional behaviors by a child, while later damage might be less important because the adult would have already acquired the necessary social skills.

To study the behavioral development of primates that might remain amnesic from infancy through adulthood, we prepared newborn monkeys with removal of the medial temporal lobe structures. We then followed in some detail the development of their cognitive and socioemotional behavior. Our experimental findings are described in the remainder of the chapter.

BEHAVIORAL CONSEQUENCES OF NEONATAL DAMAGE TO THE AMYGDALOHIPPOCAMPAL COMPLEX

Newborn rhesus monkeys sustained two-stage bilateral removals to the amygdalohippocampal complex. This included the amygdaloid nuclei, hippocampus, and adjacent cortical areas, such as the periamygdaloid cortex, the entorhinal cortex, and portions of the perirhinal cortex and parahippocampal gyrus, as shown in Figure 8.1. Operated newborn controls sustained two-stage bilateral ablations to the anterior portion of the inferior temporal cortex (area TE, a higher-order cortical area of the visual system from which visual inputs reach the limbic structures). Reasons for selecting cortical area TE as the site of the comparison lesion have been described in detail elsewhere (Bachevalier, 1991). Operated animals were age-matched with unoperated controls and all infant

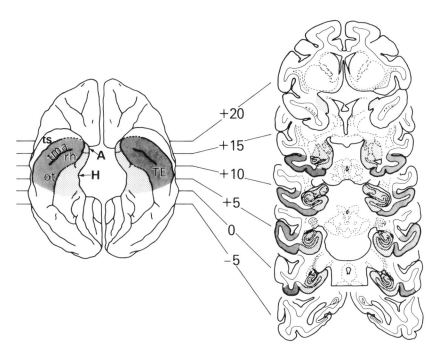

Figure 8.1. Ventral surface and coronal sections illustrating the intended neonatal area TE lesions (dark stippling) and amygdalohippocampal lesions (light stippling). Abbreviations: A, amygdaloid complex; H, hippocampal formation; ot, occipitotemporal sulcus; rh, rhinal sulcus; TE, anterior two-third of inferior temporal cortex; tma, anterior middle temporal sulcus; ts, superior temporal sulcus. The bilateral lesions were performed in two unilateral stages at approximately one week and three weeks of age, respectively. *Source:* Bachevalier, 1990

monkeys were raised either in dyads or triads consisting of one or two operated animals and one unoperated control.

LEARNING AND MEMORY ABILITIES

The formation of *visual discrimination habits* in these animals was measured when they were three months of age with a concurrent discrimination task with twenty-four-hour intertrial intervals (24-hr ITI). This task has been used to demonstrate the existence of preserved learning ability in amnesic monkeys with damage to the medial temporal lobe structures (Malamut et al., 1984) and can be performed by young infant monkeys (Bachevalier and Mishkin, 1984). A series of twenty pairs of objects was presented to the monkey just once a day as follows. A positive object and a negative object (i.e., one baited and one unbaited) were presented simultaneously over the lateral wells of the test tray. After the monkey made a choice by displacing one of the objects, there was a twenty-second delay, after which the second pair of objects was presented for choice. This procedure continued until all twenty pairs had been presented once each. The same series of objects was then presented for choice once every twenty-four hours; the positive and negative objects within each pair, as well as the serial order of the pairs, remained constant across sessions, but the objects' left–right positions were randomized daily. Testing was continued in this way until the monkeys attained the criterion of 90 correct responses in 100 consecutive trials with the first set of twenty object-pairs (Set A). The procedure was repeated for a second set of twenty object-pairs (Set B).

Performance of operated infant monkeys (Figure 8.2) was compared with that of monkeys that had been tested in the same way after receiving identical brain lesions when they were adults (Malamut et al., 1984; Phillips et al., 1988). The results indicated that damage to the limbic system appeared to leave formation of visual discrimination habits intact whether the lesions were made early or late, strengthening the view that this type of learning process does not depend on the integrity of the limbic structures. By contrast, lesions of area TE yielded a severe and long-lasting deficit in visual habit formation if the damage occurred late, but they produced only a mild, transitory deficit of this function if

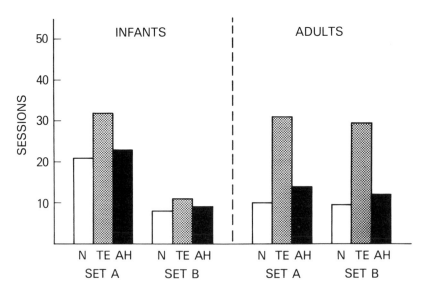

Figure 8.2. The average number of sessions to attain criterion on two consecutive sets of discriminations (Sets A and B) by three-month-old monkeys (operated neonatally) and adult monkeys. N, normal controls; TE, animals with bilateral TE lesions; AH, animals with bilateral amygdalohippocampal lesions.
Source: Bachevalier, 1990

the damage occurred early. These data suggest a functional sparing of visual habit formation after early damage to the inferior temporal cortical area TE (Bachevalier et al., 1990).

The development of *limbic-dependent memory functions* in infant monkeys was investigated by testing the same monkeys at ten months of age in an object recognition task with trial unique objects (delayed nonmatching-to-sample), a task that was used to demonstrate anterograde amnesia in adult monkeys with damage to the medial temporal lobe (Mishkin, 1978). In this task, the animal has to remember, on the basis of a single trial, whether or not an object has been seen before. Each trial consisted of two parts. First, the animal was confronted with a sample object overlying the baited central well of a test tray, which the animal removed from the well to obtain the food reward. Ten seconds later the animal was confronted with the sample object and a new object, now overlying the lateral wells of the test tray. In this second part, the monkey was rewarded for displacing the novel object. Twenty trials separated by thirty-second intervals were given daily, with each trial featuring a new pair of objects chosen from a stock of several hundred.

First, the monkey had to learn the rule of avoiding the familiar item in favor of the new one and thereby show that it could remember each sample for at least a few seconds. Then, its recognition memory was taxed further in two ways: through progressive increases of the delay between sample presentation and choice test (from the initial 10-second delay to 30-, 60-, and 120-second delays) and then through progressive increases in the number of sample items to be remembered (from the initial single object to three, five, and ten items). As shown in Figure 8.3, both early and late damage to the medial temporal lobe structures yielded severe impairment in visual recognition, reflected in drops in performance of 22 percent for the infants and 32 percent for the adults (as compared to their normal controls). By contrast, although late damage to area TE resulted in a drop in performance of 29 percent, early lesions of this cortical area resulted in a drop of only 8 percent. Thus, with regard to limbic-dependent memory, there is again evidence of a greater compensatory potential after neonatal cortical damage than after neonatal medial temporal lobe damage (Bachevalier, 1990, 1992).

Additional testing of these same monkeys when they reached adulthood (six to seven years) indicated that the effects of these early lesions were long-lasting (Bachevalier and Mishkin, 1988). For example, at this age, the monkeys with neonatal damage to area TE exhibited sparing of both habit and memory formation of the same magnitude as that found earlier when they were three and ten months old. By contrast, the monkeys with neonatal medial temporal lobe lesions resembled those with late medial temporal lobe lesions in that they were unimpaired in habit formation, but were severely impaired in recogni-

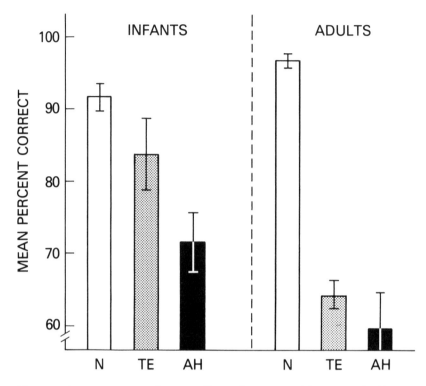

Figure 8.3. Average scores on the recognition performance task by ten-month-old monkeys (operated neonatally) and adult monkeys. Abbreviations are as in Figure 8.2. *Source:* Bachevalier, 1990

tion memory. Furthermore, the memory loss after early medial temporal lobe lesions, like that after late medial temporal lobe lesions (Murray and Mishkin, 1983; Parkinson et al., 1988), appears to involve all sensory modalities since impairment in several other memory tasks, such as tactual recognition memory and memory for spatial locations, was found in adult monkeys with early medial temporal lobe lesions (Malkova et al., 1991).

In summary, these behavioral data indicate that early damage to the amygdalohippocampal complex, like late damage, yields severe and global sensory memory loss. Nevertheless, despite the amnesia, animals with early amygdalohippocampal damage are able to learn long lists of object-pairs, indicating that some form of learning was entirely spared by the early lesions. By implication, these findings suggest that the medial temporal lobe structures are essential early in life to promote the normal development of cognitive memory functions.

SOCIOEMOTIONAL BEHAVIORS

The emotional and social development of the infant monkeys with neonatal amygdalohippocampal lesions was assessed by analyzing their interactions with their age-matched normal controls with whom they were raised, and by comparing these social interactions with those of normal infants raised together. At the ages of two and six months, two infant monkeys from the same rearing cohort (e.g., one operated and its pair-reared control or two pair-reared normal infant monkeys) were placed in a play cage containing toys and towels. The behavior of each pair was videorecorded for two periods of five minutes each, separated by a five-minute interval, for six consecutive days. The frequency and duration of behaviors for each animal on the videotapes were scored independently by two observers, who assigned the behaviors to one of seven different behavioral categories:

Approach: social contact initiated by the observed monkey.
Acceptance of approach: acceptance of social contact initiated by the other monkey.
Dominant approach: immature forms of aggression, such as snapping at the other monkey, taking toys away from the other monkey, or pushing the other monkey away.
Active withdrawal: active withdrawal from social approach initiated by the other monkey.
Inactivity: passive behavior.
Manipulation: manipulations of toys or parts of the cage with the limbs or mouth.
Locomotor stereotypies: abnormal motor behaviors, such as circling or doing somersaults.

The results indicate that, at both two and six months of age, pairs of normal animals spent most of their time in social interactions, locomotion, or manipulation. They exhibited virtually no behaviors considered to be abnormal, such as active withdrawal, locomotor stereotypies, or self-directed activities, and almost no inactivity. Between two and six months, however, the nature of social interactions between normal animals did change. Whereas at two months social behavior consisted primarily of following the other monkey and clinging to it, at six months these immature behaviors were replaced primarily by rough-and-tumble play and chasing.

Unlike normal infant monkeys, those with neonatal medial temporal lobe lesions began to show numerous socioemotional abnormalities as they matured (Figure 8.4). At two months of age, the infant monkeys with medial temporal lobe lesions showed more inactivity and manipulated objects less than did their controls.

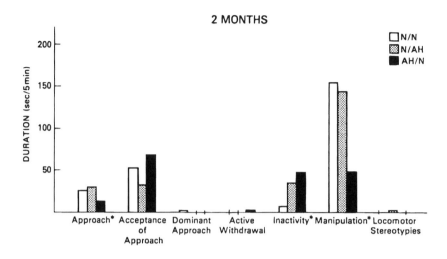

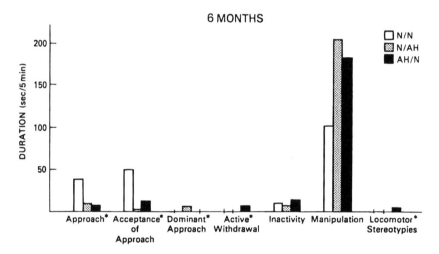

Figure 8.4. The average duration (seconds per five-minute session) of behavioral activities at two and six months of age in animals with neonatal amygdalohippocampal damage (AH/N) and their age-matched normal controls (N/AH), as compared with the average duration of behavioral activities of normal controls paired together (N/N). * statistical differences between groups ($p < .05$).

The analysis of their social interactions revealed that animals with early medial temporal lobe lesions did not initiate social contact as much as did their unoperated controls, but they did have a normal amount of accepting approach from their control, indicating that the normal animal in the pair was initiating most of the social interactions. It is interesting that at six months of age the operated monkeys displayed even more striking pathology. The amount of social interaction between the operated animals and their controls decreased dramatically as compared with animals in the normal dyads. These results indicate that animals with the amygdalohippocampal removals displayed less initiation of social approach as well as less acceptance of social contacts. In addition, the normal controls adapted to the social unresponsiveness of the animal with amygdalohippocampal damage by reducing the amount of social contact attempted. Furthermore, there were also qualitative differences in appearance and social interactions between the animals with early medial temporal lobe lesions and their controls at six months of age. They had blank, unexpressive faces and poor body expression (i.e., a lack of normal playful posturing), and they displayed very few eye contacts.

Social dominance was measured by analyzing dominant approach and active withdrawal. At two months of age, there was virtually no dominant approach or active withdrawal by any animals. At six months of age, however, there was more dominant approach in the control animals paired with the operated monkeys—even more than in animals from dyads with two normal controls—and more active withdrawal in animals with early amygdalohippocampal lesions. This is of particular interest because the increase in active withdrawal, which occurs in response to an initiation of social contact by the other animal, suggests that animals with early medial temporal lobe lesions were both uninterested in social contact and socially inept and also actively avoided social contact. Perhaps as a result of the drastic reduction in the amount of social contact, both animals with early medial temporal lobe lesions and their controls exhibited an increase in manipulation. In addition to these social disturbances, animals with early medial temporal lobe lesions developed locomotor stereotypies.

Finally, all of the socioemotional disturbances of infants with amygdalohippocampal damage were still present when these animals reached adulthood, indicating that early damage of the medial temporal lobe had long-lasting effects on socioemotional behavior.

Although the operated controls that had received early damage to area TE showed none of the disturbances seen in infant monkeys with early medial temporal lobe lesions, they did display other behavioral abnormalities such as hyperactivity and increased frequency of shifting behavioral activities resembling those of children with attention-deficit hyperactivity disorder (Merjanian et al., 1989). However, when the animals reached adulthood, these behavioral abnormalities were almost totally absent.

In summary, neonatal damage to the amygdalohippocampal complex in primates results in a profound loss of memory functions as well as severe socioemotional disorders. To learn more about the underlying neural substrate of the behavioral disorders resulting from early amygdalohippocampal damage, we investigated whether or not the full-fledged syndrome we have described could be fractionated by restricted damage to specific structures in the medial temporal lobe. This notion has been discussed by others (Zola-Morgan et al., 1991). It is possible that the pathology responsible for the socioemotional disturbances may be amygdaloid damage alone, and not combined amygdalohippocampal damage. Thompson and collaborators (1977, 1981) already reported long-lasting social disturbances in monkeys that had sustained damage to the amygdaloid complex at two months of age. Conversely, it is also possible that the amnesic syndrome after early damage to the amygdalohippocampal complex may have resulted from damage to the hippocampal formation alone. Mahut and Moss (1986) showed that damage to the hippocampal formation at two months of age yielded long-lasting memory loss. To investigate these possibilities, we prepared additional newborn monkeys with damage to either the amygdaloid complex or the hippocampal formation and began to test them in cognitive tasks and social interactions in the same way as the monkeys with neonatal damage to the amygdalohippocampal complex.

BEHAVIORAL CONSEQUENCES OF NEONATAL DAMAGE TO THE AMYGDALA OR TO THE HIPPOCAMPUS

Newborn monkeys sustained restricted bilateral damage either to the amygdala, including the amygdaloid nuclei, the periamygdaloid cortex, and the rostral portion of the entorhinal cortex (and probably part of the axons from neurons in perirhinal cortical area), or to the hippocampal formation, including the hippocampus and a portion of the parahippocampal gyrus. Again, the lesions were done in two stages at the ages of approximately one and three weeks. Testing of learning and memory abilities was done at three months of age for visual habit formation and at ten months of age for visual recognition memory. Social interactions were videorecorded at two and six months of age. Behavioral responses of infant monkeys with partial limbic lesions were compared to those of unoperated infant monkeys as well as to those of infant monkeys with combined amygdalohippocampal complex lesions described in the previous section of this chapter.

VISUAL HABIT FORMATION AND VISUAL RECOGNITION MEMORY

As expected, like infant monkeys with the combined amygdalohippocampal damage, those with damage to the amygdaloid complex or to the hippocampal formation were clearly able to form visual habits at three months of age (Table 8.1). In addition, like selective amygdalar and hippocampal damage in adult monkeys (Mishkin, 1978), neonatal

Table 8.1 Object Discrimination and Object Recognition

Task	Age	N	AH	A	H
24-hr ITI	3 months	9 + 3.4	14 + 4.3	15 + 4.2	12 + 3.02
	3-4 years	11 + 2.8	12 + 3.4	Not tested	Not tested
DNMS	10 months	88.7 + 3.9	71.7 + 3.9**	80.1 + 5.9*	88.1 + 4.5
	3-4 Years	95.1 + 2.9	59.6 + 5.1**	90.7 + 2.4*	87.9 + 5.3*

Note: Scores are the mean number of sessions to attain criterion in the three sets of concurrent discriminations (24-hr ITI) and the average correct responses across all delays and lists in the visual recognition task (DNMS). Infant groups included six to eight monkeys and adult groups included three to four monkeys. Abbreviations: N, unoperated controls; AH, animals with combined amygdalohippocampal removals; A, animals with amygdalar lesions; H, animals with hippocampal lesions.
** ($p < .01$) and * ($p < .05$) as compared with unoperated controls.

damage to the amygdaloid complex or to the hippocampal formation did not yield the severe impairment in visual recognition memory seen in animals with early or late damage to the amygdalohippocampal complex (Table 8.1). In fact, whereas both amygdalar and hippocampal lesions in adulthood yielded a mild memory loss, only the neonatal amygdalar lesions produced a deficit equivalent in magnitude. By contrast, the neonatal hippocampal lesions left this ability intact (Bachevalier and Mishkin, 1991).

In conclusion, these data suggest that early in life either the amygdaloid nuclei or the cortical areas around the rhinal sulcus, or both, are involved in the development of visual recognition memory. The findings also indicate that in infancy, like in adulthood (Clower et al., 1991), the hippocampal formation does not participate in recognition memory, at least when the delays are short (i.e., less then ten minutes).

SOCIOEMOTIONAL BEHAVIOR

As in our previous study, the socioemotional behavior of infant monkeys with selective medial temporal lobe lesions was analyzed by pairing the operated infant monkeys with their normal controls in a play cage at the ages of two and six months.

At two months of age, as shown in Figure 8.5, like infant monkeys with combined amygdalohippocampal lesions, those with *amygdalar* lesions displayed more inactivity and less manipulation than their normal controls; unlike the former, however, they showed no obvious impairment in initiation of social contact, but they did show more social withdrawal and more dominant approach than did their normal controls. At six months of age, again like animals with combined amygdalohippocampal lesions, those with neonatal amygdalar lesions displayed less initiation of social contact and more social withdrawal than did their controls, indicating significant changes in social relationships. However, unlike infant monkeys with amygdalohippocampal damage, those with

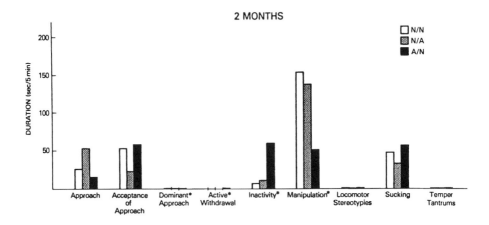

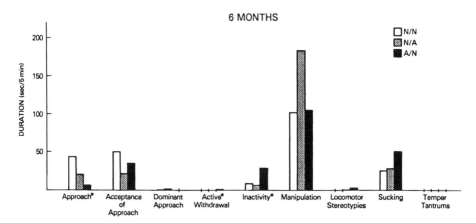

Figure 8.5. The average duration (seconds per five-minute session) of behavioral activities at two and six months of age in animals with neonatal amygdalar lesions (A/N) and their age-matched normal controls (N/A), as compared with the average duration of behavioral activities of normal controls paired together (N/N).
* statistical differences between groups ($p < .05$).

amygdalar lesions did not display less acceptance of approach, more manipulation, stereotypic behaviors, or loss of facial and body expressions, but they were more passive.

At two months of age, as shown in Figure 8.6, the animals with early damage to the *hippocampal* formation showed some degree of socioemotional disturbances (e.g., a reduction in initiation of social contacts, more inactivity, and less manipulation than normal controls). These behavioral disturbances, however, were not apparent when these animals

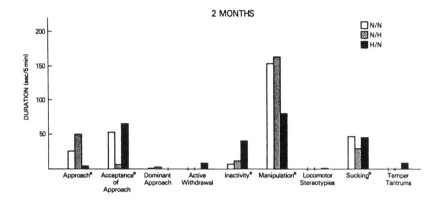

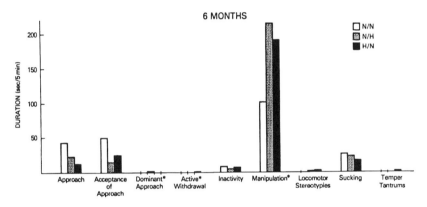

Figure 8.6. The average duration (seconds per five-minute session) of behavioral activities at two and six months of age of animals with neonatal hippocampal lesions (H/N) and their age-matched normal controls (N/H), as compared with the average duration of behavioral activities of normal controls paired together (N/N).
* statistical differences between groups (p <.05).

reached six months of age. At this age, the amount of social interaction with the control animals was only slightly reduced as compared to that found in normal animals. Furthermore, animals with neonatal hippocampal lesions did not display stereotypic behaviors. Thus, it seemed that the behavioral disturbances of infants with early damage to the hippocampal formation appeared negligible.

In summary, the behavioral data thus far indicate that early damage to the amygdaloid nuclei and cortical areas around the rhinal sulcus yields mild deficits in memory function and moderate disturbances in social interactions. By contrast, early damage to the hippocampal formation yields a sparing of memory and only mild socioemotional disturbances. Because infant monkeys with selective medial temporal lobe lesions have not been retested as adults, we do not yet know the long-term behavioral consequences of these early selective lesions. Nevertheless, it appears that both the nature and the developmental time course of the behavioral disturbances depend greatly on the specific limbic structure involved in the neonatal lesions.

The recent discovery that ento- and perirhinal cortical areas contribute both to memory (Murray et al., 1989; Zola-Morgan et al., 1989; Meunier et al., 1993) and to emotional responses (Meunier et al., 1991) raises the question of whether partial damage to these cortical areas that occurred during amygdalar resections may have contributed to the mild impairment in recognition memory as well as to the socioemotional abnormalities. Further studies of the behavioral consequences of restricted neonatal damage either to the ento- and perirhinal cortex or to the amygdaloid nuclei are clearly warranted.

RELATIONSHIP TO INFANTILE AUTISM

To recapitulate, our studies of behavioral development in infant monkeys with neonatal damage to the medial temporal lobe structures have indicated that the same neonatal damage that leads to severe cognitive memory disorder can also have extremely serious consequences for personality and social development; in part, perhaps, because the cognitive memory disorder is present from infancy onward (see also DeLong, 1992), *but also* because of the direct effect of the medial temporal lobe lesions on mechanisms of emotionality and social interactions.

The experimental work described in this chapter is promising from the standpoint of the similarities between the behavioral syndrome seen in infant monkeys with neonatal damage to the amygdalohippocampal complex and autistic children (70 percent of the autistic children have social disorders associated with mental retardation). They share the symptoms of abnormalities in social interactions, absence of facial and body expressions as well as the development of stereotypic behaviors. Both disorders are characterized by memory deficits despite normal learning abilities in certain kinds of learning tasks. There is an early onset of symptoms in both cases, although the complete syndrome is not apparent in early infancy. Thus, the time course as well as the nature of the socioemotional disturbances and the cognitive impairment observed in monkeys with early damage to the medial temporal lobe structures strongly suggest that autism too may result from early dysfunction of the medial temporal lobe. Direct support for this proposal has been provided by recent reports of neuropathological abnormalities in the medial temporal lobe structures of mentally retarded autistic subjects (Bauman and Kemper, 1985, 1988, this volume; Hof et al., 1991; Hoon and Reiss, 1992). It is also of interest that, like autistic children, monkeys with early amygdalohippocampal damage exhibit considerable variability of specific symptoms. This suggests that autism too may result from a common locus of pathology that produces multiple phenotypic displays rather than resulting from multiple pathologies that each yield a particular subset of autistic symptoms.

The extent of the medial temporal lobe involved in the disease may also be of great significance. Indeed, the pattern of disturbances differed greatly according to the medial temporal lobe structures involved in the lesion. For example, although early damage to the amygdaloid complex and portion of the cortical areas around the rhinal sulcus yielded a pattern of disturbances similar to that described for the combined amygdalohippocampal lesions, the magnitude of these disturbances was much smaller. In addition, early damage to the hippocampal formation yielded a different pattern of disturbances. These animals had no memory deficits—at least for retention intervals up to three minutes—and negligible socioemotional disturbances. So far, contrary to recent proposals (DeLong, 1992; Chapter 9), the results indicate that early damage to the amygdaloid complex and the surrounding rhinal cortex appears to be more closely related to the emergence of autisticlike behavior in the monkeys than early damage to the hippocampal formation. Furthermore, because our neonatal lesions of the amygdaloid complex included the amygdaloid nuclei and a portion of the rhinal cortical areas, it is still possible that the mild memory impairment seen in monkeys with early amygdalar lesions may have resulted from this additional cortical damage (Zola-Morgan et al., 1989; Murray, 1991; Meunier et al., 1993). If this were to be the case, it will indicate that the socioemotional disturbances and the cognitive impairments may be related to the extent of damage to the amygdaloid nuclei and the ento- and perirhinal cortical areas, respectively. It is interesting, therefore, to consider the possibility that these patterns of behavioral disturbances in monkeys with early selective medial temporal lobe lesions might also be found in some cases of autism, thus suggesting that the different patterns of behavioral symptomatology in autism may result from neuropathology in restricted and different parts of the medial temporal lobe.

Although we acknowledge that the neuropathology found in medial temporal lobe structures in autistic children is entirely different from the destructive brain lesions we inflicted to the infant monkeys, we believe that the resemblance between monkeys with neonatal medial temporal lobe lesions (more specifically the amygdaloid complex and surrounding ento- and perirhinal cortical areas), and autistic children is sufficiently close to encourage further study of this putative animal model of infantile autism. While the discussion in this chapter has focused on the evidence for temporal-lobe involvement in the autistic syndrome, our model does not preclude the involvement of other neural structures (Bauman and Kemper, 1988; Courchesne et al., 1988; Prior and Hoffmann, 1990; Holroyd et al., 1991; Minshew, 1991; Bishop, 1993), either as alternative or additional loci of neuropathology. Indeed, it could be argued that any kind of *early* dysfunction in the medial temporal lobe structures is likely to impinge on the neuroanatomic and neurochemical organization as well as on the functioning of subcortical and cortical areas, such as the neostriatum, the prefrontal, cingulate, and parietal cortices, which share strong anatomical connections with the medial temporal lobe structures.

ACKNOWLEDGMENTS

We gratefully acknowledge the contributions of our colleagues Karen Pettigrew and Mimi Brickson. We thank Corinne Hagger, Mortimer Mishkin, and Elisabeth A. Murray for their valuable comments on an earlier version of this chapter. We also thank Mortimer Mishkin for his support throughout all phases of this work.

REFERENCES

Aggleton, J. P., and Mishkin, M. 1986. The amygdala: Sensory gateway to the emotions. In R. Plutchik and H. Kellerman, eds., *Emotion: Theory, Research, and Experience.* 281–99. Vol. 3 of *Biological Foundations of Emotion.* New York: Academic Press.

Aggleton, J. P., and Passingham, R. E. 1981. Syndrome produced by lesions of the amygdala in monkeys (*Macaca mulatta*). *Journal of Comparative and Physiological Psychology* 95:961–77.

Ameli, R., Courchesne, E., Lincoln, A., Kaufman, A. S., and Grillon, C. 1988. Visual memory processes in high-functioning individuals with autism. *Journal of Autism and Developmental Disorders* 18:601–15.

Bachevalier, J. 1990. Ontogenetic development of habit and memory formation in primates. In A. Diamond, ed., *Development and Neural Bases of Higher Cognitive Functions.* 457–84. Vol. 608 of *Annals of the New York Academy of Sciences.* New York: New York Academy of Sciences.

Bachevalier, J. 1991. An animal model for childhood autism: Memory loss and socioemotional disturbances following neonatal damage to the limbic system in monkeys. In C. A. Tamminga and S. C. Schulz, eds., *Advances in Neuropsychiatry and Psychopharmacology.* Vol. 1 of Schizophrenia Research. 129–40. New York: Raven Press.

Bachevalier, J. 1992. Cortical versus limbic immaturity: Relationship to infantile amnesia. In M. R. Gunnar and C. A. Nelson, eds., *Developmental Behavioral Neuroscience.* 130–53. Vol. 24 of *The Minnesota Symposia on Child Psychology.* Hillsdale, NJ: Lawrence Erlbaum Associates.

Bachevalier, J., Brickson, M., Hagger, C., and Mishkin, M. 1990. Age and sex differences in the effects of selective temporal lobe lesions on the formation of visual discrimination habits in rhesus monkeys (*Macaca mulatta*). *Behavioral Neuroscience* 104:885–99.

Bachevalier, J., and Mishkin, M. 1984. An early and a late developing system for learning and retention in infant monkeys. *Behavioral Neuroscience* 98:770–78.

Bachevalier, J., and Mishkin, M. 1988. Long-term effects of neonatal temporal cortical and limbic lesions on habit and memory formation in rhesus monkeys. *Society for Neuroscience Abstracts* 14:1.

Bachevalier, J., and Mishkin, M. 1991. Effects of neonatal lesions of the amygdaloid complex or hippocampal formation on the development of visual recognition memory. *Society for Neuroscience Abstracts* 17:338.

Bauman, M. L., and Kemper, T. L. 1985. Histoanatomic observations of the brain in early infantile autism. *Neurology* 35:866–74.

Bauman, M. L., and Kemper, T. L. 1988. Limbic and cerebellar abnormalities: Consistent findings in infantile autism. *Journal of Neuropathology and Experimental Neurology* 47:369.

Bishop, D. V. M. 1993. Annotation: Autism, executive functions, and theory of mind: A neuropsychological perspective. *Journal of Child Psychology and Psychiatry* 34:279–93.

Boucher, J. 1981. Immediate free recall in early childhood autism: Another point of behavioral similarity with amnesic syndrome. *British Journal of Psychology* 72:211–15.

Boucher, J., and Warrington, E. K. 1976. Memory deficits in early infantile autism some similarities to the amnesic syndrome. *British Journal of Psychology* 67:73–87.

Brooks, D. N., and Baddeley, A. D. 1976. What can amnesic patients learn? *Neuropsychologia* 14:111–22.

Brown, S., and Schafer, E. A. 1888. An investigation into the functions of the occipital and temporal lobes of the monkey's brain. *Philosophical Transactions of the Royal Society of London* 179B:303–27.

Clower, R. P., Alvarez-Royo, P., Zola-Morgan, S., and Squire, L. R. 1991. Recognition memory impairment in monkeys with selective hippocampal lesions. *Society for Neuroscience Abstracts* 17:338.

Cohen, N. J., and Squire, L. R. 1980. Preserved learning and retention of pattern-analyzing skill in amnesia: Dissociation of "knowing how" and "knowing that." *Science* 210:207–9.

Corkin, S. 1968. Acquisition of motor skill after bilateral medial temporal-lobe excision. *Neuropsychologia* 6:255–66.

Courchesne, E., Yeung-Courchesne, R., Press, G. A., Hesselink, J. R., and Jernigan, T. L. 1988. Hypoplasia of cerebellar vermal lobules VI and VII in autism. *New England Journal of Medicine* 318:1349–54.

Damasio, A. R., Eslinger, P. J., Damasio, H., Van Hoesen, G. W., and Cornell, S. 1985. Multimodal amnesic syndrome following bilateral temporal and basal forebrain damage. *Archives of Neurology* 42:252–59.

Damasio, A. R., and Maurer, R. G. 1978. A neurological model for childhood autism. *Archives of Neurology* 35:777–86.

Deonna, T., Ziegler, A. L., Moura-Serra, J., and Innocenti, G. 1993. Autistic regression in children: Relationship to limbic pathology and epilepsy. Report of 2 cases. *Developmental Medicine and Child Neurology* in press.

DeLong, G. R. 1978. A neuropsychological interpretation of infantile autism. In M. Rutter and E. Schopler, eds., *Autism.* 207–18. New York: Plenum Press.

DeLong, G. R. 1992. Autism, amnesia, hippocampus, and learning. *Neuroscience and Behavioral Reviews* 16:63–70.

DeLong, G. R., and Bauman, M. L. 1987. Brain lesions in autism. In E. Schopler and G. B. Mesibov, eds., *Neurobiological Issues in Autism*. 229–42. New York: Plenum Press.

Fein, D., Pennington, B., and Waterhouse, L. 1987. Implications of social deficits in autism for neurological dysfunction. In E. Schopler and G. B. Mesibov, eds., *Neurobiological Issues in Autism*. 127–44. New York: Plenum Press.

Freeman, J. H., and Stanton, M. E. 1991. Fimbria–fornix transections disrupt the ontogeny of delayed alternation but not position discrimination in the rat. *Behavioral Neuroscience* 105:386–95.

Friedman, H. M., and Allen, N. 1969. Chronic effects of complete limbic lobe destruction in man. *Neurology* 19:679–90.

Gascon, G. G., and Gilles, F. 1973. Limbic dementia. *Journal of Neurology, Neurosurgery, and Psychiatry* 36:421–50.

Hebben, N., Shedlack, K., Eichenbaum, H., and Corkin, S. 1981. The amnesic patient H. M.: Diminished ability to interpret and report internal states. *Society for Neurosciences Abstracts* 7:235.

Hetzler, B. E., and Griffin, J. L. 1981. Infantile autism and the temporal lobe of the brain. *Journal of Autism and Developmental Disorders* 9:153–57.

Hirsh, R. 1974. The hippocampus and contextual retrieval of information from memory: A theory. *Behavioral Biology* 12:421–45.

Hof, P. R., Knabe, R., Bovier, P., and Bouras, C. 1991. Neuropathological observations in a case of autism presenting with self-injury behavior. *Acta Neuropathologica* 82:321–26.

Holroyd, S., Reiss, A. L., and Bryan, R. N. 1991. Autistic features in Joubert syndrome: A genetic disorder with agenesis of cerebellar vermis. *Biological Psychiatry* 29:287–94.

Hoon, A. H., and Reiss, A. L. 1992. The mesial-temporal lobe and autism: Case report and review. *Developmental Medicine and Child Neurology* 34:252–65.

Horel, J. A., Keating, E. G., and Misantone, L. J. 1975. Partial Klüver–Bucy syndrome produced by destroying temporal neocortex or amygdala. *Brain Research* 94:347–59.

Iwai, E., Nishio, T., and Yamaguchi, K. 1986. Neuropsychological basis of a K–B sign in Klüver–Bucy syndrome produced following total removal of inferotemporal cortex of macaque monkeys. In Y. Oomura, ed., *Emotion: Neural and Chemical Control*. 299–311. Tokyo: Japan Scientific Society Press.

Kling, A. 1972. Effects of amygdalectomy on social-affective behavior in nonhuman primates. In B. E. Eleftheriou, ed., *The Neurobiology of the Amygdala*. 511–36. New York: Plenum Press.

Klüver, H., and Bucy, P. C. 1938. An analysis of certain effects of bilateral temporal lobectomy in the rhesus monkey, with special reference to "psychic blindness." *Journal of Psychology* 5:33–54.

Klüver, H., and Bucy, P. C. 1939. Preliminary analysis of function of the temporal lobe in monkeys. *Archives of Neurology* 42:979–1000.

Lilly, R., Cummings, J. L., Benson, F., and Frankel, M. 1983. The human Klüver–Bucy syndrome. *Neurology* 33:1141–45.

Mahut, H., and Moss, M. 1986. The monkey and the sea horse. In R. L. Isaacson and K. H. Pribram, eds., *The Hippocampus*, Vol. 4. 241–80. New York: Plenum Press.

Malamut, B. L., Saunders, R. C., and Mishkin, M. 1984. Monkeys with combined amygdalo-hippocampal lesions succeed in object discrimination learning despite 24-hour intertrial intervals. *Behavioral Neuroscience* 98:759–69.

Malkova, L., Bachevalier, J., and Mishkin, M. 1991. Long-term effects of neonatal limbic lesions on tactile recognition in rhesus monkeys. *Society for Neuroscience Abstracts* 17:338.

Marlowe, W. B., Mancall, E. L., and Thomas, J. J. 1975. Complete Klüver–Bucy syndrome in man. *Cortex* 11:53–59.

Merjanian, P. M. 1985. Involvement of the hippocampus and amygdala in autism. Thesis. University of California, Irvine.

Merjanian, P. M., Bachevalier, J., Crawford, H., and Mishkin, M. 1986. Socioemotional disturbances in the developing rhesus monkey following neonatal limbic lesions. *Society for Neuroscience Abstracts* 12:23.

Merjanian, P. M., Bachevalier, J., Pettigrew, K. D., and Mishkin, M. 1988. Developmental time course as well as nature of socio-emotional disturbances in rhesus monkey following neonatal limbic lesions resemble those in autism. *Society for Neuroscience Abstracts* 14:2.

Merjanian, P. M., Bachevalier, J., Pettigrew, K. D., and Mishkin, M. 1989. Behavioral disturbances in the developing rhesus monkey following neonatal lesions of inferior temporal cortex (area TE) resemble those in attention-deficit hyperactivity disorder. *Society for Neuroscience Abstracts* 15:302.

Merjanian, P. M., and Nadel, L. 1993. A review of temporal lobe involvement in autism. *Neuroscience and Biobehavioral Reviews* in press.

Merjanian, P. M., Nadel, L., Jans, D. D., Granger, D. A., Lott, I. T., and Kean, M. L. 1984. Involvement of the hippocampus and amygdala in classical autism: A comparative neuropsychological study. *Society for Neuroscience Abstracts* 10:524.

Meunier, M., Bachevalier, J., Murray, E. A., Merjanian, P. M., and Richardson, R. 1991. Effects of rhinal cortical or limbic lesions on fear reactions in rhesus monkeys. *Society for Neuroscience Abstracts* 17:337.

Meunier, M., Bachevalier, J., Mishkin, M., and Murray, E. A. 1993. Effects on visual recognition memory of combined and separate ablations of the entorhinal and perirhinal cortex in rhesus monkeys. *Journal of Neuroscience* in press.

Milner, B. 1962. Les troubles de la mémoire accompagnant des lésions hippocampiques bilatérales. In P. Passouant, ed., *Physiologie de l'hippocampe.* 257–72. Paris: Centre de la Recherche Scientifique.

Minshew, N. J. 1991. Indices of neural function in autism: Clinical and biological implications. *Pediatrics* 87 (Suppl.):774–80.

Minshew, N. J., and Goldstein, G. 1993. Is autism an amnesic disorder? Evidence from the California Verbal Learning Test. *Neuropsychology* 7:209–16.

Mishkin, M. 1978. Memory in monkeys severely impaired by combined but not separate removal of amygdala and hippocampus. *Nature* 273:297–98.

Mishkin, M. 1982. A memory system in the monkey. *Philosophic Transaction of the Royal Society of London* B298:85–95.

Mishkin, M., and Appenzeller, T. 1987. The anatomy of memory. *Scientific American* 256:80–89.

Mishkin, M., Malamut, B. L., and Bachevalier, J. 1984. Memories and habits: Two neural systems. In G. Lynch, L. McGaugh, and N. M. Weinberger, eds., *Neurobiology of Learning and Memory.* 65–77. New York: Guilford Press.

Mishkin, M., and Petri, H. L. 1984. Memories and habits: Some implications for the analysis of learning and retention. In N. Butters and L. Squire, eds., *Neuropsychology of Memory.* 287–96. New York: Guilford Press.

Murray, E. A. 1991. Medial temporal lobe structures contributing to recognition memory: The amygdaloid complex versus the rhinal cortex. In J. P. Aggleton, ed., *The Amygdala: Neurobiological Aspects of Emotion, Memory, and Mental Dysfunction.* 453–70. New York: Wiley-Liss, Inc.

Murray, E. A., and Mishkin, M. 1983. Severe tactual memory deficits in monkeys after combined removal of the amygdala and hippocampus. *Brain Research* 270:340–44.

Murray, E. A., Bachevalier, J., and Mishkin, M. 1989. Effects of rhinal cortical lesions on visual recognition memory in rhesus monkeys. *Society for Neuroscience Abstracts* 15:342.

Obrador, S. 1947. Temporal lobotomy. *Journal of Experimental Neurology* 6:185–93.

Ornitz, E. M. 1983. The functional neuroanatomy of infantile autism. *International Journal of Neuroscience* 19:85–124.

Overman, W. H. 1990. Performance on traditional match-to-sample, nonmatch-to-sample, and object discrimination tasks by 12 to 32 month-old children: A developmental progression. In A. Diamond, ed., *The Development and Neural Bases of Higher Cognitive Functions*. 365–83. Vol. 608 of The New York Academy of Sciences. New York: New York Academy of Sciences.

Overman, W. H., Bachevalier, J., Turner, M., and Peuster, A. 1992. Object recognition *vs* object discrimination: Comparisons between human infants and infant monkeys. *Behavioral Neuroscience* 106:15–29.

Parkinson, J. K., Murray, E. A., and Mishkin, M. 1988. A selective mnemonic role for the hippocampus in monkeys: Memory for the location of objects. *Journal of Neuroscience* 8:4159–67.

Phillips, R. R., Malamut, B. L., Bachevalier, J., and Mishkin, M. 1988. Dissociation of the effects of inferior temporal and limbic lesions on object discrimination learning with 24-hr intertrial intervals. *Behavioral Brain Research* 27:99–107.

Pool, J. L. 1952. The visceral brain of man. *Journal of Neurosurgery* 96:209–48.

Prior, M., and Hoffmann, W. 1990. Brief report: Neuropsychological testing of autistic children through an exploration with frontal lobe tests. *Journal of Autism and Developmental Disorders* 20:581–90.

Rosvold, H. E., Mirsky, A. F., and Pribram, K. 1954. Influence of amygdalectomy on social behavior in monkeys. *Journal of Comparative and Physiological Psychology* 47:173–78.

Rumsey, J. M., and Hamburger, S. D. 1988. Neuropsychological findings in high-functioning men with infantile autism, residual state. *Journal of Clinical and Experimental Neuropsychology* 10:201–21.

Rutter, M. 1978. Diagnosis and definition. In M. Rutter and E. Schopler, eds., *Autism: A Reappraisal of Concepts and Treatment*. 1–26. New York: Plenum Press.

Saunders, R. C., Murray, E. A., and Mishkin, M. 1984. Further evidence that amygdala and hippocampus contribute equally to recognition memory. *Neuropsychologia* 22:785–96.

Scoville, W. B., and Milner, B. 1957. Loss of recent memory after bilateral hippocampal lesions. *Journal of Neurology, Neurosurgery, and Psychiatry* 20:11–21.

Spiegler, B. J., and Mishkin, M. 1979. Associative memory severely impaired by combined amygdalo-hippocampal removals. *Society for Neuroscience Abstracts* 5:323.

Squire, L. R., Cohen, N. J., and Zouzounis, J. A. 1984. Preserved memory in anterograde amnesia: Sparing of a recently acquired skill. *Neuropsychologia* 22:145–52.

Terzian, H., and Delle Ore, G. 1955. Syndrome of Klüver and Bucy reproduced in man by bilateral removal of the temporal lobes. *Neurology* 5:373–80.

Thompson, C. I. 1981. Long-term behavioral development of rhesus monkeys after amygdalectomy in infancy. In Y. Ben-Ari, ed., *The Amygdaloid Complex*, INSERM Symposium No. 20. 259–70. Amsterdam: Elsevier/North-Holland Biomedical Press.

Thompson, C. I., Bergland, R. M., and Towfighi, T. J. 1977. Social and nonsocial behaviors of adult rhesus monkeys after amygdalectomy in infancy and adulthood. *Journal of Comparative and Physiological Psychology* 91:533–48.

Wang, J., Aigner, T., and Mishkin, M. 1990. Effects of neostriatal lesions on visual habit formation in rhesus monkeys. *Society for Neuroscience Abstracts* 16:617.

Warrington, E. K., and Weiskrantz, L. 1968. New method of testing long-term retention with special reference to amnesic patients. *Nature* (Lond.) 217:972–74.

Weiskrantz, L. 1956. Behavioral changes associated with ablations of the amygdaloid complex in monkeys. *Journal of Comparative and Physiological Psychology* 49:381–91.

Zola-Morgan, S., and Squire, L. R. 1985. Complementary approaches to the study of memory: Human amnesia and animal models. In N. W. Weinberger, J. L. McGaugh, and L. Lynch, eds., *Memory Systems of the Brain: Animal and Human Cognitive Processes*. 463–77. New York: Guilford Press.

Zola-Morgan, S., Squire, L. R., and Amaral, D. G. 1986. Human amnesia and the medial temporal region: Enduring memory impairment following a bilateral lesion limited to field CA1 of the hippocampus. *Journal of Neuroscience* 6:2950–67.

Zola-Morgan, S., Squire, L. R., Alvarez-Royo, P., and Clower, R. P. 1991. Independence of memory functions and emotional behavior: Separate contributions of the hippocampal formation and the amygdala. *Hippocampus* 1:207–20.

Zola-Morgan, S., Squire, L. R., Amaral, D. G., and Suzuki, W. 1989. Lesions of perirhinal and parahippocampal cortex that spare the amygdala and hippocampal formation produce severe memory impairment. *Journal of Neuroscience* 9:4355–70.

9

MEMORY FUNCTION AND AUTISM

Ronald J. Killiany, Ph.D.
Mark B. Moss, Ph.D.

Since the mid 1980s increasing evidence has emerged to demonstrate that infantile autism may reflect morphologically distinct alterations in the central nervous system and, in particular, the temporal lobe limbic system (see Chap. 7). Indeed, it had long been suspected that autism and autisticlike disorders may be caused by temporal lobe dysfunction (Hetzler and Griffin, 1981), and neuropathologic studies are now providing evidence in support of this hypothesis. The presence and extent of involvement of the central nervous system in autism have also provided a new focus for the behavioral and neuropsychologic assessment of higher cortical function of children with this disorder. Accordingly, in view of the role of the temporal lobe in behavior, one of the domains coming under close examination is memory function.

The neural system or systems underlying memory function are responsible for receiving, storing, and making available vast quantities of diverse information. However, the exact processes through which this function is accomplished are not fully understood. There is no consensus among cognitive psychologists and neurobiologists as to how many different neural systems subserve memory or, within each system, how many stages are involved. However, workers in the field generally accept that memory is not a unitary phenomenon.

It is beyond the scope of this chapter to review the entire literature on memory function. However, the basic concepts, much of the current thinking on the dissociation of memory function, and the literature relevant to autism will be covered in some detail. The chapter will conclude with approaches to the assessment of memory in autism.

170

COMPONENTS OF MEMORY FUNCTION

AMNESIA

Amnesia is a condition characterized by the inability to acquire new information despite normal attention, relatively intact recall of previously learned material, and preservation of certain perceptual and intellectual functions. Amnesia can result from a wide variety of etiologies, which include anoxia, alcoholic neurotoxicity, cerebrovascular accident, closed head injury, nutritional deficiency, surgical intervention, or tumor. Patients who have been rendered amnesic appear to share three common features. First, all amnesic persons have some form of anterograde amnesia. This means that they are unable to learn and retain certain types of new information after the onset of amnesia. Patient H. M., who was inadvertently rendered amnesic during surgery to relieve debilitating epileptic seizures in 1953, is perhaps the best-studied case of anterograde amnesia. Testing of H. M., thirty-one years after surgery, illustrates the magnitude of his anterograde memory impairment. When asked the current year, he is wrong by as much as forty-three years, while he underestimates his age by ten to twenty-six years (Corkin, 1984). In 1973, H. M. was unable to correctly identify Watergate, John Dean, or San Clemente, even though he was exposed to this information as he watched the news on television every night (reported in Corkin, 1984).

The second feature shared by patients with amnesia is a varying amount of retrograde memory loss. *Retrograde memory dysfunction* is defined by the inability to recall information acquired before the onset of the intervening event. For example, it is not uncommon for survivors of serious auto accidents to have vivid recollections of the events that led up to the accident, yet be unable to recall the actual accident. Although H. M. exhibits a retrograde memory impairment, the severity and extent are unclear, but reports suggest a range of months to years.

The third feature shared by patients with amnesia is a residual capacity to learn and retain certain types of information. For example, when H. M. was repeatedly presented with a mirror tracing task, he performed the task with ever-increasing accuracy even though he denied having seen the task before (Milner et al., 1968). Similarly, patients in the early stages of Alzheimer disease appear to have an equivalent sparing of the capacity to learn and retain perceptual motor skills or tasks.

Examination of both amnesic patients and nonhuman primates rendered amnesic has provided a great deal of insight into which anatomical structures subserve mnemonic functions. In this chapter, we will use anatomic information as our guide to the various components of memory as we look at the process through which information travels in the memory system. For our purposes, we will consider memory to have five stages: registration, short-term storage, consolidation, long-term storage, and retrieval. Each of the stages is temporally continuous and subserved by anatomically distinct regions of the nervous system.

REGISTRATION

For information to be processed by the memory system, an individual must be physically exposed to it in one form or another. As with all information, that used by the memory system is taken in through the senses. Each sensory modality independently forms a memory of every stimulus impinging upon it. This modality-specific "sensory memory" contains the full perceptual information generated by the stimulus for the modality. Sensory memory is stored as a trace of neuronal activation which decays rapidly over time. Each sensory modality has a different rate of decay for its memory trace. For the visual modality, sensory memory (referred to as iconic memory) lasts for about 200 milliseconds (Neisser, 1967). For the auditory modality, sensory memory (referred to as echoic memory) lasts from two to ten seconds. For the tactual modality, sensory memory lasts for about four seconds. For the kinesthetic or motoric modality, the sensory memory may last as long as eighty seconds. The duration of the sensory memory for either the olfactory modality or the gustatory modality is unknown.

When a new stimulus impinges upon a modality, the previous sensory memory is lost as it becomes overwritten with a new neuronal trace. It is not clear where sensory memory takes place (i.e., central nervous system versus receptor site for each modality) or to what extent we have any conscious control over the content of the sensory memories.

IMMEDIATE MEMORY

The duration of sensory memory is very short, yet by rehearsing we are able to hold spans of auditory and visual information for relatively long periods of time. This is accomplished through a component of the memory system referred to as "immediate memory." The ability to concentrate, rehearse, and recall a span of digits, words, or visual features is perhaps the best example of this capacity. Any disruption to the rehearsal process results in the loss of the information from immediate memory. For example, if you are repeating a phone number to yourself and become distracted, the information you were trying to retain is forgotten. Experiments by Petersen and Petersen (1959) demonstrated that normal subjects forget a significant proportion of what they referred to as meaningless information in less than one minute in the presence of a distraction.

Immediate memory is limited in terms of the amount of information that it can store, ranging from about five to seven items. However, this limit may be misleading, for what actually constitutes an item is variable. If you were asked to remember the string of randomly generated numbers 2 5 8 9 3 7 4, each number would constitute an item and the string of numbers would presumably fill the immediate memory capacity. Similarly, if you were asked to remember the string of letters Z Q P M T X G, each letter would constitute an item and the string of letters would presumably fill the immediate memory capacity. However, if you were asked to remember the string of letters F O O L I S H, the string of letters would be "chunked" into a single word, which would presumably occupy only one item in immediate memory. Through this process of chunking, we are able to reorganize material, give it meaning, and thus seemingly exceed the seven-item limit of immediate memory. In addition, the ability to chunk material improves with practice. Ericsson and Chase (1982) reported on a case in which an individual's auditory digit span was extended to as high as eighty-two items through 200–300 hours of extensive training and practice.

As with other components of memory, impairments of immediate memory coexist with spared learning and memory capacities. Patient K. F., as a result of both a motorcycle accident and surgery to remove a left parietal subdural hematoma, displays this type of memory impairment (Warrington and Shallice, 1969). When repeatedly tested on a digit span test, K. F. had a reliable digit span of one, yet he had no difficulty with either verbal learning tasks or the retention of visually presented material (Shallice and Warrington, 1970). In addition, patient H. M., though unable to recall current events he has just been exposed to on the television news, had a normal forward digit span of six items through 1977 (reported in Corkin, 1984).

Anatomically, the structures responsible for mediating immediate memory have not been fully defined. It appears, however, that the mediating structure is somewhat specific to the type of information being processed. Auditory immediate memory for verbal material is thought to be mediated by the inferior parietal lobe of the left or language hemisphere (Warrington et al., 1971) at the level where the parietal lobe conjoins the left temporal lobe (Saffran and Marin, 1975; McCarthy and Warrington, 1984). Visual immediate memory may be mediated by more than one structure. The rehearsal of visually presented verbal material is thought to be mediated by the left occipital lobe (Kinsbourne and Warrington, 1962, 1963; Warrington and Rabin, 1971), while it is less clear where the rehearsal of visually presented spatial information is mediated. Both the right occipital–parietal regions (Alajouanine, 1960) and the parietal regions alone (Warrington and James, 1967; DeRenzi et al., 1977) have been suggested as the subserving structures for spatial information in immediate memory that has been presented visually.

Finally, it is unclear whether or not immediate memory should even be considered a form of memory. A digit span subtest is used in the Wechsler tests (the intelligence scales and the Wechsler Memory Scale), though not necessarily as a means to assess mnemonic ability. Immediate memory as we described it here requires a large amount of concentration on the part of the individual. Thus, Spitz (1972) argued that the digit span subtest is actually a measure of the efficiency of attention rather than a test of memory.

RECENT MEMORY

Sensory memory is modality-specific and decays rapidly with time. Immediate memory requires conscious effort to hold over time and is lost with distraction. How then are we able to take in and recall so much material with so little effort? Information from sensory memory is assembled into multimodal units and placed in short-term storage while it is being further processed. The duration of this short-term storage or "recent memory" is highly variable, ranging from minutes to hours. Neither rehearsal nor conscious awareness is required to retain information in recent memory. Information in short-term storage that we are consciously aware of is referred to as explicit memory, while that which we are not consciously aware of is referred to as *implicit memory*. For example, if you were mentally putting together a list of items to pick up later in the day, continual rehearsal of the information would be impractical. Yet, by studying the list you incorporate it into recent memory in a conscious or explicit manner. On the other hand, information concerning the plot of a television show viewed last night has been obtained in an implicit manner. When the show was viewed, no active attempt was being made to learn and retain this information.

Of all the theoretical components to the memory system, no other component has received as much attention as recent memory. In addition to the implicit–explicit subdivision we just described, countless other subdivisions have been proposed to further subdivide this component of the memory system (see Table 9.1). These subdivisions are based on the residual learning and memory capacities found in patients with amnesia. While Table 9.1 is not an exhaustive list of all the proposed subdivisions, it is representative. Each of these theories makes the same general claim that there is more than one type of short-term storage; however, each also contains subtle differences from the others. Perhaps the earliest of these subdivisions to be proposed was "Knowing How versus Knowing That" (Ryle, 1949), which has evolved into the most widely known subdivision, "Procedural versus Declarative" (Cohen and Squire, 1980). These theories basically suggested that recent memory was actually composed of two distinct subdivisions. Damage to one subdivision would cause an impairment of one type of memory while

Table 9.1. Some of the Theoretical Divisions of Recent Memory

Classification	Reference
Knowing How versus *Knowing That*	Ryle, 1949
Association versus *Recognition* Memory	Gaffan, 1974
Habit versus *Contextual Retrieval*	Hirsh, 1974
Stimulus-Response versus *Representational* versus *Organized*	Ruggerio and Flagg, 1976
Taxon versus *Locale*	O'Keefe and Nadel, 1978
Reference versus *Working* Memory	Olton, Becker, and Handelman, 1979
Procedural versus *Declarative* Knowledge	Cohen and Squire, 1981
Association versus *Representational* versus *Abstract*	Oakley, 1981
Semantic versus *Cognitive Mediation*	Warrington and Weiskrantz, 1982
Incidental versus *Intentional* Retrieval	Jacoby, 1984
Procedural versus *Propositional* Knowledge	Tulving, 1984
Early versus *Late* Systems	Schacter and Moscovitch, 1984
Procedural versus *Semantic* versus *Episodic*	Tulving, 1985
Declarative versus *Nondeclarative* Knowledge	Squire and Zola-Morgan, 1991

sparing the other type of memory. For the purposes of this chapter, we will consider the various subdivisions to be virtually synonymous with each other.

Procedural Memory. The "Knowing How" or "Procedural" subdivision is thought to be implicit and accessible only through the performance of a task or by engaging in the skill in which the knowledge is embedded (Squire, 1986). For example, most of us are unable to verbally describe in detail how to tie a shoe, yet we easily perform this task daily. This subdivision of recent memory has also been described as "associative memory," which involves producing the same response to a stimulus both at the time of original learning and at later times (Oakley, 1981). In other words, because you were originally taught to answer the telephone when it rings, you pick up the receiver each time you hear the telephone ringing virtually without thought.

An impairment of the procedural subdivision of recent memory has been described in patients with Huntington disease. These patients have relatively intact language skills and mild deficits on constructional and visuospatial tasks (Butters et al., 1978; Caine et al., 1978; Josiassen et al., 1982; Brandt et al., 1984). However, they are significantly impaired in the acquisition of both a pursuit rotor tracking task (Heindel et al., 1988) and a mirror reading skill (Martone et al., 1984).

The specific anatomy of this procedural subdivision is not fully known. Evidence from patients with Huntington disease suggests that the neostriatum seems to be associated with the acquisition of motor skills (Heindel et al., 1988). Evidence from animal experiments is also somewhat in accord with this view of the neostriatum (Mahut and Moss, 1984; Mishkin et al., 1984; Mishkin and Petri, 1984). Thus, it seems reasonable to conclude that the capacity to obtain and store procedural knowledge is based on subcortical structures and not lost as a result of cortical damage. This conclusion has actually been stretched to include more than just regions of the neostriatum. There is also evidence from the animal literature that the ability to associate a stimulus with a response (a procedural task) may even be mediated by residual neural tissue down to the spinal cord level (Oakley, 1981).

Declarative Memory.   The "Knowing That" or "Declarative" subdivision may be either explicit or implicit and is accessible to conscious awareness. It contains facts, episodes, lists, and routes of everyday life. Unlike procedural knowledge, declarative information can be brought to mind verbally as a proposition or nonverbally as an image (Squire, 1986). This subdivision was thought to mediate such behaviors as being able to find your car in a parking lot (trial unique recognition), knowing what you had for dinner last night, and being able to recall anything from the past moments of your life. This subdivision has also been referred to as "representational memory" and assigned the responsibility of allowing for the ability to act on the basis of a representation or image of a prior event. The ability to base our responses on representations of events is highly important to our everyday activities. For example, when you attempt to find your car in a parking lot, you are forced to rely on a representation or image of where you parked the car. The actual stimulus of parking the car is no longer available upon which to base a decision. Information in representational memory includes that from a single unique event as well as the organization of the traces of such events into a framework or map that preserves their relationship (serial memory) and allows for the retrieval of each event within a precise spatiotemporal context (Oakley, 1981). If you think back to all the events that occurred yesterday before dinner, you will come up with a temporally organized continuum of events, not a list of unconnected single events.

Several examples of patients with impairment of the declarative subdivision of recent memory have been identified. There is the classic case of patient H. M., who, as we already mentioned, became profoundly amnesic after surgery to relieve debilitating epileptic seizures. There are also reports of two patients who developed this type of memory disorder after either an ischemic episode or repetitive generalized seizures (Zola-Morgan et al., 1986; Victor and Agamanolis, 1990). In addition, patients in the initial stages of Alzheimer disease also typically display this type of memory impairment. One of the earliest symptoms generally noted by patients suspected of having Alzheimer disease is an inability to learn and retain new information (Moss and Albert, 1988). Additionally, these patients have a great deal of difficulty retaining information across delays as short as two minutes when they are not allowed to rehearse (Moss et al., 1986). However, in contrast to the patients we have discussed with Huntington disease, those with this type of memory impairment appear to possess an intact capacity to acquire and retain procedural knowledge. When patients with Alzheimer disease were given the same pursuit rotor task on which patients with Huntington disease were found to be impaired, they performed the task with normal levels of accuracy (Eslinger and Damasio, 1986).

The specific anatomy of the declarative subdivision of recent memory is still being debated. As early as 1957, Scoville and Milner concluded that damage to the hippocampal formation bilaterally results in this type of deficit. They examined eight patients who had undergone bilateral excisions of the amygdaloid nuclei and found memory impairment only in the patients whose excisions extended far enough caudally to damage portions of the hippocampal formation. No memory deficit was seen after excisions limited to the uncus or amygdala. Similarly, investigators using nonhuman primates found that lesions of the hippocampal formation and overlying cortex result in an impairment of declarative or representational memory (Mahut et al., 1982; Zola-Morgan and Squire, 1986). It was alternatively demonstrated in the nonhuman primate that only combined lesions of the amygdala, hippocampus, and overlying cortexes result in a significant memory impairment (Mishkin, 1978). Further studies of the nonhuman primate have indicated that while the amygdala itself does not contribute to the declarative memory process, the cortical areas overlying the amygdala and typically damaged in performing an amygdalectomy (removal of the amygdala) do contribute to this memory process (Zola-Morgan et al., 1989a, 1989b; Zola-Morgan et al., 1989).

Interactions of the Recent Memory Subdivisions. The two subdivisions of recent memory that we have just described presumably work together in the adult to produce what we consider a normal mnemonic capacity. At least four possibilities exist as to how these subdivisions interact:

(1) they may represent two completely separate subdivisions;
(2) the two subdivisions may be distinct but interact with one another;
(3) one subdivision may be subservient to the other for its source of information; and
(4) the two subdivisions may be completely dependent upon each other.

Looking at patients with impairments of recent memory provides insight into the relationship between the two subdivisions. Patients with an impairment of procedural memory, such as those with Huntington disease, are impaired at acquiring new skills yet have a relatively spared capacity for representational knowledge. Conversely, patients with an impairment of declarative memory, such as those in the early stages of Alzheimer disease, are unable to learn and retain representational knowledge yet easily acquire new skills. This suggests that the two subdivisions are neither dependent upon each other nor subservient to each other in the adult.

Hence we are left to determine whether the procedural and declarative memory subdivisions interact with or are independent of each other. If the subdivisions are independent, damage to one should not affect the performance of the other. However, the clinical evidence does not support this view. While patients with Huntington disease are not as impaired as those with Alzheimer disease on verbal memory tasks, they are nonetheless impaired in comparison to control subjects on this task (Heindel et al., 1988). In addition, it has been noted that while patients with impairments of the declarative memory subdivision do learn and retain certain skills, the information that they retain is hyperspecific and not generalizable to changes in the skill (Glisky et al., 1986). Therefore, by the process of elimination we are left with the conclusion that the two recent memory subdivisions interact to produce "normal" mnemonic functions.

Developmental work has shed some light on the nature of these interactions. Work with human infants has shown that the procedural memory subdivision appears to be functional shortly after birth. Infants as young as two months of age are capable of forming specific memories for nominal stimuli. These memories are imbedded in both the context and the environmental surroundings in which training of this skill took place (Rovee-Collier, 1991). It is interesting that these very early memories appear to be highly specific, much like those of patients with impairments of declarative memory.

Further insights have been provided by developmental studies of nonhuman primates. In the infant rhesus macaque, procedural memory or habit learning appears to be not only mature at three months of age (Bachevalier and Mishkin, 1984) but also enhanced with respect to the adult capacity (Mahut and Killiany, 1990). In contrast, the declarative memory subdivision appears to mature more slowly over time. For the time period of the first two years of life in the infant rhesus macaque, varying reports have been made as to whether this capacity can mediate performance at adult levels (Mahut and Killiany, 1990) or cannot mediate behavior at adult levels (Bachevalier and Mishkin, 1984; Killiany and Mahut, 1991). In addition, at about one year of age, infant monkeys that had previously acquired procedural skills more rapidly than adults became retarded in acquiring additional procedural skills (Killiany and Mahut, 1990).

Taken together, the clinical and experimental work suggests that the two subdivisions of recent memory are distinct subdivisions that interact in the adult. The procedural system either develops rapidly after birth or is functional at birth, while the declarative memory system develops more gradually. Furthermore, the procedural memory system appears to be able to mediate the rapid formation of highly specific memories until the declarative system functionally matures, at which time more adult-like memories are formed.

CONSOLIDATION

The storage of information by the memory system appears to take place differentially. That is, some information appears to be concretely held, while other information is more fluid. Information in recent memory is rather fluid in nature. It can be lost by traumatic events such as automobile accident, electroconvulsive therapy, or epileptic seizure. Information in remote memory, as we will discuss in the next section, appears to be rather concrete in nature and thus less susceptible to loss than that in recent memory.

As early as 1949, Hebb postulated that two processes were necessary for the brain to retain information. The first process, analogous to what we have termed recent memory, required the continual reverberation of a neural circuit. The second process, analogous to what we will discuss in the next section, required an actual structural change in the neural pattern of the central nervous system. Consolidation thus consisted of the transformation of this temporary reverberating circuit into a permanent memory trace. If there were a disruption of the system before a permanent memory trace could be consolidated, then the information in the reverberating process would be either lost or damaged. Little has changed since Hebb's early postulations on the concept of consolidation.

Isolated aspects of the consolidation process are uniquely intriguing. Though rehearsal undoubtedly plays a role, it is unclear why certain information is consolidated while other information is not. The duration of the consolidation process similarly remains undefined. Evidence from both animal and clinical studies indicated that there is a period of seconds to hours in which a memory is fragile and thus susceptible to permanent loss. Furthermore, in humans there is a longer period of time during which the memory is consolidated but is impaired (Albert, 1984). However, it is unclear whether consolidation is actually completed at the end of this period. McGaugh and Gold (1976) suggested that the impairments of memory measured during these periods are actually indicators of the effectiveness of a given treatment under the particular experimental conditions rather than a reflection of the state of consolidation.

Squire et al. (1984) expanded the concept of consolidation to include a period of years after initial learning. They based this view on studies of retrograde amnesia in psychiatric patients receiving bilateral electroconvulsive therapy. These studies found that while one- or two-year-old memories are selectively impaired, older memories appear unaffected (Cohen and Squire, 1981; Squire and Cohen, 1979; Squire et al., 1976; Squire et al., 1975). This expanded view of the consolidation process also accounts for the retrograde memory impairments found in patients rendered amnesic by traumatic events (patient H. M.—Scoville and Milner, 1957; patient N. A.—Teuber et al., 1968; patient R. B.—Zola-Morgan et al., 1986). However, there are two problems associated with this view of consolidation. First, it is unlikely that reverberation in a neural circuit could accommodate such a long consolidation process. Second, as McGaugh and Gold (1976) suggested, the impairments of memory found in these cases may indicate only the magnitude of the traumatic event rather than reflect on the state of consolidation. Thus, even this expanded view may underestimate the true duration of the consolidation process.

It is difficult to identify patients with only a selective deficit of the consolidation process. As we have already mentioned, patients H. M., N. A., and R. B. have a selective retrograde amnesia that can be interpreted as resulting from a single disruption of the consolidation process. It is less clear in these patients whether or not consolidation still takes place. H. M., though rendered amnesic in 1953, has demonstrated at times evidence of recall and recognition of postoperative events. For example, when shown a half dollar, he correctly identified the figure on it as President Kennedy (Milner et al., 1968). Similarly, it has been demonstrated that H. M.'s performance on tests of remote memory improves with prompts (Marslen-Wilson and Teuber, 1975). These findings suggest that H. M. may still be consolidating information for storage in remote memory.

Anatomically, the same medial temporal structures that subserve recent memory have been proposed to function in the consolidation process. Squire et al. (1984) postulated the following sequence of events. Stimuli are perceived and analyzed by the primary, secondary, and association cortexes. Next, from the multimodal association areas information is transferred through the medial temporal regions to the hippocampus, which acts as a reverberating circuit with diffuse connections back to the cortical regions. The information is then "held" briefly by the hippocampus until neuronal changes occur in the original cortical regions and store the information. Consolidation consists of interaction between the cortex and the hippocampus. Therefore, damage to the same structures that result in an impairment of recent memory may also result in an impairment of the consolidation process.` Unfortunately, it has proven to be difficult to dissociate the process of consolidation from either recent or remote memory. One is therefore left to infer that these processes overlap. All information in recent memory may be in the process of being consolidated into remote memories, a process that is time- dependent, variably susceptible to disruption, and completed only by a portion of the original information.

REMOTE MEMORY

As we have already mentioned, some of the information we retain appears to be concretely held, while other information is more susceptible to being lost. The most recent information we have incorporated into the memory system is typically the most vulnerable because it has not been fully encoded in the central nervous system as a long-term record. The remote memory component of the memory system represents the long-term storage unit of the system. Information is encoded in remote memory through the process of consolidation in such a manner that it can be accessed later. Remote memory classically has been thought of as a static, unchanging component of the memory system that functioned much like a data base. However, there appears to be more taking place in remote memory than was originally thought.

Even in remote memory there appears to be a differential in the susceptibility of information to being lost. Information stored most recently is more vulnerable to being lost than information stored in the more remote past. This phenomenon was first described in 1882 by Ribot and has since been referred to as *Ribot's law*. While it is possible that some loss of more recent memories is due to a disruption of the consolidation process, this cannot fully account for the findings. Albert et al. (1979) found a temporal gradient to the memory impairment of Korsakoff patients on a remote memory battery. The gradient spanned thirty years, with patients being most impaired on information from the most recent decade and least impaired on information from the most distant decade tested. This span of thirty years cannot be accounted for solely by a deficit of consolidation.

Tulving (1972) suggested that remote memory should be subdivided into episodic and semantic components. The episodic component contains a personalized account of specific events that we have experienced. As such, these memories are rich in detail and contain material that is extraneous to the actual event being recalled. For example, if you were asked when the war in the Persian Gulf began, whether or not you could correctly answer February 24, 1992, related information such as what you were doing at the time you first heard about the war would also come to mind. The semantic component, on the other hand, contains personalized interpretations of general knowledge, principles, associations, and rules. Material stored in semantic remote memory basically contains facts without extraneous material. For example, if you were asked who was the first president of the United States, whether or not you could correctly answer George Washington, related information such as where you first learned George Washington was the first president does not typically come to mind.

There is clinical evidence to support the view of remote memory as two subdivisions. Kinsbourne and Wood (1975) asked amnesic patients both to identify an item, such as a railroad ticket, and to describe an instance in which they had used that particular item. The amnesic patients were unimpaired at identifying common items (semantic memory); however, they could not describe any episodes in which they had personally used the items (episodic memory). Similarly, while amnesic patients display memory impairments, they perform normally on tests of general knowledge (semantic memory) such as the intelligence tests. In fact, patient H. M.'s full-scale IQ score actually increased, from a preoperative score of 104 to a high postoperative score of 118 in 1962 and 1977 (Corkin, 1984).

Events are initially encoded into remote memory as an episodic event. Over time, the number of associations to the memory diminish as forgetting of the extraneous information surrounding the event occurs. The memory either is gradually completely forgotten or becomes semantic in nature. The normal rate of forgetting information in remote memory is quite high and, as suggested by Ribot's law, is a function of the age of the event. Bahrick, et al., (1975) found a decline with a negative rate of acceleration by 60 percent in the free recall of names over a range of two weeks to fifty-seven years. Accordingly, remote memory for episodic events that occurred in the distant past may be a personalized general knowledge of an event rather than an actual episodic memory of the event.

There is presently no clear answer as to how we decide what information is designated "to be retained" and what information is determined to be extraneous. One hypothesis that is frequently advanced is that the process depends on the frequency of use (i.e., rehearsal). That is, information that is ultimately retained in the memory system is what we use. The memory may initially be stored as an episodic event, but each time it is recalled less and less of it is relevant, until only semantic information remains.

The shift in remote memory from being episodic-based to being semantic-based would account for the differential susceptibility to loss. Information stored in a semantic manner would have a low susceptibility to loss, while that stored in an episodic manner would be more vulnerable. Thus, the amount of detail present in a memory as well as the vulnerability of that memory to loss are both a function of the age of the memory. However, this may not always appear to hold true. For example, elderly individuals when talking about the "good old days" provide exquisite detail to these recollections. In this case it is uncertain how much of the detail is factual and how much was learned as the recollection gets repeated over time. The notion of a shift from episodic information to semantic information is a convenient summary of the sequence that takes place in remote memory, but it may fall short of fully explaining remote memory.

Gade and Mortensen (1990) described three patterns of remote memory loss. The first, as we already discussed, is relatively short and affects only a few years before the onset of amnesia. This type of remote memory loss is typically seen after trauma such as a severe automobile accident or after electroconvulsive therapy. In addition, patients H. M., N. A., and R. B. display this type of remote memory loss. The second pattern of remote memory loss is time-graded corresponding to Ribot's law. That is, recent events are more poorly recalled than more distant events. For example, a patient with this type of memory loss may have vivid recollections of childhood, but not be able to recall who was the previous president. This pattern of remote memory loss is typically seen in patients with Wernicke–Korsakoff disease (we will discuss more about this later). Finally, the third pattern of remote memory loss is a flat loss, where information is lost across all time periods. Albert et al. (1981) compared the performance of patients with Huntington disease to control subjects and found that the Huntington disease patients were impaired and that this loss was equal at all time intervals.

The anatomical basis for remote memory has not been fully determined. One theory is that it is a widely distributed cortical event. Squire et al. (1984) suggested that the same cortical regions that are responsible for initially perceiving a stimulus are those that eventually store the memory of it. Patients with losses of remote memory, as described earlier, have diverse etiology, which neither confirms nor conflicts with this cortical model. Thus, further study is needed before we can more fully understand this component of the memory system.

An intriguing phenomenon associated with remote memory is flashbulb memory. Many people have vivid recollections of the circumstances in which they learned of major events. For example, where were you when you learned or the assassination of John F. Kennedy, Malcolm X, or Martin Luther King? What were you doing when either President Ronald Reagan or John Lennon was shot? What were your first thoughts upon hearing of the explosion of the space shuttle Challenger or the nuclear disaster in Chernobyl? Flashbulb memories appear to be different from memories for other events that occurred in approximately the same time period because of the degree of extraneous information that remains associated with flashbulb memories over time. Brown and Kulik (1977) suggested that for flashbulb memories to occur there must be both a high level of surprise to the event and a strong emotional response to it.

Several issues remain unresolved with respect to flashbulb memory. First, not everyone agrees that it even exists. Several investigators (Neisser, 1982; Rubin and Kozin, 1984) noted examples of inaccuracy in flashbulb memories and thus questioned whether there is a difference between flashbulb memories and other autobiographical memories. Additionally, it is unclear how flashbulb memories are stored. Based on the amount of detail present in flashbulb memory, Brown and Kulik (1977) theorized that it must be subserved by a separate special memory mechanism. Conversely, noting the rate of forgetting and the degree of inaccuracy in flashbulb memory, McCloskey et al. (1988) concluded that it is a product of ordinary memory mechanisms. Therefore, until these issues are resolved, flashbulb memory remains merely an interesting notion.

RETRIEVAL OF INFORMATION

To this point the various components of the memory system that are responsible for the storage of information have been discussed. However, storage represents only one function of the memory system. Another important function is providing access to the information in a meaningful manner. For information to be retrieved from memory, a search must take place to find the appropriate information. A key feature to the search is the way in which information is organized in the memory system. Just as our homes are all organized by addresses and as books in the library are organized by a code, the information in the memory system appears to be organized by category. Loftus (1972) found that when subjects were asked to list items based on a given property such as yellow, they tend to group their listings based on categories. For example, first they list birds that are yellow, then they list flowers that are yellow, and so on.

Retrieval consists of first finding the appropriate category followed by searching that category for the desired information. This is analogous to looking up a word in the dictionary. First we determine the correct letter the word begins with and then we look up the word among other words that begin with the same letter. Loftus and Cole (1974) further showed that when two searches are conducted of the same category, the second takes place more rapidly than if it were independent of the first. Thus, once a category has been found, it would appear that accessing information in that category is easier than if the category has not yet been located.

Patients who have developed amnesia as a result of Korsakoff disease are especially impaired at retrieving previously learned material. An example of this type of memory loss is patient P. Z. (see Butters and Miliotis, 1985, for a review), who developed Wernicke–Korsakoff syndrome three years after completing his autobiography. When tested on autobiographical information, P. Z. was unable to recall information that he previously considered to be most prominent in his professional and personal life.

The neurologic circuitry that subserves retrieval, like that of all the components of the memory system, has not been fully determined. The etiology of Korsakoff disease suggests that the dorsal medial thalamic nuclei and the mammillary bodies play a role. Furthermore, both tumors of these regions and shrapnel wounds of these regions (Kahn and Crosby, 1972) result in a Korsakoff-like amnesic disorder. However, it is unclear whether this deficit is a direct result of damage to these regions or secondary to the insult.

IS THERE A MEMORY DISORDER ASSOCIATED WITH AUTISM?

Overall, the population of individuals with autism represents a heterogeneous group in terms of the severity of impairment, the overt behavioral profile, and the presence of any "special talents." According to the DSM-III-R (American Psychiatric Association, 1987), the symptoms of autism are characterized by impairment of three types. First, there is an impairment of reciprocal social interaction, illustrated by a lack of awareness of the existence of others. Second, there is an impairment of communication, which includes both verbal dysfunctions such as a lack of speech or echolalia and an impairment of nonverbal communication such as facial gestures. Third, the behavioral repertoire of an autistic child is characterized by repetitive perseverations such as stereotyped body movement. In addition to the criteria listed in the DSM-III-R, Rutter (1978) included an insistence upon sameness and an age of onset before thirty months in the diagnosis of infantile autism. However, the inclusion or not of age remains somewhat controversial.

It has been speculated that at least some of the symptomatology of autism could be explained in terms of a memory deficit. For example, off-topic comments made by an autistic individual may occur simply because he or she cannot recall the topic of the conversation. Similarly, the repetitive perseverations could be explained by an inability to recall previously performing an activity. Investigators comparing the performance of autistic children to adult patients with amnesia due to either Korsakoff disease or medial temporal lobe damage (hippocampus) have found the following: Autistic children, like amnesic patients, display an intact immediate memory, relatively good performance on tests of visual spatial reasoning (Bartak, Rutter, and Cox, 1975), preserved capacity to learn and retain motor skills (Goldstein, 1959; Hermelin and O'Conner, 1970), and an impairment of recent memory, as evidenced by their inability to verbally report activities in which they participated (Boucher, 1981). However, the impairment of recent memory found in autistic children appears to be relatively specific to verbal material, while that in amnesic adults is more global. Autistic children are impaired at recalling auditory–verbal material after a filled delay (Boucher and Warrington, 1976), yet are unimpaired at recent memory for static visual stimuli (Selfe, 1983). Similarly, even though autistic children display an intact immediate memory, their span for words differs more from their span for digits than is the case in other groups of children (Boucher, 1978).

At least two possibilities exist to account for the discrepancies found in the behavioral profiles of autistic children and adult amnesic patients. First, the adult who develops amnesia has a vast store of information from which to draw, including a working understanding of language. However, if there is a memory impairment associated with autism, then the child developing autism by thirty months of age would presumably be impaired at learning all new information, including language. Second, the etiology of the two disorders may be completely different. Unfortunately, little is known about the etiology of autism at this time. Pneumoencephalograms of patients with autism have demonstrated ventricular enlargement of the left temporal horn, which was attributed in part to a distinct flattening of the normal hippocampal contour (Hauser et al., 1975). It is interesting that Milner (1970) reported that while isolated left mesial temporal lesions in the adult do not produce a global amnesia, they do produce a memory impairment that is relatively specific for verbal material. Autopsy reports on autistic individuals have shown bilaterally symmetrical abnormalities confined primarily to the hippocampal complex and closely associated areas as well as to the cerebellum (Bauman and Kemper, 1985, 1986, 1987). Hippocampal damage of this type would be consistent with an impairment of recent memory. However, because of the extreme heterogeneity of symptoms among the autistic population, further studies need to be completed to determine if these findings are representational of the entire autistic population.

Bachevalier (1991) suggested an animal model for childhood autism based on work with infant monkeys that sustained damage to the limbic cortices thought to subserve recent memory functions. She found that infant monkeys with combined, bilateral, neonatal ablations of the amygdala, hippocampus, and overlying cortices display a severe memory deficit (Bachevalier and Mishkin, 1988) accompanied by socioemotional abnormalities that are similar to those seen in autistic children

(Merjanian et al., 1986). It is interesting that subsequent work has failed to demonstrate a memory deficit in infant monkeys after bilateral neonatal ablations limited to the hippocampus and overlying cortices (Bachevalier and Mishkin, 1991). Thus, even the proposed animal model of autism does not give us a clear indication of the presence or absence of a memory deficit in autism.

RECENT APPROACHES TO THE STUDY
OF MEMORY FUNCTION IN AUTISM

Data have accumulated to suggest that most cases of autism and autistic-like disorders evidence marked dysfunction of the central nervous system. One of the challenges that has always faced behavioral psychologists and neuropsychologists is finding appropriate instruments to assess behavior in patients or clients with marked language disturbance or severe retardation. This is particularly true in designing experiments to assess the memory functions of children with autism.

In assessing memory function it is necessary to keep in mind all domains of cognitive function that are engaged in performing the task. It is important to be aware of the possibility that deficits in another cognitive domain may confound or significantly interact with mnemonic test variables.

For example, one must be aware of the degree to which autistic children are perseverative, circumstantial, and stimulus-bound. These tendencies can alter a response in such a way that tasks designed to assess memory may not produce responses that accurately reflect the child's true ability. For example, in paradigms that rely on continuous yes–no recognition, one cannot be sure if any given response is simply a perseveration of a previous response or is one specific to the stimulus provided. Similarly, the extent to which a task relies on naming ability or verbal skills in general makes it less applicable to the autistic population.

One memory task developed in our laboratory adapted for use in severely retarded and autistic populations (Mackay and Ratti, 1990) overcomes some of these problems. The delayed recognition span test requires a simple response, has a gamelike quality that makes it more appealing and nonthreatening, and permits tracking and quantification of memory function over time. This task measures the subject's memory span by requiring the identification of a new stimulus presented among an increasing set of previously presented familiar stimuli (Moss et al., 1986). Stimuli are placed one at a time on a board in a series of increasing length (see Figure 9.1). Each new stimulus is added after a fixed delay interval (during which the subject cannot see the board). The subject's task is merely to point to the new stimulus that was just added during the delay. A variety of stimulus classes can be used (e.g., colors,

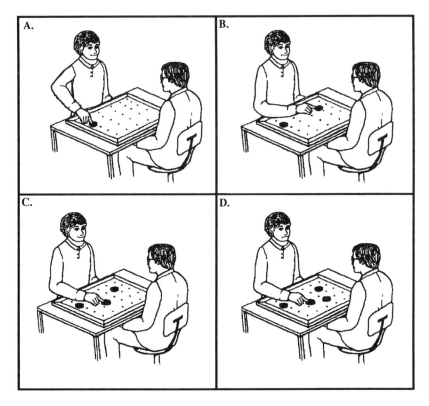

Figure 9.1. The Delayed Recognition Span Test apparatus, showing the manner in which patients respond in the testing situation. A: The patient points to a disk on the tray. B: The patient points to the new disk on the tray. C: The patient again points to the new disk on the tray. D: The patient fails to point to the new disk on the tray.

pictures, objects, spatial positions, or words), so that stimulus-specific recognition memory can be assessed. When colors, pictures, or objects are used, the stimuli are moved randomly during the delay intervals so the position of the stimulus does not provide an additional cue. When the stimulus parameter being tested is the spatial position of the stimuli (all the stimuli are identical), there is, of course, no alteration in their position during the delay interval.

CONCLUSION

More work is clearly needed in the development of behavioral instruments to assess memory function as well as other cognitive domains in childhood autism and autism-related disorders. A finer-grained analysis of the acquisition and retention of stimulus–stimulus and stimulus–response relations, together with the further delineation of patterns and types of neuropathologic changes and the development of animal models in autism (Bachevalier, 1991; Chap. 8), will significantly shorten the path leading to the understanding of the neurobiologic basis of this disorder.

REFERENCES

Alajouanine, T. 1960. *Les Grandes Activites du Lobe Occipital.* Paris: Masson.

Albert, M. S. 1984. Implications of different patterns of remote memory loss for the concept of consolidation. In H. Weingartner and E. Parker, eds. *Memory Consolidation.* Hillsdale, NJ: Erlbaum, pp. 211–30.

Albert, M. S., Butters, N., and Brandt, J. 1981. Patterns of remote memory in amnesic and demented patients. *Archives of Neurology* 38:495–500.

Albert, M. S., Butters, N., and Levin, J. 1979. Temporal gradients in the retrograde amnesia of patients with alcoholic Korsakoff's disease. *Archives of Neurology* 36:211–16.

American Psychiatric Association. 1987. *Diagnostic and Statistical Manual of Mental Disorders.* 3rd edition, revised. Washington, D.C.: American Psychiatric Association.

Bachevalier, J. 1991. An animal model for childhood autism. In C. A. Tamminga and S. C. Schulz, eds. 129–40. *Advances in Neuropsychiatry and Psychopharmacology.* New York: Raven Press.

Bachevalier, J., and Merganian, P. M. 1993. The contribution of medial temporal lobe structures in infantile autism: A neurobehavioral study in primates. In M. L. Bauman and T. L. Kemper, eds. 146–169. *The Neurobiology of Autism.* Baltimore: Johns Hopkins University Press.

Bachevalier, J., and Mishkin, M. 1984. An early and a late developing system for learning and retention in infant monkeys. *Behavioral Neuroscience* 98:770–78.

Bachevalier, J., and Mishkin, M. 1988. Long-term effects of neonatal temporal cortical and limbic lesions on habit and memory formation in rhesus monkeys. *Society for Neuroscience Abstracts* 14:1.

Bachevalier, J., and Mishkin, M. 1991. Effects of neonatal lesions of the amygdaloid complex or hippocampal formation on the development of visual recognition memory. *Society for Neuroscience Abstracts* 17:338.

Bahrick, H. P., Bahrick, P. O., and Wittlinger, R. P. 1975. Fifty years of memory for names and faces. *Journal of Experimental Psychology: General* 104:54–75.

Bartak, L., Rutter, M., and Cox, A. 1975. A comparative study of infantile autism and specific developmental receptive language disorder—I. The children. *British Journal of Psychiatry* 126:127–45.

Bauman, M. L., and Kemper, T. L. 1985. Histoanatomic observations of the brain in early infantile autism. *Neurology* 35:866–74.

Bauman, M. L., and Kemper, T. L. 1986. Developmental cerebellar abnormalities: A consistent finding in early infantile autism. *Neurology* 36:190.

Bauman, M. L., and Kemper, T. L. 1987. Limbic involvement in a second case of early infantile autism. *Neurology* 37:147.

Bauman, M. L., and Kemper, T. L. 1993. Neuroanatomic observations of the brain in autism. In M. L. Bauman and T. L. Kemper, eds. 119–145. *The Neurobiology of Autism.* Baltimore: Johns Hopkins University Press.

Boucher, J. 1978. Echoic memory capacity in autistic children. *Journal of Child Psychology and Psychiatry* 19:161–66.

Boucher, J. 1981. Immediate free recall in early childhood autism: Another point of behavioral similarity with amnesic syndrome. *British Journal of Psychology* 72:211–15.

Boucher, J., and Warrington, E. K. 1976. Memory deficits in early infantile autism: Some similarities to the amnesic syndrome. *British Journal of Psychology* 67:73–87.

Brandt, J., Strauss, M. E., Larus, J., Jensen, B. A., Folstein, S. E., and Folstein, M. F. 1984. Clinical correlates of dementia and disability in Huntington's disease. *Journal of Clinical and Experimental Neuropsychology* 6:401–12.

Brown, R., and Kulik, J. 1977. Flashbulb memories. *Cognition* 5:73–99.

Butters, N., and Miliotis, P. 1985. Amnesic disorders. In K. Heilman and E. Valenstein, eds. *Clinical Neuropsychology*. New York: Oxford, pp. 403–52.

Butters, N., Sax, D., Montgomery, K., and Tarlow, S. 1978. Comparison of the neuropsychological deficits associated with early and advanced Huntington's disease. *Archives of Neurology* 35:585–89.

Caine, E., Hunt, R., Weingartner, H., and Ebert, M. 1978. Huntington's dementia: Clinical and neuropsychological features. *Archives of General Psychiatry* 35:377–84.

Cohen, N. J., and Squire, L. R. 1980. Preserved learning and retention of pattern analyzing skill in amnesia: Dissociation of knowing how and knowing that. *Science* 210:207–10.

Cohen, N., and Squire, L. R. 1981. Retrograde amnesia and remote memory impairment. *Neuropsychologia* 19:337–56.

Corkin, S. 1984. Lasting consequences of bilateral medial temporal lobectomy: Clinical course and experimental findings in H. M. *Seminars in Neurology* 4:249–59.

De Renzi, E., Faglioni, P., and Previdi, P. 1977. Spatial memory and hemispheric locus of lesion. *Cortex* 13:424–33.

Ericsson, K. A., and Chase, W. G. 1982. Exceptional memory. *American Scientist* 70:607–15.

Eslinger, P. J., and Damasio, A. R. 1986. Preserved motor learning in Alzheimer's disease: Implication for anatomy and behavior. *Journal of Neuroscience* 6:3006–9.

Gade, A., and Mortensen, E. L. 1990. Temporal gradient in the remote memory impairment of amnesic patients with lesions in the basal forebrain. *Neuropsychologia* 28:985–1001.

Gaffan, D. 1974. Recognition impaired and association intact in the memory of monkeys after transection of the fornix. *Journal of Comparative and Physiological Psychology* 86:1100–09.

Glisky, E. L., Schacter, D. L., and Tulving, E. 1986. Computer learning by memory-impaired patients: Acquisition and retention of complex knowledge. *Neuropsychologia* 24:313–28.

Goldstein, K. 1959. Abnormal mental conditions in infancy. *Journal of Nervous and Mental Disorders* 128:538–57.

Hauser, S. L., DeLong, G. R., and Rosman, N. P. 1975. Pneumographic findings in the infantile autism syndrome. *Brain* 98:667–88.

Hebb, D. O. 1949. *The Organization of Behavior*. New York: Wiley.

Heindel, W. C., Butters, N., and Salmon, D. P. 1988. Impaired learning of a motor skill in patients with Huntington's disease. *Behavioral Neuroscience* 102:141–47.

Hermelin, B., and O'Connor, N. 1970. *Psychological Experiments with Autistic Children*. Oxford: Pergamon Press.

Hetzler, B. E., and Griffin, J. L. 1981. Infantile autism and the temporal lobe of the brain. *Journal of Autism and Developmental Disorders* 9:153–57.

Hirsh, R. 1974. The hippocampus and contextual retrieval of information from memory: A theory. *Behavioral Biology* 12:421–44.

Jacoby, L. L. 1984. Incidental versus intentional retrieval: Remembering and awareness as separate issues. In L. R. Squire and N. Butters, eds. *Neuropsychology of Memory*. New York: Guilford Press, pp. 145–56.

Josiassen, R., Curry, L., Roemer, R., DeBease, C., and Mancall, E. 1982. Patterns of intellectual deficit in Huntington's disease. *Journal of Clinical and Experimental Neuropsychology* 4:173–83.

Kahn, E. A., and Crosby, E. 1972. Korsakoff's syndrome associated with surgical lesions involving the mammillary bodies. *Neurology* 22:317–25.

Killiany, R. J., and Mahut, M. 1990. Hippocampectomy in infant rhesus monkeys facilitates object–reward association learning but not memory for conditional object–object associations. *Society for Neuroscience Abstracts* 16:847.

Killiany, R. J., and Mahut, M. 1991. Ontogenetic development of recognition memory span in rhesus macaques. *Third IBRO World Congress of Neuroscience Abstracts* 165.

Kinsbourne, M., and Warrington, E. K. 1962. A disorder of simultaneous form perception. *Brain* 85:461–86.

Kinsbourne, M., and Warrington, E. K. 1963. The localizing significance of limited simultaneous form perception. *Brain* 85:697–702.

Kinsbourne, M., and Wood, F. 1975. Short-term memory processes and the amnesic syndrome. In D. Deutsch and J. A. Deutsch, eds. *Short-Term Memory*. New York: Academic Press, pp. 258–291.

Loftus, E. F. 1972. Nouns, adjectives, and semantic memory. *Journal of Experimental Psychology* 96:213–15.

Loftus, E. F., and Cole, W. 1974. Retrieving attribute and name information from semantic memory. *Journal of Experimental Psychology* 102:1116–22.

McCarthy, R. A., and Warrington, E. K. 1984. A two route model of speech production: Evidence from aphasia. *Brain* 107:463–85.

McCloskey, M., Wible, C. G., and Cohen, N. J. 1988. Is there a special flashbulb-memory mechanism? *Journal of Experimental Psychology: General* 117:171–81.

McGaugh, J., and Gold, P. E. 1976. Modulation of memory by electrical stimulation of the brain. In M. R. Rosensweig and E. L. Bennett, Eds. *Neural Mechanisms of Learning and Memory*. Cambridge, MA: MIT Press, pp. 135–42.

Mackay, H. A., and Ratti, C. A. 1990. Position-numeral equivalences and delayed position recognition span. *American Journal on Mental Retardation* 95:271–82.

Mahut, H., and Killiany, R. J. 1990. Ontogeny of object-reward association learning and trial-unique object recognition memory: Effects of early hippocampectomy on the two capacities in rhesus macaques. *Society for Neuroscience Abstracts* 16:847.

Mahut, M., and Moss, M. B. 1984. Consolidation of memory: The hippocampus revisited. In L. R. Squire and N. Butters, eds.*Neuropsychology of Memory* . New York: Guilford Press 297- 315

Mahut, M., Zola-Morgan, S., and Moss, M. B. 1982. Hippocampal resections impair associative learning and recognition memory in the monkey. *Journal of Neuroscience* 2:1214–29.

Marslen-Wilson, W. D., and Teuber, H. L. 1975. Memory for remote events in anterograde amnesia: Recognition of public figures from news photographs. *Neuropsychologia* 13:347–52.

Martone, M., Butters, N., Payne, M., Becker, J., and Sax, D. S. 1984. Dissociations between skill learning and verbal recognition in amnesia and dementia. *Archives of Neurology* 41:965–70.

Merjanian, P. M., Bachevalier, J., Crawford, H., and Mishkin, M. 1986. Socioemotional disturbances in the developing rhesus monkey following neonatal limbic lesions. *Society for Neuroscience Abstracts* 12:23.

Milner, B. 1970. Memory and the medial temporal regions of the brain. In K. H. Pribram and D. E. Broadbent, eds. *Biology of Memory*. New York: Academic Press, pp. 29–50.

Milner, B., Corkin, S., and Teuber, H. L. 1968. Further analysis of the hippocampal amnesic syndrome. *Neuropsychologia* 6:215–34.

Mishkin, M. 1978. Memory in monkeys severely impaired by combined but not separate removal of amygdala and hippocampus. *Nature* 273:297–98.

Mishkin, M., Malamut, B. L., and Bachevalier, J. 1984. Memories and habits: Two neural systems. In G. Lynch, L. McGaugh, and N. M. Weinberger, eds. 65–77. *Neurobiology of Learning and Memory*. New York: Guilford.

Mishkin, M., and Petri, H. L. 1984. Memories and habits: Some implications for the analysis of learning and retention. In N. Butters and L. Squire, eds. 287–96. *Neuropsychology of Memory*. New York: Guilford.

Moss, M. B., and Albert, M. S. 1988. Alzheimer's disease and other dementing disorders. In M. S. Albert and M. B. Moss, eds. 145–78. *Geriatric Neuropsychology*. New York: Guilford.

Moss, M. B., Albert, M. S., Butters, N., and Payne, M. 1986. Differential patterns of memory loss among patients with Alzheimer's disease, Huntington's disease, and alcoholic Korsakoff's syndrome. *Archives of Neurology* 43:239–46.

Neisser, U. 1967. *Cognitive Psychology*. New York: Appleton.

Neisser, U. 1982. *Memory Observed*. San Francisco: Freeman.

Oakley, D. A. 1981. Brain mechanisms of mammalian memory. *British Medical Bulletin* 37:175–80.

O'Keefe, J., and Nadel, L. 1978. *The Hippocampus as a Cognitive Map*. Oxford: Clarendon Press.

Olton, D. S., Becker, J. T., and Handelman, G. E. 1979. Hippocampus, space and memory. *Behavioral and Brain Sciences* 2:313–17.

Petersen, L. R., and Petersen, M. J. 1959. Short term retention of individual items. *Journal of Experimental Psychology* 91:341–43.

Ribot, T. 1882. *Diseases of Memory*. New York: Appleton.

Rovee-Collier, C. 1991. The "memory system" of prelinguistic infants. In A. Diamond, ed. *The Development and Neural Basis of Higher Cognitive Functions*. New York: Academic Press, pp. 517–42.

Rubin, D. C., and Kozin, M. 1984. Vivid memories. *Cognition* 16:81–95.

Ruggiero, F. T., and Flagg, S. F. 1976. Do animals have memory? In D. L. Medin, W. A. Roberts, and R. T. Davis, eds. *Processes of Animal Memory*. Hillsdale, NJ: Erlbaum, pp. 212–23.

Rutter, M. 1978. Diagnosis and definition. In M. Rutter and E. Schopler, eds. *Autism: A Reappraisal of Concepts and Treatment*. New York: Plenum Press, pp. 1–25.

Ryle, G. 1949. *The Concept of Mind*. London: Hitchinson.

Saffran, E. M., and Marin, O. S. M. 1975. Immediate memory for word lists and sentences in a patient with a deficient auditory short-term memory. *Brain and Language* 2:420–33.

Schacter, D. L., and Moscovitch, M. 1984. Infants, amnesics and dissociable memory systems. In M. Moscovitch, ed. *Infant Memory*. New York: Plenum, pp. 173–216.

Scoville, W. B., and Milner, B. 1957. Loss of recent memory after bilateral hippocampal lesions. *Neuropsychologia* 20:11–21.

Selfe, L. 1983. *Normal and Anomalous Representational Drawing Ability in Children.* London: Academic Press.

Shallice, T., and Warrington, E. K. 1970. Independent functioning of the verbal memory stores: A neuropsychological study. *Quarterly Journal of Experimental Psychology* 22:261–73.

Spitz, H. H. 1972. Note on immediate memory for digits: Invariance over the years. *Psychological Bulletin* 78:183–85.

Squire, L. R. 1986. Mechanisms of memory. *Science* 232:1612–19.

Squire, L. R., Chace, P. M., and Slater, P. C. 1976. Retrograde amnesia following electroconvulsive therapy. *Nature (London)* 260:775–77.

Squire, L. R., and Cohen, N. 1979. Memory and amnesia: Resistance to disruption develops for years after learning. *Behavioral and Neural Biology* 25:115–25.

Squire, L. R., Cohen, N. J., and Nadel, L. 1984. The medial temporal region and memory consolidation: A new hypothesis. In H. Weingartner and E. Parker, eds. *Memory Consolidation.* Hillsdale, NJ: Erlbaum, pp. 185–209.

Squire, L. R., Slater, P. C., and Chace, P. M. 1975. Retrograde amnesia: Temporal gradient in very long term memory following electro-convulsive therapy. *Science* 187:77–79.

Squire, L. R., and Zola-Morgan, S. 1991. The medial temporal lobe memory system. *Science* 253:1380–86.

Teuber, H. L., Milner, B., and Vaughan, H. G. 1968. Persistent anterograde amnesia after stab wound of the basal brain. *Neuropsychologia* 6:267–82.

Tulving, E. 1972. Episodic and semantic memory. In E. Tulving and W. Donaldson, eds. 381–403. *Organization of Memory.* New York: Academic Press.

Tulving, E. 1984. Precis of elements of episodic memory. *Behavioral and Brain Sciences* 7:223–68.

Tulving, E. 1985. How many memory systems are there? *American Psychologist* 40:385–98.

Victor, M., and Agamanolis, D. 1990. Amnesia due to lesions confined to the hippocampus: A clinical-pathologic study. *Journal of Cognitive Neuroscience* 2:246–57.

Warrington, E. K., and James, M. 1967. Disorders of visual perception in patients with localised cerebral lesions. *Neuropsychologia* 5:253–66.

Warrington, E. K., Logue, V., and Pratt, R. T. C. 1971. The anatomical localisation of selective impairment of auditory verbal short-term memory. *Neuropsychologia* 9:377–87.

Warrington, E. K., and Rabin, P. 1971. Visual span of apprehension in patients with cerebral lesions. *Quarterly Journal of Experimental Psychology* 23:423–31.

Warrington, E. K., and Shallice, T. 1969. The selective impairment of auditory verbal short-term memory. *Brain* 92:885–96.

Warrington, E. K., and Weiskrantz, L. 1982. Amnesia: A disconnection syndrome? *Neuropsychologia* 20:233–48.

Zola-Morgan, S., and Squire, L. R. 1986. Memory impairment in monkeys following lesions limited to the hippocampus. *Behavioral Neuroscience* 100:155–60.

Zola-Morgan, S., Squire, L. R., and Amaral, D. G. 1986. Human amnesia and the medial temporal region: Enduring memory impairment following a bilateral lesion limited to field CA1 of the hippocampus. *Journal of Neuroscience* 6:2950–67.

Zola-Morgan, S., Squire, L. R., and Amaral, D. G. 1989a. Lesions of the amygdala that spare adjacent cortical regions do not impair memory or exacerbate the impairment following lesions of the hippocampal formation. *Journal of Neuroscience* 9:1922–36.

Zola-Morgan, S., Squire, L. R., and Amaral, D. G. 1989b. Lesions of the hippocampal formation but not lesions of the fornix or the mammillary nuclei produce long-lasting memory impairment in monkeys. *Journal of Neuroscience* 9:898–913.

Zola-Morgan, S., Squire, L. R., Amaral, D. G., and Suzuki, W. 1989. Lesions of perirhinal and parahippocampal cortex that spare the amygdala and hippocampal formation produce severe memory impairment. *Journal of Neuroscience* 9:4355–70.

10

THE CEREBELLUM IN AUTISM:
CLINICAL AND ANATOMIC PERSPECTIVES

Jeremy D. Schmahmann, M.D.

It may appear surprising that there is a discussion of the cerebellum in this book on early infantile autism because these patients have no clinical deficits suggestive of cerebellar disease. However, neuroimaging studies (Chap. 4) and neuroanatomical observations (Chap. 7) have revealed a number of abnormalities of the cerebellum in this condition. What could be the significance of these observations? What do we presently know about cerebellar function that could permit speculation about the relevance of these observations? These neuroimaging and pathologic findings in autism come at a fortuitous time in the re-evaluation of our understanding of cerebellar function. Whereas the role of the cerebellum in the coordination of equilibrium, posture, gait, and appendicular movements is well established, the possibility that there is a cerebellar contribution to higher function has begun to attract attention.

CLINICAL AND LABORATORY OBSERVATIONS

Prominent neuropsychiatric manifestations such as schizophrenia, manic depression, and poor intellect have been recorded since the last century in association with cerebellar agenesis and dysgenesis. In many of the early studies, patients with hereditary ataxia were described as suffering from mental deficiency, dementia, and psychosis, and characterizations of these deficits included emotional lability, irritability, loss of comprehension, poverty of association, and general intellectual impairment. The relevance to contemporary neurologic thought of these incompletely studied early cases is debatable, as discussed more fully and referenced in Schmahmann (1991).

Neuropsychologic tests in patients with olivopontocerebellar degeneration have revealed deficits in verbal and nonverbal intelligence, memory, and frontal system function in proportion to the severity of ataxia (Kish et al., 1988), and patients with cerebellar atrophy have demonstrated slowed speed of information processing, disorganization in visuospatial skills and memory, and poor planning and programming abilities (Botez et al., 1985, 1989). Studies in patients with discrete cerebellar lesions such as unilateral cerebellar hemispheric infarction have revealed neuropsychologic deficits including impaired mental imagery and anticipatory planning (Leiner et al., 1986) as well as prolonged reaction times and inability to use temporal clues correctly, apparently independent of their motor incapacity (Keele and Ivry, 1990). The advent of PET and SPECT scanning has permitted the observation that inferolateral neocerebellar areas are metabolically active during language processes performed in the absence of movement (Petersen et al., 1989), and vermal and paravermal structures are metabolically active during panic and anxiety states (Reiman et al., 1989). These observations supplement the demonstrations of crossed cerebellar diaschisis following lesions of cerebral association cortexes (Pantano et al., 1986), including those associated primarily with aphasia (Metter et al., 1987). In an evaluation of a patient following surgical excision of the posterior inferior cerebellar vermis and adjacent parts of the hemispheres, abnormalities were noted in visuospatial skills and in abstract thinking and concept formation, as well as with paired word associations and naming. The SPECT scan of the brain in that patient showed hypoperfusion particularly in the left temporal and parietal lobes, consistent with reversed cerebellar diaschisis (Schmahmann, 1991). Another patient was recently observed to have difficulty with word generation tasks and in word and pattern discrimination following a right lateral cerebellar infarct (Petersen and Fieze, 1993). Patients with acquired damage to neocerebellar structures are impaired in their ability to shift direction of attentional focus, a deficit closely matched by patients with early infantile autism (Akshoomoff and Courchesne, 1992). Thus, the evaluation of the putative causal association between disturbances of higher function and lesions of the cerebellum has begun to be reappraised critically with the help of contemporary techniques, and with the necessary caution that this novel concept demands (Schmahmann, 1992).

Stimulation of the cerebellar cortex by chronically implanted subdural electrodes has been shown to be effective in controlling seizures, depression, anger, and aggression in patients (Heath, 1977; Cooper et al., 1978). Moreover, highly aggressive rhesus monkeys that received lesions in the neocerebellar hemispheres, or incomplete lesions of the vermis, showed no change in their aggressive behavior even at the time of maximal neurological impairment. By contrast, animals that received lesions of the vermis, flocculonodular lobe, part of the lobulus simplex, and the paramedian lobule became quite docile and showed no signs of aggression in the confrontation situation even after their ataxia had subsided (Peters and Monjan, 1971; Berman et al., 1973).

Electric stimulation of the rostral fastigial nucleus of unanesthetized cats has produced a variety of nonmotor effects including hypertension, tachycardia, alerting and grooming responses, self-stimulation, predatory attack, and sham rage (Moruzzi, 1947; Zanchetti and Zoccolini, 1954; Berntson et al., 1973; Reis et al., 1973; Ball et al., 1974; Martner, 1975). These behaviors, generally considered to be represented in the hypothalamus and limbic system (Kaada, 1972), prompted Reis et al. (1973) to suggest that the fastigial nucleus may function in the behavioral realm primarily as a modulator of emotional and visceral reaction patterns.

The cerebellum also appears to participate in conditioned learning, as exemplified by the acoustic startle response in the rat (Leaton and Supple, 1986) and the classically conditioned eyelid and nictitating membrane response in rabbit (Thompson, 1988). Sanes et al. (1990) demonstrated that patients with hemispheric cerebellar degeneration have impaired learning of skilled movements, consistent with the observation that cerebellar mutant mice (Lalonde et al., 1987), or rats subjected to cerebellar hemispherectomy (Molinari, 1991), have impaired spontaneous alternation and habituation, and deficits of visuospatial memory.

ANATOMIC SUBSTRATES

To postulate that the cerebellum could contribute to nonmotor activity, and specifically to higher-order behavior, there must be an anatomical substrate that could support such a role. The contribution of the motor and sensory cortices to the cerebellum by way of the basis pontis is well known, as is the feedback system to the "motor" thalamus and cerebral cortex from the cerebellar nuclei. What anatomical information is there, however, that could be compatible with this putative behavioral role of the cerebellum?

CEREBRAL ASSOCIATION CORTEX PROJECTIONS TO PONS

In an attempt to address the question whether the cerebellum receives the type of information from the cerebral cortex that could facilitate a cerebellar modulation of cognitive ability, recent studies evaluated the projections to the pons from the cerebral association areas. The association areas in the parietal, temporal, and frontal lobes are responsible for integrative, complex, motivational activity, and when lesioned in humans and animals result in a variety of syndromes that are now part of classic neurologic teaching (Mesulam, 1985). After synapsing in the pons, these cortical projections traverse the contralateral middle cerebellar peduncle and terminate as mossy fibers in the granule cell layer of the (mostly contralateral) cerebellar cortex. This corticopontocerebellar pathway is the principal means whereby information from the associative cerebral cortex is conveyed to the cerebellum. The inferior olive, which sends its climbing fiber efferents to the dendritic trees of Purkinje cells of the cerebellar cortex, receives afferents from the cerebral cortex indirectly through the central tegmental tract originating mostly in the red nucleus, and possibly directly from the cerebral cortex. The associative cortical regions, however, have not been observed to contribute efferents either to the red nucleus or to the inferior olive in earlier studies or in our own analyses. Thus, the corticopontocerebellar pathway is unrivaled in importance in conveying processed, multimodal cortical information to the cerebellum (Figure 10.1). The neurons of the basis pontis project upon the cerebellar cortex, although the presence of GABAergic neurons in the basilar pons raises the possibility of a local intrapontine circuitry as well (Thier and Koehler, 1987). There is also a minor reciprocal projection to the pons from all the deep cerebellar nuclei. We do not know how the basilar pons influences the information it receives from the cerebral cortex before transmitting it to the cerebellum. Nevertheless, there is ample precedent in the neuroscience literature to draw certain conclusions with respect to the functions of the pons and cerebellum by virtue of the nature of the information conveyed to these regions from the cerebral cortex. As a result, defining the nature and topographical organization of the behaviorally relevant projections from the cerebral hemispheres to the pons would potentially provide at least partial anatomical support for this postulated association between cerebellar function and higher order behavior. A conservative view of this corticopontocerebellar relationship is that higher-order cerebral areas provide information to the cerebellum necessary for the production of skilled movements, but that there is no cerebellar contribution to the organization and development of strategies for higher-order integrated actions. Whereas this conclusion may be correct, there is substantial information derived from an increasing number of sources, which suggests that this view does not sufficiently account for the anatomical circuitry described shortly.

These connectivity studies have been performed in the rhesus monkey brain, which, while considerably simpler and smaller than the human brain, nevertheless has many analogous architectonic areas as defined by Brodmann (1909), and has been extensively studied with respect to anatomical connections and behavioral and physiological properties.

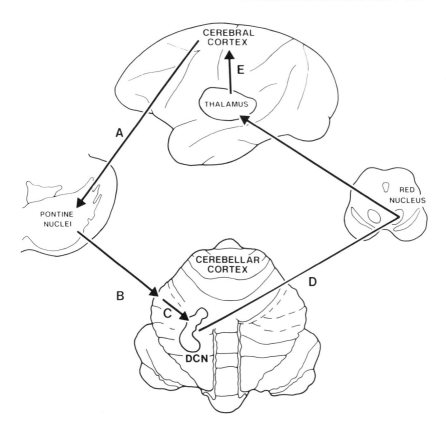

Figure 10.1. Diagram of the anatomic circuitry linking the association areas of the cerebral hemispheres with the cerebellum. The corticopontine projection (A) carries higher-order, multimodal information to the nuclei of the basis pontis, from where it is conveyed via the pontocerebellar pathway (B) to the cerebellar cortex. The cerebellar corticonuclear projection (C) allows the deep cerebellar nuclei (DCN) to send their axons to the thalamus (the cerebellothalamic projection, D) via the red nucleus, to which *en passant* terminals are distributed. The thalamic projection to the association cortices (E) completes the feedback circuit. This schematic view of the cerebrocerebellar link does not imply a closed-loop system, and the multiple details of each of the projection systems mentioned are not shown here.

THE BASILAR PONS

Based in part upon its cellular architecture, the basilar pons has been divided into various nuclei depicted in Figure 10.2A. The boundaries between individual nuclei may be ascertained with some degree of certainty, and vary slightly between cases. This subdivision on anatomic grounds appears to be reflected to some extent also in the pontine connections of the different cerebral cortical fields. The terminations in the pons of the corticopontine projection are distributed in discrete clusters that sometimes coalesce forming continuous bands, and they may be arranged in lamellae concentric to the traversing corticofugal fibers (Figure 10.2B–D). These clusters frequently branch and converge, although some have described them as isolated bands or columns.

PARIETOPONTINE CONNECTIONS

The association areas of the posterior parietal cortex have been shown to play a role in complex functions, integrating information from different sensory modalities, and regulating coordinated behavioral responses to environmental and internal stimuli. Clinical observations have demonstrated that posterior parietal lesions are associated with disturbances of complex visuospatial integration, neglect of the contralateral body and extrapersonal space, impaired language, apraxia, and agnosia. The multimodal and motivationally relevant properties of the posterior parietal neurons have also been shown in behavioral and electrophysiological studies (for review and references, please see Hyvarinen, 1982; Pandya et al., 1988; Mesulam, 1985).

Both the superior and inferior parietal lobules are thought to be involved in the sequential processing of somatotopically organized information received from the adjacent primary somatosensory cortices. Cortical architectonic and connectional studies reveal two rostrocaudal trends in the posterior parietal cortex (Figure 10.3). One trend begins in the dorsal postcentral gyrus where the trunk and lower limb are represented in the primary somatic sensory cortex, and continues caudally in the superior parietal lobule (SPL). The other trend begins in the ventral postcentral gyrus containing the head, neck, and arm representations, and continues caudally in the inferior parietal lobule. The banks of the intraparietal sulcus also differ from each other in that the cortex in the upper bank appears to be part of the somatic sensory association area, whereas the lower bank is concerned with the somatosensory modality as well as with visual and vestibular information.

The most caudal regions of the superior parietal lobule (area PGm) and inferior parietal lobule (areas PG and Opt) have been regarded as

---

Figure 10.2. A: Diagram of the subdivisions of the pontine nuclei in the transverse plane (perpendicular to the long axis of the pons, as shown at upper left). The roman numerals I-IX represent the rostrocaudal levels at approximately equal intervals through the pons. B: Diagram of the lateral surface of the cerebral hemisphere of a representative case in which the isotope injection (shaded black area) was placed in architectonic area PEa in the upper bank of the intraparietal sulcus. The resulting anterogradely transported label (black dots) is observed throughout the pons, as shown in the transverse sections labeled I-IX, corresponding to the pontine levels shown in A. The dots reflect the location of terminal label in the pons, and their density is an attempt to convey the relative strength of projection. The cortical projection to the pontine nuclei is ipsilateral,

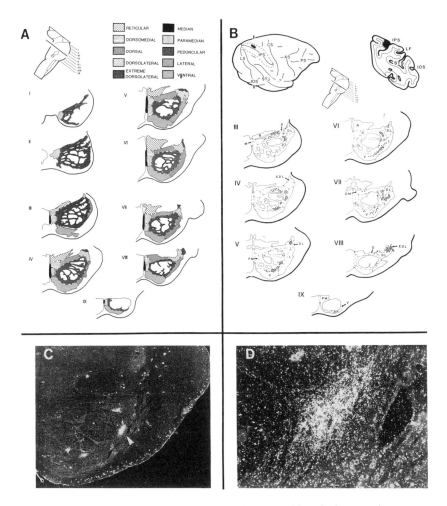

and thus only one side of the pons is shown. The dashed lines in the pons demarcate the different pontine nuclei. C: Low-power (X 30) and D: High-power (X 55) darkfield photomicrographs show terminations in the peripeduncular and intrapeduncular pontine nuclei of anterogradely transported isotope label from the rostral inferior parietal lobule injection in another case.

The abbreviations used to label the cerebral hemisphere in this and subsequent figures are: AS, arcuate sulcus; CING S, cingulate sulcus; CC, corpus callosum; CS, central sulcus; IOS, inferior occipital sulcus; IPS, intraparietal sulcus; LF, lateral (Sylvian) fissure; LS, lunate sulcus; OTS, occipitotemporal sulcus; POMS, parieto-occipital medial sulcus; PS, principalis sulcus; STS, superior temporal sulcus. The abbreviations for the pontine nuclei in this and subsequent figures are: D, dorsal; DL, dorsolateral; DM, dorsomedial; EDL, extreme dorsolateral; L, lateral; M, median; P, peduncular (intrapeduncular versus peripeduncular not specified); PM, paramedian; R, nucleus reticularis tegmenti pontis; V, ventral.

Source: After Nyby and Jansen, 1951, with modifications according to our observations (Schmahmann and Pandya, 1989)

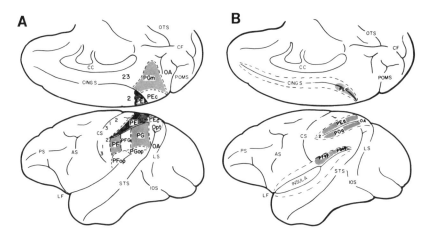

Figure 10.3. Diagram of the lateral and medial surfaces of the cerebral hemispheres in the rhesus monkey, showing the architectonic parcellation of the posterior parietal cortex, according to Pandya and Seltzer (1982). In A the zones lying on the exposed surfaces of the hemispheres, and in B the intraparietal, lateral, and cingulate sulci are opened to show the location of the zones lying within the sulci.
Source: Pandya and Seltzer, 1992

polymodal association areas by virtue of their connections and functional properties. Thus, area PGm has been shown to be a site of convergence of somatosensory, kinesthetic, visual, and auditory information. It also has connections with the prefrontal cortex and the cingulate gyrus. Areas PG and Opt have prominent reciprocal connections with paralimbic cortices (parahippocampal gyrus, presubiculum, perirhinal cortex, and cingulate gyrus) and multimodal zones in the temporal and frontal lobes. Unlike the rostral part of the superior and inferior parietal lobules which are connected with modality-specific thalamic nuclei, areas PGm and PG/Opt have thalamic connections predominantly with associative thalamic nuclei. Area Opt alone has connections with the lateral dorsal nucleus, as well as with the anterior nucleus of thalamus which are considered part of the limbic system circuitry. These caudally located multimodal zones in PG/Opt, and to a lesser degree in PGm, subserve highly complex, nonmodality specific functions which are invested with emotional and motivational significance (for review and references, please see Pandya and Yeterian, 1985; Schmahmann and Pandya, 1990).

The pontine projections from the posterior parietal cortex are directed most heavily towards the peripeduncular and lateral pontine nuclei (Figures 10.2B–D; Figure 10.4). There are lesser but nevertheless substantial projections to other nuclei including the intrapeduncular, ventral, dorsolateral, extreme dorsolateral, and dorsal nuclei. Differences in pontine terminations are dependent upon the site of origin of the projection. In general, however, projections arising from multimodal regions in both trends in the posterior parietal cortex are more strongly represented and more laterally placed within the pontine nuclei than are projections arising from more rostral, unimodal regions (for review and references, please see Schmahmann and Pandya, 1989).

TEMPOROPONTINE CONNECTIONS

The role of the temporal lobe with respect to language, memory, and complex behaviors has been well established, and confusional states, highly structured visual hallucinations and the Klüver–Bucy syndrome consequent upon lesions in this area are also acknowledged (Mesulam, 1985). In the monkey, anatomic and physiologic observations have shown that the temporal lobe contains unimodal and multimodal areas that appear to contribute differentially to the organization of behavior. Architectonic areas TPO and PGa in the upper bank of the superior temporal sulcus (Figure 10.5) have been shown to be association areas concerned with multiple sensory modalities (i.e., vision, somatic sensation, and audition). They have connections with association areas of the frontal and parietal cortexes, as well as with limbic related structures at the medial and inferior frontal convexity and parahippocampal and cingulate gyri, and contain neurons which respond preferentially to more than one modality and to complex stimuli such as faces. In contrast, the superior temporal gyrus appears to be an association area confined to the auditory realm; and the depth of the superior temporal sulcus, area IPa, appears to be an important association area for the somatosensory modality. The inferotemporal region and the lower bank of the superior temporal sulcus that are strongly interconnected, contain neurons that are functionally unimodal within the visual system, subserve central vision, and seem to be involved in object discrimination (for review and references, please see Mishkin et al., 1983; Van Essen, 1985; Desimone and Ungerleider, 1986; Pandya et al., 1988).

The projections from temporal lobe to the basis pontis are derived predominantly from the upper bank of the superior temporal sulcus, areas TPO and PGa, with a lesser contribution from the superior temporal region. The extreme dorsolateral, dorsolateral, and lateral nuclei are the major recipients of efferents from each of the TPO subdivisions (see, e.g., Figure 10.6A), with the most caudal part of the upper bank of the superior temporal sulcus also projecting to the peripeduncular, ventral, and rostral intrapeduncular nuclei. Pontine projections from the superior temporal gyrus and the medial portion of the supratemporal plane including the second auditory area, AII are less intense than from the upper bank of the superior temporal sulcus, and they are directed

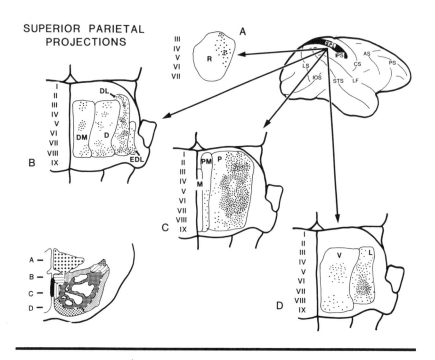

SUPERIOR PARIETAL
PROJECTIONS

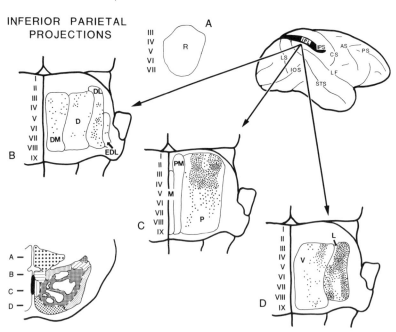

INFERIOR PARIETAL
PROJECTIONS

Figure 10.4. Summary diagrams of the distribution of the projections (black dots) from the posterior parietal cortices to the individual pontine nuclei in the rhesus monkey. The entire rostrocaudal extent of the pontine nuclei has been reconstructed in the frontal plane in four dorsoventral groupings (A to D), corresponding to the levels shown in the lower left diagram. The sum of the projections to the pontine nuclei from the superior parietal lobule are seen in A, and from the inferior parietal lobule in B.
Source: Schmahmann and Pandya, 1989

mainly to the peripeduncular, dorsolateral, and lateral nuclei (Schmahmann and Pandya, 1991).

The lower bank of the superior temporal sulcus is quite different from the upper bank and the supratemporal plane because, with the exception of the caudally located area MT (Ungerleider et al., 1984), it contributes no projections to the basis pontis (Figure 10.6B) (Glickstein et al., 1985; Schmahmann and Pandya, 1991).

The anatomic connections from the multimodal temporal areas to the pons are therefore intriguing because, to reiterate, these regions of the cerebral cortex are concerned with higher-order functions, not with motor control, and have now been shown to transmit this information to the cerebellum via the corticopontocerebellar system.

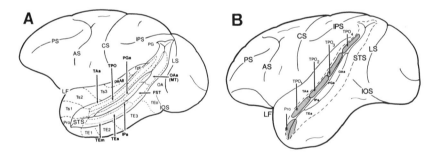

Figure 10.5. A: Diagram of the lateral surface of the cerebral hemisphere of a rhesus monkey, showing the architectonic parcellation of the superior temporal gyrus (areas TS1, TS2, TS3, paAlt, and Tpt); the inferotemporal region (areas TE1, TE2, and TE3); and the cortex lying within the superior temporal sulcus, according to Seltzer and Pandya (1978). In the superior temporal sulcus, the multimodal areas TPO and PGa are located in the upper bank. The surrounding unimodal association area for the auditory realm (area TAa) is situated in the upper bank of the superior temporal sulcus and the superior temporal gyrus; the somatosensory associated area IPa is located at the fundus of the superior temporal sulcus; and the visual association areas (areas TEa, TEm, and OAa [FST and MT]) occupy the lower bank of the superior temporal sulcus and the inferotemporal region. B: The four rostrocaudal subdivisions of the multimodal area TPO in the upper bank of the superior temporal sulcus, according to Seltzer and Pandya (1989b).
Source: A: Seltzer and Pandya, 1978. B: Seltzer and Pandya, 1989.

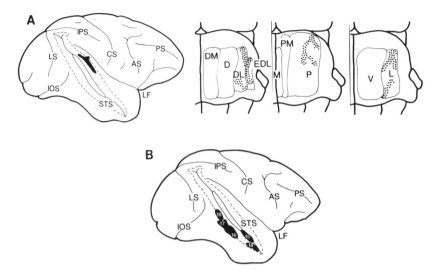

Figure 10.6. A: Diagram of the rostrocaudal and mediolateral extents of the projections (black dots) to the individual pontine nuclei, shown in the frontal plane, from areas TPO3 of the superior temporal sulcus, and area TAa. B: Diagram of the lateral surface of the cerebral hemisphere of a rhesus monkey, showing the sites of injection of isotope in the unimodal association areas of the lower bank (visual) and depth (somatosensory) of the superior temporal sulcus in five cases, involving areas TEa, TEm, TE2, and rostral FST. None of the injections in these cases resulted in anterograde termination in the basis pontis.
Source: Schmahmann and Pandya, 1991

FRONTOPONTINE CONNECTIONS

The prefrontal cortex (Figure 10.7) has been shown to be concerned with the highest levels of behavioral organization and integration in patients as well as in nonhuman primates. These prefrontal areas are not primarily concerned with motor activity, but rather are concerned with a variety of complex cognitive processes. These include planning, sequencing, and strategy formation in time and space, orientation, attention, personality, emotionality, behavioral adjustment, and inhibition of behavior. It has been suggested that the supplementary motor area at the dorsal aspect of the medial convexity, which is reciprocally interconnected with the anterior cingulate gyrus, focuses limbic outflow onto motor executive regions and links intention formation to the programming and execution of specific actions. The cortex located in the arcuate concavity (area 8) is a zone of converging inputs from different sensory modalities, including visual, auditory, and somatosensory systems. Apart from its recognized importance in eye movements, this region is crucial for the planning of sequenced movements and for the initiation and suppression of voluntary action (for review and refer-

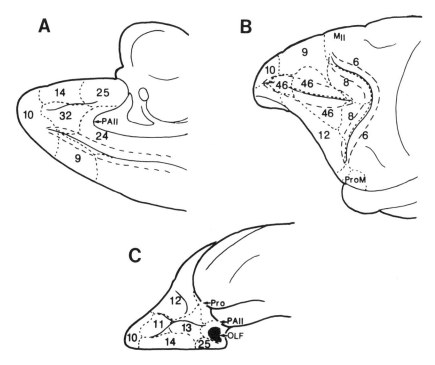

Figure 10.7. Diagrams of the medial (A), lateral (B), and ventral (C) surfaces of the cerebral hemisphere of a rhesus monkey, showing the subdivisions of the prefrontal cortex based on cytoarchitectonic criteria.
Source: Barabas and Pandya, 1989

ences, please see Goldberg, 1985; Stuss and Benson, 1986; Pandya and Yeterian, 1991).

Connectivity studies in nonhuman primates have revealed pontine projections from the supplementary motor area—area 8, area 46, and area 9—and from the prefrontal cortex anterior to a plane joining the rostral tips of the superior and inferior rami of the arcuate sulcus. The details of the termination patterns of these projections vary according to the site of origin. The medial, paramedian, dorsal, and ventral pons are favored, but the lateral pons is also implicated in some cases (Kuypers and Lawrence, 1967; De Vito and Smith, 1964; Kürnzle and Akert, 1977; Stanton et al., 1988a, 1988b; Shook et al., 1990). Our own preliminary observations reveal that the doral lateral prefrontal convexity (areas 46, 8B, 9, and 10) and the medial prefrontal cortex (areas 8 and 32) provide the majority of the prefrontal pontine efferents, whereas the ventral lateral and orbitofrontal cortexes provide sparse, or no, pontine terminations. There is a differential organization of the prefrontopontine projections, including area 10 at the frontal pole, both in terms of the cortical derivation as well as with respect to the rostrocaudal extent and the mediolateral/dorsoventral arrangement of the terminations in the pons (Schmahmann and Pandya, 1993a). The projection from these regions via the pons to the cerebellum (and the feedback to them from cerebellum via thalamus, as will be discussed shortly) has functional implications in the consideration of the role of the cerebellum in the realm of higher-order behavior.

OCCIPITOTEMPORAL PROJECTIONS TO PONS

There is a striking dichotomy of pontine projections from the occipitotemporal region. These cortical areas have been studied with respect to their participation in the dual visual streams arising in the occipital lobe and coursing through the parastriate regions to either the parietal cortex or the temporal lobe (Figure 10.8). The former, passing through successive stages of architectonic, connectional, and physiologic differentiation, includes the dorsal part of the prelunate gyrus, the caudal part of the lower bank of the superior temporal sulcus (area MT), the polymodal convergence zones in the lower bank of the intraparietal sulcus, and the polymodal parts of the caudal inferior parietal lobule. The other visual stream is directed inferiorly from the parastriate zone into the ventral prelunate gyrus, the rostral lower bank of the superior temporal sulcus, and the middle and inferior temporal gyri. Whereas the dorsal stream is mainly concerned with the spatial features of objects or events in the periphery of the visual field, the ventral stream is more in-

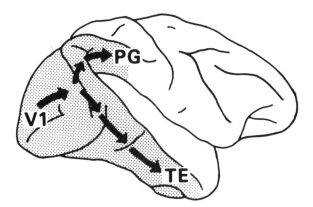

Figure 10.8. Diagram of the two major processing systems within the visual system. The dorsal pathway is directed into the parietal lobe and is concerned with spatial perception and visuomotor performance; the ventral pathway is directed into the temporal lobe and is important for object recognition.
Source: Mishkin et al., 1983

volved with the identification of objects and their characteristics such as form, color, and orientation, and is more concerned with stimuli occurring in the central part of the visual field (for review and references, please see Mishkin et al., 1983; Van Essen, 1985; Desimone and Ungerleider, 1989).

Pontine projections are derived from the dorsal stream regions (Figure 10.9) and are distributed in the lateral, peripeduncular, and dorsolateral nuclei. The medial prelunate region projects to their rostral half,

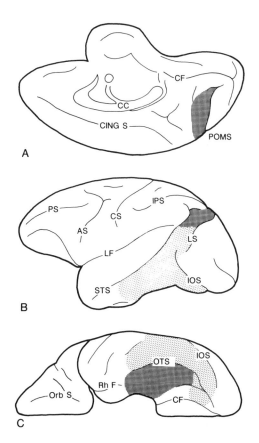

Figure 10.9. Diagrams of the medial (A), lateral (B), and ventral (C) surfaces of the cerebral hemisphere of a rhesus monkey, showing the differential origins of projection to the basis pontis from the occipitotemporal regions. Injections of radioisotope tracers in the areas shaded with solid lines resulted in terminations in the pons, whereas injections in those areas shaded by the stippled lines did not. The occipitotemporal projections appear to be derived from the medial and dorsal prelunate gyri as well as the mid- and caudal parahippocampal region, whereas the ventral prelunate and inferotemporal cortices do not have connections with the basilar pons.
Source: Schmahmann and Pandya, 1993b

whereas the dorsal prelunate gyrus projects throughout their rostrocaudal extent, as well as to the extreme dorsolateral nucleus and, to a lesser extent, to the nucleus reticularis tegmenti pontis. In contrast, the ventral trend (ventral prelunate gyrus, inferotemporal region and inferior temporal gyrus as well as the lower bank of the superior temporal sulcus) has no pontine connections (Schmahmann and Pandya, 1993b).

Furthermore, the posterior parahippocampal region, which is concerned with spatial aspects of memory (Nadel, 1991) and events in the periphery of the visual field, also has projections to the lateral, dorsolateral, and peripeduncular pontine nuclei, similar to those seen from the dorsal prelunate gyrus (Schmahmann and Pandya, 1993b). Thus these findings extend a dichotomy in the pattern of pontine projections to the occipitotemporal and posterior parahippocampal regions that has previously been suggested for the occipital cortex (Brodal, 1978; Glickstein et al., 1985). That is, visual cortical areas (primary or associative) that are concerned with the peripheral visual field, visual spatial parameters, and visual motion project to the pons, whereas regions concerned with the central visual field and visual object identification do not. In addition, the pontine afferents from the posterior parahippocampal gyrus may facilitate a cerebellar contribution to visual spatial memory, particularly when invested with motivational valence.

PARALIMBIC AND AUTONOMIC CONNECTIONS WITH PONS

Vilensky and Van Hoesen (1981) speculated on the potential influence of the limbic system on the cerebellum and its many functional roles in motor behavior by virtue of their demonstration of pontine projections from the cingulate gyrus. Projections were distributed in a ring around the periphery of the pontine grey matter, the rostral cingulate (areas 35, 25, and 24) projecting to the dorsomedial, medial and ventromedial parts, and the caudal cingulate gyrus (areas 23 and the retrosplenial cortex) sending efferents to the lateral and ventrolateral aspects. This cingulopontine projection has been observed in the cat as well (Aas and Brodal, 1988), and the pontine terminals appear to converge upon the same ventromedial part of the rostral pons favored by the medial mammillary nucleus.

Hypothalamic inputs to pons in the cat are derived from the posterior and dorsal hypothalamic regions that project medially and dorsomedially within the caudal third of the pontine nuclei, and with a more sparse projection seen laterally (Aas and Brodal, 1988). In monkey a direct and reciprocal hypothalomocerebellar projection has been identified. The ansiform and paramedian lobules and the paraflocculus are connected with the lateral and posterior hypothalamic areas, and the anterior lobe is connected with these foregoing regions as well as with the ventromedial, dorsomedial and dorsal hypothalamic nuclei. All the deep cerebellar nuclei project to the contralateral posterior and lateral hypothalamic nuclei (Haines and Dietrichs, 1984).

The medial mammillary bodies implicated in the amnestic syndrome of Korsakoff project not only to the pons but also directly to the cerebellum. In the cat, the medial mammillary nucleus projects ventromedially at all rostrocaudal levels of the pontine nuclei (Aas and Brodal, 1988). In the monkey the lateral mammillary and supramammillary nuclei project to the cerebellar ansiform and paramedian lobules, paraflocculus, and anterior lobe, whereas the medial mammillary nucleus receives projections from all the contralateral cerebellar nuclei (Haines and Dietrichs, 1984). Our own observations in the monkey (Schmahmann and Pandya, 1992, 1993b) also reveal projections to pons from the posterior parahippocampal regions which have been implicated particularly in the spatial aspects of memory. This anatomical data is complemented by physiological observations suggesting the existence of pathways linking components of the limbic system with the cerebellum (Anand et al., 1959; Snider and Maiti, 1976), and by the reciprocal connections between cerebellum and the brainstem catecholaminergic and serotoninergic nuclei that have widespread projections to the cerebral cortex including the higher order areas (Dempsey et al., 1983; Marcinkiewicz et al., 1989).

These findings may help to explain the generation of autonomic phenomena produced in animals by cerebellar stimulation, because, as suggested by Haines and Dietrichs (1984), these pathways may permit the cerebellum to have a relatively direct influence on visceral centers in the brainstem and spinal cord. In conjunction with the observations of Berger et al., (1986) with respect to the subicular–retrosplenial–pontine projections in rabbit, these findings could perhaps also be consistent with a cerebellar involvement in certain aspects of memory or learning, such as the apparent importance of the cerebellar component of the memory trace for classic conditioning.

A NOTE ON THE COURSE OF THE FIBER PATHWAYS TO THE PONS

The fibers destined for the basis pontis travel from their sites of origin through the white matter of the cerebral hemispheres toward the cerebral peduncle, and assume a characteristic trajectory (Schmahmann and Pandya, 1992). As the fibers progress toward the cerebral peduncle, they converge from all areas (rostral, middle, and caudal in the postrolandic parasensory association areas), and are situated in the white matter of the posterior limb of the internal capsule above the midpoint of the lateral geniculate nucleus (LGN), and at the medial aspect of the LGN (Figure 10.10). They also demonstrate a certain degree of topographic organization in the posterior limb of the capsule above the LGN as well as in the cerebral peduncle. Taken together

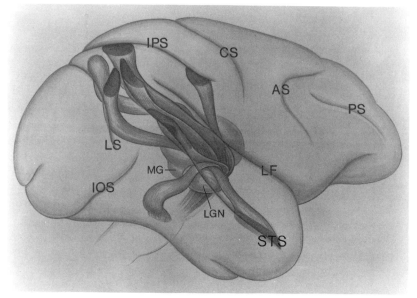

Figure 10.10. Composite summary diagram of the trajectory and organization of fibers from the parietal, temporal, and occipital association areas as they course toward the critical point in the white matter above and medial to the midportion of the lateral geniculate nucleus before descending into the cerebral peduncle.
Source: Schmahmann and Pandya, 1992

with the observations concerning termination patterns of these associative corticopontine projections, it would appear that the corticopontine system consists of segregated and partially overlapping pathways, which are to some extent distinguishable anatomically at each stage of their trajectory from origin to destination. Furthermore, the existence of a common area through which all parasensory associative input to pons is transmitted suggests that a precisely located lesion in this part of the corticopontocerebellar circuit may disrupt the cerebellar access to higher-order information derived from the parasensory associative regions.

Abnormalities of higher function are described in patients following infarction in the distribution of the anterior choroidal artery (AChA) that supplies this critical white matter region. Hemiparesis, hemianopsia, and hemisensory deficits are seen in these patients (Masson et al., 1983). In addition, however, severe visual neglect, constructional apraxia, alexia due to disorders of visuospatial strategy, anosognosia and motor impersistence have been described following infarction of the right AChA involving the posterior limb of the internal capsule, and aphasia with impaired fluency, semantic paraphasias, perseveration and decreased psycho-linguistic ability were noted following a similar lesion on the left (Cambier et al., 1983; Hommel et al., 1985; Helgason et al., 1986). Whereas disruption of the thalamocortical circuitry is generally assumed to be the essential element in the development of these behavioral manifestations of subcortical lesions, the anatomic observations concerning the course of the fiber pathways to the pons from the parasensory association cortices raise the possibility that the corticopontocerebellar system may also be relevant in this regard.

A MULTIMODAL CONVERGENCE ZONE WITHIN THE BASILAR PONS?

It is of some interest to note that there is a region in the lateral basis pontis in the monkey that receives projections from the association areas of the parietal and temporal lobes, as well as from the cingulate gyrus and the posterior parahippocampal region. This suggests that perhaps there is at least one locus in the lateral pons that contains neurons responsive to multiple modalities. Electrophysiological recording of neurons in the dorsolateral pons reveals direction-specific visual responses (Mustari et al., 1988; May et al., 1988); however, the nature of the response properties of neurons in the lateral nucleus remains to be determined.

CEREBROCEREBELLAR AFFERENT CONNECTIONS

Precisely where in cerebellum these associative and limbic inputs are distributed still needs to be elucidated, although certain principles of organization have been established. For example, it is known from physiological studies that the parietal and frontal cortices are functionally related to the neocerebellar hemispheres, and auditory and visual inputs are received in vermal lobules VI and VII (Allen and Tsukuhara, 1974). Anatomic investigations have revealed that the dorsolateral pontine region is connected with audiovisual parts of the cerebellar vermis in monkey, and with the paraflocculus and paramedian lobes in cat (Hoddevik et al., 1977; Robinson et al., 1984; Frankfurter et al., 1977). In the monkey the anterior lobe receives projections from the caudal pons; the paramedian lobule from the rostral two thirds; crus I afferents are from the rostromedial, and crus II from the medial, ventral, and lateral parts. The vermal visual area (vermal lobules VII and VIIIa) receives projections from the dorsomedial and dorsolateral pons. Afferents to the flocculus are derived from the lateral and dorsomedial pontine nuclei; those to the uvula from the dorsolateral and medial regions (Brodal, 1979, 1982). The anatomic evaluation of the cerebrocerebellar communication has been more completely studied in the cat than in the monkey, and it is apparent that species differences limit the validity of these findings with respect to the organization of these pathways in man. In cat, area 6 has strong connections with crus II; the sensorimotor cortex with the anterior lobe and somewhat less with the paramedian lobule; the second somatosensory cortex with the paramedian lobule and the paraflocculus; the parietal association cortex with the posterior lobe; the visual cortex with most of the lateral intermediate zone of the posterior lobe and particularly the dorsal paraflocculus; and the auditory cortex (mostly auditory association area AII) with crus II and the dorsal paraflocculus (Brodal, 1987). Based on the divergent and convergent patterns of corticopontine and pontocerebellar projections, Brodal concluded that information from one small part of the cerebral cortex is distributed to numerous discrete sites in the cerebellar cortex, where it is combined with other, specific kinds of information. It remains to be determined whether this pattern of projections could be consistent with one or more, possibly multimodal, pontine regions projecting to widespread but specific parts of the cerebellum.

CEREBELLAR EFFERENT CONNECTIONS

Cerebellar feedback to the cerebral cortex originates in the deep cerebellar nuclei (Figure 10.1), and although the cerebellothalamic pathway is generally regarded as arising in the dentate and interpositus nuclei, the fastigial nucleus also contributes [to nucleus X and the pars oralis of the ventral posterolateral nucleus (VPLo), according to the terminology of Olszewski, 1952]. The cerebellar efferents contribute projections to the red nucleus as they traverse it, and then they terminate in the thalamus. The cerebellar-recipient thalamic nuclei, especially different aspects of the ventrolateral nucleus, have traditionally been regarded as the motor thalamus. Indeed, the caudal and pars postrema aspects of the ventrolateral nucleus (VLc and VLps) are prime cerebellar targets, but so are nucleus X and the VPLo nucleus (Stanton, 1980; Thach and Jones, 1979).

Two additional facts, however, are of substantial interest. First, these motor thalamic nuclei have projections to regions of the cerebral cortex outside the primary motor areas (Figure 10.11). In the monkey, the supplementary motor area receives somatotopically organized projections from the dentate and interpositus posterior nuclei via the VPLo and VLc nuclei, nucleus X and also from the pallidal recipient pars oralis of the ventrolateral nucleus (VLo) (Schell and Strick, 1984; Wiesendanger and Wiesendanger, 1985; Orioli and Strick, 1989). In addition the prefrontal periarcuate areas are reciprocally interconnected with nucleus X (Kievit and Kuypers, 1977; Stanton et al., 1988a), VLc (Kievit and Kuypers, 1977), and VPLo (Kürnzle and Akert, 1977). The temporal and posterior parietal lobes have also been shown to receive projections from these cerebellar-recipient thalamic nuclei. The upper bank of the superior temporal sulcus receives projections from the VLc and VLps nuclei (Yeterian and Pandya, 1989), the posterior parietal cortex from all the motor nuclei. Nucleus VLps has the strongest poste-

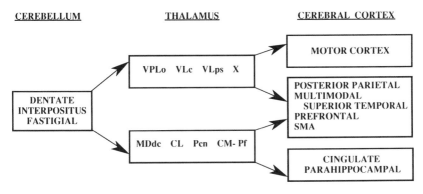

Figure 10.11. Summary diagram of the cerebellothalamocortical pathways that may be relevant in redirecting information from the cerebellum back to the higher-order areas of the cerebral cortex. The traditionally motor cerebellar-recipient thalamic nuclei (VPLo, VLc, VLps, and X) not only project to the motor and premotor cortex but also in varying degrees of strength are connected with the supplementary motor area (SMA), the prefrontal (area 8), posterior parietal (superior and inferior parietal lobules), and multimodal temporal regions (area TPO in the upper bank of the superior temporal sulcus) Furthermore, the intralaminar and medial dorsal thalamic nuclei that are known to project in varying combinations to the association and limbic cortices (MDdc, CL, Pcn, CM-Pf) have been shown to receive projections from the deep cerebellar nuclei. The CL nucleus projections, in particular, are widespread and include the primary motor cortex (projection not shown here). See text for references.

rior parietal projections, being directed to all aspects of the superior parietal lobule (gyral, sulcal, lateral, and medial convexities) and to the caudal aspects of the inferior parietal lobule including the lower bank of the intraparietal sulcus. The VLc projections are similar to those of VLps, although more restricted and less intense. Nucleus X projects to both the upper and lower banks of the intraparietal sulcus; and VPLo projects to both the gyral and sulcal cortices of the superior parietal lobule at the lateral convexity of the hemisphere (for references and review, please see Schmahmann and Pandya, 1990).

The second anatomic observation of some considerable interest in this discussion is the other "nonmotor" thalamic nuclei that have been shown to receive cerebellar afferents (Figure 10.11). These include the intralaminar nuclei, particularly centralis lateralis (CL), as well as the paracentralis (Pcn) and centromedian-parafascicular (CM-Pf) complex, and the medial dorsal nucleus (Ilinsky and Kultas–Ilinsky, 1987; Wiesendanger and Wiesendanger, 1985; Orioli and Strick, 1989; Thach and Jones, 1979; Stanton, 1980; Kalil, 1981; Batton et al., 1977; Strick, 1976). The CL nucleus, like other intralaminar nuclei, has widespread cortical connections including the posterior parietal cortex, the multimodal regions of the upper bank of the superior temporal sulcus, the prefrontal cortex, the cingulate gyrus, and the primary motor cortex (Kievit and

Kuypers, 1977; Yeterian and Pandya, 1985, 1989, 1991; Schmahmann and Pandya, 1990; Siwek and Pandya, 1991; Vogt et al., 1987), and the Pcn nucleus projections include the parahippocampal gyrus (Blatt, G., Rosene, D. L., Pandya, D. N., 1991, personal communication).

The cerebellar nuclei project to the medial dorsal (MD) thalamic nucleus which has generally been regarded as the major site of thalamic connections with the frontal lobe. The MD receives projections from the cerebellum mainly in its paralaminar parts, that is, in the laterally situated pars multiformis (MDmf), and more caudally in the pars densocellularis (MDdc) (Stanton, 1980; Ilinsky and Kultas-Ilinsky, 1987). The cerebellar-recipient paralaminar MDmf and MDdc have reciprocal connections with area 8, area 46 at both banks of the principal sulcus, and area 9 in the frontal lobe (for review and references please see Siwek and Pandya, 1991), but also with the cingulate gyrus, posterior parietal cortex, and multimodal parts of the superior temporal sulcus (Yeterian and Pandya, 1985; Vogt et al., 1987; Schmahmann and Pandya, 1990).

It is interesting to note that those regions of the temporal lobe that have pontine projections are also connected with cerebellar-recipient thalamic nuclei. Thus the upper bank of the superior temporal sulcus and the superior temporal regions that have pontine efferents also have reciprocal connections with the cerebellar-recipient CL, Pcn, and MDdc thalamic nuclei, as well as with VLc and VLps to a smaller extent. In contrast, the lower bank of the rostral superior temporal sulcus and the middle temporal gyrus which have no pontine connections are connected with the pulvinar medialis, suprageniculate and limitans nuclei which have no afferents from the cerebellum (Yeterian and Pandya, 1989, 1991; Schmahmann and Pandya, 1990, 1991).

The demonstration of the cortical projections from these cerebellar-recipient thalamic nuclei adds a new dimension to our understanding of the nature of the feedback from cerebellum upon the cerebral cortex. It seems to suggest a feed-forward and feedback circuit linking the cerebellum with nonmotor cerebral cortical areas, including the associative and paralimbic regions.

CONCLUSIONS AND HYPOTHESIS

MECHANISMS OF CEREBELLAR MODULATION OF HIGHER FUNCTION

The mechanisms whereby the cerebellum may influence higher-order behavior are not known. Heath (1977) expressed the view that the cerebellum could accomplish this through its influences on structures associated with expressions of emotions, feelings, levels of awareness, and motor function, whereas Keele and Ivry (1990) believe that the observations with respect to classic conditioning may be accounted for by disturbances of timing. It has been suggested that cerebellar corticonuclear microcomplexes serve as the basic functional units of the cerebellum with each microcomplex interacting with, and influencing, the extracerebellar motor or autonomic systems with which it is matched (Oscarsson, 1979; Ito, 1982). It is therefore possible to imagine that these putative mechanisms may also apply to the modulation of cognitively relevant information received from the cerebral cortex by the anatomic pathways discussed earlier. Thus, after information from the limbic system or association areas arrives in cerebellum it may be acted upon in ways we do not yet fully understand, and then be redirected in its modified form back to the brainstem, thalamus, and cerebral cortex, and so express its influence upon higher function. Experimental work in the monkey in both the sensory and motor cortexes has demonstrated the importance of cerebrocerebellar interactions in recovery from cerebellar injury (Mackel, 1987; Growdon et al., 1967). When the sensory cortex was removed subsequent to a cerebellar lesion and after recovery from the cerebellar deficits, the initially recovered cerebellar deficits became much worse again. Furthermore, removal of the sensory cortex prior to a cerebellar lesion exaggerated the cerebellar deficits and severely limited their recovery. In addition, the effects of combined sequential cerebellar and sensory cortical lesions were much worse than expected if the two lesions were merely additive. This indicated to Mackel (1987) that there was some functional interrelationship between the sensory cortex and the cerebellum that promoted compensation. These sensorimotor interrelationships with the cerebellum may serve as a paradigm for the understanding of the anatomically and physiologically defined relationships between association and paralimbic cortices and the cerebellum.

NATURE OF THE PUTATIVE CEREBELLAR CONTRIBUTION TO BEHAVIOR

The nature of the cerebellar contribution to behavior, if indeed present, remains to be determined. One possibility is that the cerebellum serves to correlate motor acts with mood states and unconscious motivation, thus facilitating nonverbal communication. It may also transpire that in the same way as the cerebellum regulates the rate, force, rhythm, and accuracy of movements, so it may regulate the speed, capacity, consistency, and appropriateness of mental or cognitive processes. It may not then be unreasonable to suggest that dysmetria of movement is matched by an unpredictability and illogic to social and societal interaction. The overshoot and inability in the motor system to check parameters of movement may thus be equated, in the cognitive realm, with a mismatch between reality and perceived reality, and erratic attempts to correct the errors of thought or behavior. Hence, perhaps, dysmetria of thought.

Frontal pseudocerebellar ataxia is a clinical entity that has long been recognized. The explanation of this phenomenon has relied upon the frontopontocerebellar pathway. It may thus be hypothesized that this system may function in reverse. That is, cerebellar lesions may result in a pseudofrontal, pseudoparietal, or even pseudotemporal lobe syndrome for reasons outlined in the anatomical discussion. The delineation of the precise neuropsychological manifestations of different cerebellar lesions therefore will be important in order to substantiate and further develop this hypothesis. The variety of multimodal projections to cerebellum from the different associative cortices may also predict and explain different syndromes arising following lesions of the cerebral cortex.

TOPOGRAPHIC ORGANIZATION OF BEHAVIORAL FUNCTIONS IN THE CEREBELLUM

Based on the clinical and experimental work discussed, the hypothesis is offered here that there is a topography within the cerebellum of these behavior-related functions. The paradigm for this localizationist approach stems from the early demonstration of the localization of different motor-related functions within the cerebellum and the resultant division of the cerebellum into three major areas. The archicerebellum in conjunction with the vermis and fastigial nucleus is responsible for the control of equilibrium and posture; the paravermal regions receiving input from spinal cord centers coordinate truncal posture and gait and integrate spinal sensory mechanisms with the control of movement; and the neocerebellar regions and their outflow dentate nucleus are involved in the coordination of rapid movements of the extremities (Larsell, 1937; Brodal, 1981). This tripartite subdivision of motor-related cerebellar function remains in clinical use, although the concept has undergone some elaboration with the description of anatomically and connectionally definable parasagittal zones within the cerebellar cortex and white matter (Voogd, 1964; Dore et al., 1990).

In the current schema it is postulated that the cerebellar contribution to higher function may also be organized in a mediolateral manner, with different types of behavioral activity being modulated by different cerebellar regions. Thus, the older cerebellar regions consisting of the flocculonodular lobe, vermis and associated fastigial, and, to a lesser degree, globose nuclei, could perhaps be considered as the equivalent of the limbic cerebellum. These regions would then be concerned with primitive defense mechanisms including the autonomic manifestations of the fight or flight response, as well as with emotion, affect, and sexuality, and possibly also with affectively important memory. This would provide a partial explanation of the vermal or midline cerebellar nuclear abnormalities in autism, schizophrenia, and some patients with psychosis. It would also be in agreement with experiments by Berman et al. (1973) on aggressive monkeys, and the sham rage, predatory attack, and pleasure seeking behavior elicited by manipulation of the vermis or fastigial nuclei in other experimental animals. In contrast, it is hypothesized that the lateral cerebellar hemispheres and their associated dentate and emboliform nuclei have different functional properties. It is suggested that these areas may be concerned with the modulation of thought, planning, strategy formation, spatial and temporal parameters, learning, memory, and perhaps language.

RELEVANCE TO AUTISM

The experimental and behavioral observations described in this chapter do not explain the reasons for the existence of cerebellar findings in early infantile autism. They do, however, allow these observations to be seen in a novel context. In this view, the absence of cerebellar motor abnormalities in autism does not automatically imply that the observed histologic abnormalities of the cerebellum are of no consequence. Rather, the cerebellar abnormalities may be considered as representing an abnormality in one component of a neural network underlying the appropriate modulation and organization of higher order behavior including emotion, language, societal interaction, and appropriate psychological behavior. The findings in autism provide important neuropathologic support for the notion that behavioral or psychiatric conditions may be associated with cerebellar pathology. It is argued here that these findings are not simply epiphenomena but may be seen as contributing to the clinical manifestations. The cerebellar nuclear abnormalities may contribute to the affective disturbances in autism, and the lateral and inferior cerebellar pathology may be linked with the delay in language development and the inappropriate social and psychological reaction patterns. In this vein, it has been postulated that the cerebellar abnormalities render patients incapable of coordinating voluntary shifts of attention, thereby compromising their ability to engage in joint social attention and to participate in social communication (Courchesne, 1987).

FUTURE DIRECTIONS

The hypothesis concerning the topographic organization of the putative contribution of the cerebellum to higher-order behavior is offered as a framework in an attempt to better understand the functions of the cerebellum. This framework needs to be tested by clinical and clinicopathological studies, as well as by physiologic, anatomic, and behavioral investigations in the laboratory. It will be useful to evaluate the pathology of neuropsychiatric conditions not previously felt to be related to the cerebellum, as has been done in autism. Conversely, it will be helpful to determine whether diseases of the cerebellum that may be associated with behavioral or cognitive abnormalities can also be shown to demonstrate neuropathologic changes in other behaviorally relevant areas, such as hippocampus or association cortexes. It is also critically important to re-evaluate altered behavior patterns in diseases of the cerebellum such as those observed in stroke, or following discrete surgical removal of parts of the cerebellum, or in well-documented instances of degenerative diseases shown to be confined to the cerebellum. This would help ascertain whether the disturbed behaviors are a result of the cerebellar lesions, or whether they are merely epiphenomena. Further investigation with PET scanning of cerebellar activation by nonmotor tasks will be helpful in testing the hypotheses discussed here, and in defining the nature and extent of the cerebellar involvement in cognitive processes.

Anatomic studies should continue to be directed at the further delineation of the channels of communication in the cerebrocerebellar feed-forward and feed-back loops. A greater understanding of the prefrontopontine connections is awaited. The question of overlap in the pontine nuclei of projections from different cortical areas has relevance for the concept of multimodal convergence in the pons. There is need for greater precision in the understanding of the pontocerebellar pathway in the monkey. Exactly which cerebellar areas receive projections from precisely which pontine nuclei? What is the detailed relationship between the architectonically defined association areas of the cerebral cortex, the pontine nuclei, and the cerebellum? Is there a relationship between the recently defined parasagittal zones in cerebellum and the corticopontine projection? How do the nonspecific thalamic nuclei differ from the motor thalamic nuclei with respect to the origin of their cerebellar afferents?

Physiological studies are needed to address the functional properties of the pontine nuclei, as defined now by architectonic as well as geographic location in the basilar pons. Are neurons in the basis pontis responsive to stimuli dependant upon cognitive processing or emotional valence? It would be valuable to use contemporary physiologic techniques to perform simultaneous electrode recording in the cerebellum, cerebral cortex, and other regions such as thalamus or limbic cortexes in order to evaluate functional interactions between these areas in tasks that study, for example, visuospatial, attentional, or motivational behaviors. It would also be of great interest to perform behavioral studies in nonhuman primates subjected to ablative procedures of the cerebellum, or, as suggested by Dr. Hans Kuypers (personal communication, 1987), to perform ablative procedures of the middle cerebellar peduncle in order to evaluate the behavior of an animal deprived of its neocortical input.

ACKNOWLEDGMENTS

The author gratefully acknowledges the ongoing support, encouragement, and collaboration of Deepak N. Pandya, M.D., in pursuing the studies described herein. Dr. Pandya and Anne B. Young, M.D., Ph.D., critically reviewed the manuscript. The technical assistance of Ms. Mary Chiavaras is much appreciated.

REFERENCES

Aas, J. E, and Brodal, P. 1988. Demonstration of topographically organized projections from the hypothalamus to the pontine nuclei: An experimental study in the cat. *Journal of Comparative Neurology* 268:313–28.

Akshoomoff, N. A., and Courchesne, E. 1992. A new role for the cerebellum in cognitive operations. *Behavioral Neuroscience.* 106:731–38.

Allen, G. I., and Tsukuhara, N. 1974. Cerebrocerebellar communication systems. *Physiological Reviews.* 54:957–1008.

Anand, B. K., Malhotra, C. L., Singh, B., and Dua, S. 1959. Cerebellar projections to the limbic system. *Journal of Neurophysiology* 22:451–58.

Ball, G., Micco, D., Jr., and Berntson, G. 1974. Cerebellar stimulation in the rat: Complex stimulation bound oral behaviors and self-stimulation. *Physiology and Behavior* 13:123–27.

Barbas, H., and Pandya, D. N. 1989. Architecture and intrinsic connections of the prefrontal cortex in rhesus monkey. *Journal of Comparative Neurology* 286:353–75.

Batton, R. R., III, Jayaraman, A., Ruggiero, D., and Carpenter, M. B. 1977. Fastigial efferent projections in the monkey: An autoradiographic study. *Journal of Comparative Neurology* 174:281–306.

Berger, T. W., Weikart, C. L., Bassett, J. L., and Orr, W. B. 1986. Lesions of the retrosplenial cortex produce deficits in reversal learning of the rabbit nictitating membrane response: Implications for potential interactions between hippocampal and cerebellar brain systems. *Behavioral Neuroscience* 100:802–9.

Berman, A. F., Berman, D., and Prescott, J. W. 1973. The effect of cerebellar lesions on emotional behavior in the rhesus monkey. In I. S. Cooper, M. Riklan, and R. S. Snider, eds. *The Cerebellum, Epilepsy and Behavior.* 277–84. New York: Plenum Press.

Berntson, G., Potolicchio, S., Jr., and Miller, N. 1973. Evidence for higher functions of the cerebellum: Eating and grooming elicited by cerebellar stimulation in cats. *Proceedings of the National Academy of Sciences* 70:2497–99.

Botez, M. I., Gravel, J., Attig, E., and Vezina, J.-L. 1985. Reversible chronic cerebellar ataxia after phenytoin intoxication: Possible role of cerebellum in cognitive thought. *Neurology* 35:1152–57.

Botez, M. I., Botez, T., Elie, R., and Attig, E. 1989. Role of the cerebellum in complex human behavior. *Italian Journal of Neurological Science* 10:291–300.

Brodal, A. 1981. *Neurological Anatomy in Relation to Clinical Medicine.* Third edition. New York: Oxford University Press.

Brodal, P. 1978. The corticopontine projection in the rhesus monkey. *Brain* 101:251–83.

Brodal, P. 1979. The pontocerebellar projection in the rhesus monkey: An experimental study with retrograde axonal transport of horseradish peroxidase. *Neuroscience* 4:193–208.

Brodal, P. 1982. Further observations on the cerebellar projections from the pontine nuclei and the nucleus reticularis tegmenti pontis in the rhesus monkey. *Journal of Comparative Neurology* 204:44–55.

Brodal, P. 1987. Organization of cerebropontocerebellar connections as studied with anterograde and retrograde transport of HRP-WGA in the cat. *New Concepts in Cerebellar Neurobiology* 151–82. Ed. JS King. New York. Liss Publisher.

Brodmann, K. 1909. *Vergleichende Lokalisationslehre der Grosshirnrinde in inhren Prinzipien dargestellt auf Grund des Zellenbaues.* Leipzig: J.A. Barth, 1909, xii.

Cambier, J., Graveleau, P., Decroix, J. P., Elghozi, D., and Masson, M. 1983. Le syndrome de l'artère choroïdienne antérieure étude neuropsychologique de 4 cas. *Revue Neurologique (Paris)* 139:553–59.

Cooper, I. S., Riklan, M., Amin, I., and Cullinan, T. 1978. A long-term follow-up study of cerebellar stimulation for the control of epilepsy in man. In I. S. Cooper, ed. *Cerebellar Stimulation in Man.* 19–38. New York: Plenum Press.

Courchesne, E. 1987. Neurophysiological View of Autism. In E. Schopler and G.B. Mesibov, eds. *Neurobiological Issues in Autism* 285–324. New York: Plenum Press.

De Vito, J. L., and Smith, O. A. 1964. Subcortical projections of the prefrontal lobe of the monkey. *Journal of Comparative Neurology* 123:413–24.

Dempsey, C. W., Tootle, D. M., Fontana, C. J., Fitzjarrell, A. T., Garey, R. E., and Heath, R. G. 1983. Stimulation of the paleocerebellar cortex of the cat: increased rate of synthesis and release of catecholamines at limbic sites. *Biological Psychiatry.* 18:127–32.

Desimone, R., and Ungerleider, L. G. 1989. Neural mechanisms of visual processing in monkeys. In Boller, F., J. Grafman, eds. 267–99. *Handbook of Neuropsychology,* Vol. 2. Elsevier, NY.

Dore, L., Jacobson, C. D., and Hawkes, R. 1990. Organization and postnatal development of Zebrin II antigenic compartmentation in the cerebellar vermis of the grey opossum, Monodelphis domestica. *Journal of Comparative Neurology* 291:431–49.

Frankfurter, A., Weber, J. T., and Harting, J. K. 1977. Brain stem projections to lobule VII of the posterior vermis in the squirrel monkey: As demonstrated by the retrograde axonal transport of tritiated horseradish peroxidase. *Brain Research* 124:135–39.

Glickstein, M., May, J. G., and Mercier, B. E. 1985. Corticopontine projection in the macaque: The distribution of labelled cortical cells after large injections of horseradish peroxidase in the pontine nuclei. *Journal of Comparative Neurology* 235:343–59.

Goldberg, G. 1985. Supplementary motor area structure and function: Review and hypotheses. *Behavioral Brain Science* 8:567–616.

Growdon, J. H., Chamber, W. W., and Liu, C. N. 1967. An experimental study of cerebellar dyskinesia in the rhesus monkey. *Brain* 90:603–32.

Haines, D. E., and Dietrichs, E. 1984. An HRP study of hgypothalamo-cerebellar and cerebello-hypothalamic connections in squirrel monkey (Saimiri sciureus). *Journal of Comparative Neurology* 229:559–75.

Heath, R. G., Franklin, D. E., and Shraberg, D. 1979. Gross pathology of the cerebellum in patients diagnosed and treated as functional psychiatric disorders. *Journal of Nervous and Mental Disorders* 167:585–92.

Heath, R. J. 1977. Modulation of emotion with a brain pacemaker. *Journal of Nervous and Mental Disorders.* 165:300–317.

Helgason, C., Caplan, L. R., Goodwin, J., and Hedges, T., III. 1986. Anterior choroidal artery-territory infarction. Report of cases and review. *Archives of Neurology* 43:681–86.

Hoddevik, G. H., Brodal, A., Kawamura, K., and Hashikawa, T. 1977. The pontine projection to the cerebellar vermal visual area studied by means of the retrograde axonal transport of horseradish peroxidase. *Brain Research* 123:209–27.

Hommel, M., Dubois, F., Pollak, P., Francois, A., Borgel, F., Gaio, J. M., Pellat, J., and Perret, J. 1985. Syndrome de l'artere choroidienne anterieure gauche avec troubles du langage et apraxie constructive. *Revue Neurologique (Paris)* 141:137–42.

Hyvarinen, J. 1982. *The Parietal Cortex of Monkey and Man.* Berlin: Springer-Verlag.

Ilinsky, I. A., and Kultas-Ilinsky, K. 1987. Sagittal cytoarchitectonic maps of Macaca mulatta thalamus with a revised nomenclature of the motor-related nuclei validated by observations on their connectivity. *Journal of Comparative Neurology* 262:331–64.

Ito, M. 1982. Questions in modelling the cerebellum. *Journal of Theoretical Biology* 99:81–86.

Kaada, B. R. 1972. The neurobiology of the amygdala. In Eleftheriou, B.E., ed. 205–81. *Advances in Behavioral Biology, Vol. II.* New York: Plenum Press.

Kalil, K. 1981. Projections of the cerebellar and dorsal column nuclei upon the thalamus of the rhesus monkey. *Journal of Comparative Neurology* 195:25–50.

Keele, S. W., and Ivry, R. 1990. Does the cerebellum provide a common computation for diverse tasks? In E. Diamond, ed. The development and neural bases of higher cognitive functions. *Annals of the New York Academy of Sciences.* 608:179–211.

Kievit, J., and Kuypers, H.G.J.M. 1977. Organization of the thalamocortical connections to the frontal lobe in the rhesus monkey. *Experimental Brain Research* 29:299–322.

Kish, S. J., El-Awar Schut, M., Leach, L., Oscar-Berman, M., and Freedman, M. 1988. Cognitive deficits in olivopontocerebellar atrophy: Implications for the cholinergic hypothesis of Alzheimer's dementia. *Annals of Neurology* 24:200–206.

Künzle, H., and Akert, K. 1977. Efferent connections of cortical area 8 (frontal eye field) in Macaca fascicularis. A reinvestigation using the autoradiographic technique. *Journal of Comparative Neurology* 173:147–64.

Kuypers, H.G.J.M., and Lawrence, D. G. 1967. Cortical projections to the red nucleus and the brainstem in the rhesus monkey. *Brain Research* 4:151–88.

Lalonde, R., Manseau, M., and Botez, M. I. 1987. Spontaneous alternation and habituation in Purkinje cell degeneration in mutant mice. *Brain Research* 411:187–89.

Larsell, O. 1937. The cerebellum: A review and interpretation. *Archives of Neurology and Psychiatry* 38:580–607.

Leaton, R. N., and Supple, W. F. 1986. Cerebellar vermis: Essential for long-term habituation of the acoustic startle response. *Science* 232:513–15.

Leiner, H. C., Leiner, A. L., and Dow, R. S. 1986. Does the cerebellum contribute to mental skills? *Behavioral Neuroscience* 100:443–54.

Mackel, R. 1987. The role of the monkey sensory cortex in the recovery from cerebellar injury. *Experimental Brain Research.* 66:638–52.

Marcinkiewicz, M., Morcos, R., and Chretien, M. 1989. CNS connections with the median raphe nucleus: Retrograde tracing with WGA-apoHRP-gold complex in the rat. *Journal of Comparative Neurology* 289:11–35.

Martner, J. 1975. Cerebellar influences on autonomic mechanisms. *Acta Physiologica Scandanavica* (Suppl.) 425:1–42.

Masson, M., Decroix, J. P., Henin, D., Dairou, R., Graveleau, P., and Cambier, J. 1983. Syndrome de l'artere choroidienne anterieure etude clinique et tomodensitometrique de 4 cas. *Revue Neurologique (Paris)* 139:547–52.

May, J. G., Keller, E. L., and Suzuki, D. A. 1988. Smooth-pursuit eye movement deficits with chemical lesions in the dorsolateral pontine nucleus of the monkey. *Journal of Neurophysiology* 59:952–77.

Mesulam, M.-M. 1985. *Principles of Behavioral Neurology.* Philadelphia: F.A. Davis Co. 405.

Metter, E. J., Kempler, D., Jackson, C. A., Hanson, W. R., Riege, W. H., Camras, L. R., Mazziotta, J. C., and Phelps, M. E. 1987. Cerebellar glucose metabolism in chronic aphasia. *Neurology* 37:1599–1606.

Mishkin, M., Ungerleider, L. G., and Macko, K. A. 1983. Object vision and spatial vision: Two cortical pathways. *Trends in Neuroscience.* 6:414–17.

Molinari, M., Petrosini, L., Dell'Anna, M. E., and Gianetti, S. 1991. Hemicerebellectomy induces spatial memory deficits in rats. *Society for Neuroscience Abstracts* 17:919.

Moruzzi, G. 1947. Sham rage and localized autonomic responses elicited by cerebellar stimulation in the acute thalamic cat. *Proceedings of the XVII International Congress of Physiology.* Oxford: 114–15.

Mustari, M. J., Fuchs, A. F., and Wallman, J. 1988. Response properties of dorsolateral pontine units during smooth pursuit in the rhesus macaque. *Journal of Neurophysiology* 60:664–86.

Nadel, L. 1991. The hippocampus and space revisited. *Hippocampus* 1:221–29.

Nyby, O., and Jansen, J. 1951. An experimental investigation of the corticopontine projection in macaca mulatta. *Skrifter utgitt av det Norske Vedenskapsakademie: Oslo; 1. Mat. Naturv. Klasse* 3:1–47.

Olszewski, J. 1952. *The Thalamus of the Macaca Mulatta.* Basel: S. Karger.

Orioli, P. J., and Strick, P. L. 1989. Cerebellar connections with the motor cortex and the arcuate premotor area: An analysis employing retrograde transneuronal transport of WGA-HRP. *Journal of Comparative Neurology* 288:621–26.

Oscarsson, O. 1979. Functional units of the cerebellum—sagittal zones and microzones. *Trends in Neuroscience.* 2:143–45.

Pandya, D. N., and Seltzer, B. 1982. Intrinsic connections and architectorics of posterior parietal cortex in the Rhesus monkey. *Journal of Comparative Neurology* 204: 196–210.

Pandya, D. N., and Yeterian, E. H. 1985. Architecture and connections of cortical association areas. In A. Peters and E.G. Jones, (eds.) *Cerebral Cortex. Volume 4.* New York: Plenum Press, pp. 3–61.

Pandya, D. N., and Yeterian, E. H. 1991. Prefrontal cortex in relation to other cortical areas in rhesus monkey: Architecture and connections. *Progress in Brain Research.* 85:63–94.

Pandya, D. N., Seltzer, B., and Barbas, H. 1988. Input-output organization of the primate cerebral cortex. In H.D. Steklis and J. Erwin, eds. *Comparative Primate Biology, Vol. 4: Neurosciences.* 39–80. New York: Alan R. Liss, Inc.

Pantano, P., Baron, J. C., Samson, Y., Bousser, M. G., Derouesne, C., and Comar, D. 1986. Crossed cerebellar diaschisis: Further studies. *Brain* 109:677–94.

Peters, M., and Monjan, A. A. 1971. Behavior after cerebellar lesions in cats and monkeys. *Physiology and Behavior.* 6:205–6.

Petersen, S. E., and Fiez, J. A. 1993. The processing of single words studied with positron emission tomography. *Annual Review of Neuroscience.* 16:509–30.

Petersen, S. E., Fox, P. T., Posner, M. I., Mintum, M. A., and Raichle, M. E. 1989. Positron emission tomographic studies of the processing of single words. *Journal of Cognitive Neuroscience.* 1:153–70.

Reiman, E. M., Raichle, M. E., Robins, E., Mintum, M. A., Fusselman, M. J., Fox, P. T., Price, J. L., and Hackman, K. A. 1989. Neuroanatomical correlates of a lactate-induced anxiety attack. *Archives of General Psychiatry* 46:493–500.

Reis, D. J., Doba, N., and Nathan, M. A. 1973. Predatory attack, grooming and consummatory behaviors evoked by electrical stimulation of cat cerebellar nuclei. *Science* 182:845–47.

Robinson, F. R., Cohen, J. L., May, J., Sestokas, A. K., and Glickstein, M. 1984. Cerebellar targets of visual pontine cells in the cat. *Journal of Comparative Neurology* 223:471–82.

Sanes, J. N., Dimitrov, B., and Hallett, M. 1990. Motor learning in patients with cerebellar dysfunction. *Brain* 113:103–20.

Schell, G. R., and Strick, P. L. 1984. The origin of thalamic inputs to the arcuate premotor and supplementary motor areas. *Journal of Neuroscience.* 4:539–60.

Schmahmann, J. D. 1991. An emerging concept: The cerebellar contribution to higher function. *Archives of Neurology* 48:1178–87.

Schmahmann, J. D. 1992. The neuropsychology of the cerebellum—an emerging concept. Reply. *Archives of Neurology* 49:1230.

Schmahmann, J. D., and Pandya, D. N. 1989. Anatomical investigation of projections to the basis pontis from posterior parietal association cortices in rhesus monkey. *Journal of Comparative Neurology* 289:53–73.

Schmahmann, J. D., and Pandya, D. N. 1990. Anatomical investigation of projections from thalamus to the posterior parietal association cortices in rhesus monkey. *Journal of Comparative Neurology* 295:299–326.

Schmahmann, J. D., and Pandya, D. N. 1991. Projections to the basis pontis from the superior temporal sulcus and superior temporal region in the rhesus monkey. *Journal of Comparative Neurology* 308:224–48.

Schmahmann, J. D., and Pandya, D. N. 1992. Course of the fiber pathways to the pons from parasensory association cortices in rhesus monkey. *Journal of Comparative Neurology* 326:159–79.

Schmahmann, J. D., and Pandya, D. N. 1993a. Prefrontopontine projections in the Rhesus monkey. *Society for Neuroscience Abstracts.* 19:1210.

Schmahmann, J. D., and Pandya, D. N. 1993b. Prelunate, occipitotemporal, and parahippocampal projections to the basis pontis in Rhesus monkey. *Journal of Comparative Neurology.* 337:94–112.

Seltzer, B., and Pandya, D. N. 1978. Afferent cortical connections and architectonics of the superior temporal sulcus and surrounding cortex in the Rhesus monkey. *Brain Research* 149:1–24.

Seltzer, B., and Pandya, D. N. 1989. Intrinsic connections and architectonics of the superior temporal sulcus in the Rhesus monkey. *Journal of Comparative Neurology* 290:451–71.

Shook, B. L., Schlag-Rey, M., and Schlag, J. 1990. Primate supplementary eye field: I. Comparative aspects of mesencephalic and pontine connections. *Journal of Comparative Neurology* 301:618–42.

Siwek, D. F., and Pandya, D. N. 1991. Prefrontal projections to the mediodorsal nucleus of the thalamus in the rhesus monkey. *Journal of Comparative Neurology* 312:509–24.

Snider, R. S., and Maiti, A. 1976. Cerebellar contribution to the Papez circuit. *Journal of Neuroscience Research.* 2:133–46.

Stanton, G. B. 1980. Topographical organization of ascending cerebellar projections from the dentate and interposed nuclei in Macaca mulatta: An anterograde degeneration study. *Journal of Comparative Neurology* 190:699–731.

Stanton, G. B., Goldberg, M. E., and Bruce, C. J. 1988a. Frontal eye field efferents in the macaque monkey: I. Subcortical pathways and topography of striatal and thalamic terminal fields. *Journal of Comparative Neurology* 271:473–92.

Stanton, G. B., Goldberg, M. E., and Bruce, C. J. 1988b. Frontal eye field efferents in the macaque monkey: II. Topography of terminal fields in midbrain and pons. *Journal of Comparative Neurology* 271:493–506.

Strick, P. L. 1976. Anatomical analysis of ventrolateral thalamic input to primate motor cortex. *Journal of Neurophysiology* 39:1020–1031.

Stuss, D. T., and Benson, D. F. 1986. *The Frontal Lobes.* New York: Raven Press.

Thach, W. T., and Jones, E. G. 1973. The cerebellar dentatothalamic connection: Terminal field, lamellae, rods and somatotopy. *Brain Research* 169:168–72.

Thier, P., and Koehler, W. 1987. Morphology, number, and distribution of putative GABA-ergic neurons in the basilar pontine gray of the monkey. *Journal of Comparative Neurology* 265:311–22.`

Thompson, R. F. 1988. The neural basis of basic associative learning of discrete behavioral responses. *Trends in Neuroscience.* 11:152–55.

Ungerleider, L. G., Desimone, R., Galkin, T. W., and Mishkin, M. 1984. Subcortical projections of area MT in the macaque. *Journal of Comparative Neurology* 223:368–86.

Van Essen, D. C. 1985. Functional organization of primate visual cortex. In A. Peters, and E. G. Jones, eds. *Cerebral Cortex, Volume 3.* 259–329. New York: Plenum.

Vilensky, J. A., and Van Hoesen, G. W. 1981. Corticopontine projections from the cingulate cortex in the rhesus monkey. *Brain Research* 205:391–95.

Vogt, B. A., Pandya, D. N., and Rosene, D. L. 1987. Cingulate cortex of the rhesus monkey: I. Cytoarchitecture and thalamic afferents. *Journal of Comparative Neurology* 262:256–70.

Voogd, J. 1964. *The Cerebellum of the Cat.* Thesis. Assen: Van Gorcum.

Wiesendanger, R., Wiesendanger, M., and Ruegg, D. G. 1979. An anatomical investigation of the corticopontine projection in the primate (macaca fascicularis and saimiri sciureus): II. The projection from frontal and parietal association areas. *Neuroscience.* 4:747.

Yeterian, E. H., and Pandya, D. N. 1985. Corticothalamic connections of the posterior parietal cortex in the rhesus monkey. *Journal of Comparative Neurology.* 237:408–26.

Yeterian, E. H., and Pandya, D. N. 1989. Thalamic connections of the cortex of the superior temporal sulcus in the rhesus monkey. *Journal of Comparative Neurology* 282:80–97.

Yeterian, E. H., and Pandya, D. N. 1991. Corticothalamic connections of the superior temporal sulcus in rhesus monkeys. *Experimental Brain Research.* 83:268–84.

Zanchetti, A., and Zoccolini, A. 1954. Autonomic hypothalamic outbursts elicited by cerebellar stimulation. *Journal of Neurophysiology* 17:473–83.

11

STUDIES ON THE NEUROCHEMISTRY OF AUTISM

George M. Anderson, Ph.D.

Neurochemical research on autism has been performed for more than thirty years. Although few replicated neurochemical alterations have been observed, it has become increasingly apparent that a biologic basis underlies the altered behavior and development seen in individuals with autism. The early onset, pervasive nature, and chronicity of autism clearly point to brain abnormality. Twin and family studies strongly suggest that autism has a genetic basis (Rutter and Schopler, 1989; Young et al., 1989; Folstein and Piven, 1991; see also Chap. 2).

Given the apparent presence of an inherited brain alteration in autism, it is understandable that a range of neurobiologic approaches have been employed in attempting to understand the etiology and pathobiology of autism. The neurochemical research has proceeded in parallel with work in the areas of neuropharmacology, neuropathology (see Chap. 7), neuroimaging (see Chaps. 4–5), neurophysiology (see Chap. 3), and neuroimmunology. The different approaches have at times complemented one another and have served to inform and direct research in many areas.

This chapter will be concerned with the neurochemical research on the monoamine neurotransmitters and the neuropeptides. To date, the neurochemical approach has been most influenced by neuropharmacologic observations. The relevant neuropharmacologic research, as well as pertinent findings from the other areas of neurobiologic research, will be discussed when the rationale for studying each neurotransmitter is considered.

Strong cases can be made for the possible involvement of the monoamines, dopamine, norepinephrine, and serotonin, and the neuropeptides, such as opioids, in autism. The arguments are based mainly on observations of drug actions and the specific nature of the behavioral abnormalities present in autism. However, practical limitations concerning the types of measurement available have tended to limit the field of neurochemical inquiry. In addition, issues of diagnosis and subtyping have hindered the neurochemical research because it has not always been clear just how comparable and homogeneous different subject groups have been.

Finally, when discussing the rational basis for the neurochemical research, some mention of the underlying, often implicit, disease model is necessary. Much of the research appears to assume that there exists some final common pathway that causes a relatively consistent, although certainly not invariable, phenomenology. From this perspective, various trauma and inherited diatheses lead to etiologic alterations and subsequent pathobiologies, which tend to converge on systems critical to behavior that is disturbed in autism. An alternative view sees the traumatic perinatal complications sometimes associated with autism as epiphenomena related to the inherited defect. In this model a range of divergent phenotypes with varying cognitive, behavioral, and motoric aspects can arise from a single genotype.

The logical consequences of the opposing models are distinct. In the convergent model, one would hope to study those neurochemical systems that are involved at a relatively forward point in the pathobiology. Measurements made on systems not part of the final common pathway, unless very carefully related to individual history, would not reveal consistent changes in the autistic group. Conversely, the divergent model suggests that systems involved at the first stages of pathobiology would be most fruitfully studied. In all probability, the actual situation is quite complicated with a number of different genotypes, some with varying expression, as well as different insults and agents, which lead to autistic behavior.

As data from studies of inheritance and of other areas of biologic research continue to be amassed, the neurochemical studies will become more rational. It is clear that the lack of clarity regarding the genetic basis and the phenomenology of autism have handicapped the neurochemical studies performed to date. Bearing this in mind, we will review, in turn, the research on the monoamines and neuropeptides, emphasizing those areas where significant differences have been seen between autistic and control groups. We will attempt to update the research, and refer the reader to several previous reviews in this area for more complete coverage of the earlier studies (Young et al., 1982; Yuwiler et al., 1985; Anderson, 1987; Anderson and Hoshino, 1987).

DOPAMINE

Animal studies have clearly shown that dopamine neurons mediate behaviors, such as hyperactivity and stereotypies, which are often seen in autistic individuals (Moore and Bloom, 1978). Dopamine blocking agents, including the phenothiazines and haloperidol, have often proven useful for ameliorating these and other behaviors in autistic patients. In addition to this somewhat tenuous behavioral and pharmacologic evidence, the dopamine hypothesis in schizophrenia has also tended to link autism and dopamine in a round-about way.

Central dopamine functioning has been assessed in humans by postmortem studies, receptor imaging studies, neuroendocrine challenge protocols, and neurochemical measurements in bodily fluids. Much of the neurochemical research in autism has involved the measurement of the major dopamine metabolite, homovanillic acid (HVA), in urine, plasma, and cerebrospinal fluid (CSF). There are several reports of increased urinary excretion of HVA in groups of autistic individuals (see Anderson, 1987; Minderaa et al., 1989, for reviews). However, in our study of plasma and urine HVA, plasma prolactin, and urine dopamine, we found no significant differences between autistic and control groups (Minderaa et al., 1989). The normal plasma and urine metabolite data do not support the hypothesis of increased control dopamine turnover in autism. The observation of normal levels of plasma prolactin suggests that dopaminergic neurons of the tuberoinfundibular system, which exert inhibitory control on prolactin release, are unaltered in autism. Conclusions based on the HVA measurements are limited, as only about 25 percent of plasma and urine HVA appears to be derived from central dopamine turnover. Also, the peripheral measures would be capable of detecting only widespread and marked alterations in brain dopamine metabolism.

A series of studies measuring CSF HVA have been carried out and are summarized in Figure 11.1. The first studies employed probenecid to increase CSF levels of HVA by blocking the egress of acid metabolites from the CSF. Subsequent studies measured the lower levels usually present when probenecid is not used. The studies of Gillberg and colleagues (1983, 1987) indicated that group mean levels of CSF HVA were elevated approximately 50 percent in autistic subjects. However, two other studies both found normal levels of CSF HVA in autism (Ross et al., 1985; Narayan et al., 1993), which is in agreement with the earlier studies of Cohen and colleagues (1974, 1977).

At this point, it can be concluded that no replicated, significant differences have been seen between autistic and control subjects for the various neurochemical indexes of dopamine functioning.

NOREPINEPHINE

Norepinephine (NE), or noradrenaline, is an important neurotransmitter both in the brain and in the sympathetic nervous system. Central noradrenergic neurons have their cell bodies in the hindbrain and project

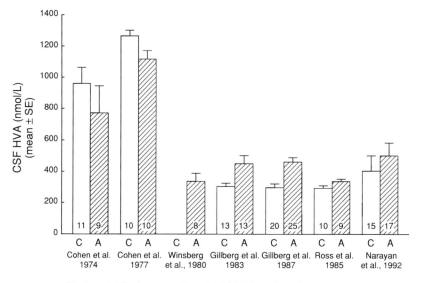

Figure 11.1. Studies of CSF homovanillic acid (HVA) in autism. Mean levels reported from control (C) and autistic (A) subjects are shown; the number of subjects studied is given within the bar.

throughout the brain (Araral and Sinnamon, 1977). Their critical role in arousal, stress response, and anxiety (Iversen and Iversen, 1985) has prompted suggestions that their functioning might be altered in autism. Treatment studies with clonidine and desipramine have also indicated that the noradrenergic system may play a role in certain autistic symptoms (Gordon et al., 1992; Fankhauser et al., 1992).

Because central and peripheral noradrenergic systems are tightly coupled, the measurement of NE and its metabolites in plasma and urine afford a fairly good perspective on central functioning (Schildkraut et al., 1978). The major central metabolite of NE, 3-methoxy-4-hydroxyphenyl-glycol (MHPG), and the predominant peripheral metabolite, vanillyl-mandilic acid (VMA), as well as NE itself, have been measured in plasma and urine. Several early studies indicated that group differences might exist, with reports of lower urinary NE and MHPG excretion, and another of increased plasma NE, in autism (see Anderson, 1987, for review). However, these and other reported differences have not been replicated. In our large study of plasma MHPG, and urinary NE, MHPG, and VMA, we saw no group differences between autistic and control subjects (Minderaa et al., 1993). In addition, the normal pattern of increased daytime versus nighttime excretion of NE was also seen in the autistic group.

The plasma and urine data strongly suggest that both central and peripheral noradrenergic functioning is unaltered in autism. The conclusion is further supported by the two reported studies of CSF MHPG (Young et al., 1981; Gillberg et al., 1987), both of which found normal CSF levels of MHPG in the autistic group.

SEROTONIN

Serotonin, or 5-hydroxytryptamine (5-HT), is the one neurotransmitter that has stimulated the most neurochemical research in autism. Initial interest in the possible role of 5-HT in autism arose from a consideration of its role in perception. The powerful effects of serotonergic hallucinogens, such as lysergic acid diethylamide (LSD), stimulated speculation around 5-HT and led to early studies of platelet 5-HT in autism (Schain and Freedman, 1961; Woolley, 1962). Although much of the work has focused on the platelet hyperserotonemia of autism, first reported in 1961 by Schain and Freedman, a number of other observations have contributed to the increasing interest in 5-HT. Reports of a critical role for 5-HT during embryogenesis (Buznikov, 1984), and in the development of the central nervous system (Lauder and Krebs, 1986; Whitaker-Aemitia et al., 1987; Zhou et al., 1987; Mayford et al., 1992) have made 5-HT of special interest in the developmental disorders such as autism. The reported (Todd and Ciarenello, 1985) presence of autoantibodies to the 5-HT$_{1A}$ receptor in autistic individuals—though not yet replicated (see Yuwiler et al., 1992)—is of particular interest, given the 5HT$_{1A}$-mediated secretion of nerve growth factors (Whitaker-Azmitia et al., 1992).

Early studies of serotonergic drugs as possible therapeutic agents were not particularly promising. More recently, the 5-HT-releasing agent fenfluramine, despite initial enthusiasm, has not been found to be of much use in treating autistic symptoms (Campbell et al., 1990). However, in the past several years a number of small treatment studies of 5-HT selective reuptake inhibitors—including clomipramine, fluvoxamine, and fluoxetine—have suggested that manipulation of the serotonergic system may be of some benefit (McDougle et al., 1990; Todd, 1991; Gordon et al., 1992; Markowitz, 1992).

Assessing central 5-HT functioning through peripheral measurements is especially difficult due to the large amounts of 5-HT produced in the enterochromaffin cells of the intestine. Although brain 5-HT is metabolized to 5-hydroxyindoleacetic acid (5-HIAA), virtually all of the 5HIAA present in plasma and urine is derived from 5-HT produced by the intestine with relatively little brain derived 5HIAA entering the circulation. Neurochemical assessment of brain 5-HT functioning has therefore depended upon CSF measurements and neuroendocrine challenge studies.

As seen in Figure 11.2, the studies of CSF 5-HIAA have been consistent in showing no differences between autistic and control groups

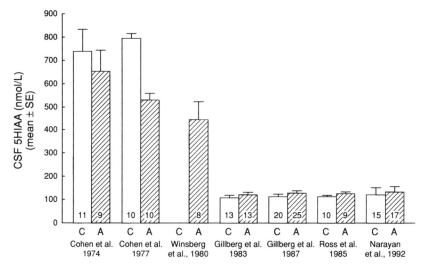

Figure 11.2. Studies of CSF 5-hydroxyindoleacetic acid (5-HIAA) in autism. Mean levels reported for control (C) and autistic (A) subjects are shown; the number of subjects studied is given within the bar.

(Narayan et al., 1992). These observations suggest that if a central 5-HT abnormality is present in autism it does not involve a widespread and marked change in 5-HT turnover. The CSF studies, therefore, are not necessarily in conflict with neuroendocrine challenge studies, which have observed relatively smaller fenfluramine-induced release of prolactin in autism (McBride et al., 1989). The neuroendocrine results are intriguing, both in terms of what central differences might be responsible for the blunted response and because of a possible link between the central abnormality and the platelet hyperserotonemia of autism.

The research on the hyperserotonemia can be grouped into three main areas. Most of the studies have involved replicating the hyperserotonemia and further characterizing the basic observation. A second area of research includes studies on the synthesis and catabolism of peripheral 5-HT. These studies bear on the important issue of whether the platelet elevation is due to an increased exposure of the platelet to 5-HT. A final group of studies have investigated the platelet itself in the hopes of finding a platelet alteration responsible for the increased storage of 5-HT. We will review the research in these three areas in some detail, with special attention to the possible strategies for elucidating the apparent platelet alteration.

As has been reviewed (Anderson, 1987; McBride et al., 1990), previous studies have consistently reported elevated platelet 5-HT in groups of autistic individuals. The results of our study (Anderson et al., 1987), which employed an HPLC–fluorometric method to determine whole blood 5-HT, are shown in Figure 11.3. The robust group mean increase of 50 percent observed in unmedicated autistic subjects was seen across the age range examined, and was apparent whether 5-HT concentration was expressed as nanograms per milliliter (as shown) or nanograms per 10^9 platelets. The magnitude of the elevation that we observed was in the midrange of the reported differences. We also observed a marked effect of neuroleptic and anticonvulsant medication on platelet 5-HT. In medicated autistic subjects, mean levels were actually slightly lower than those in normal subjects. The drug effect was also apparent when examined within individuals, and significantly lower whole blood 5-HT levels were observed when subjects were medicated. In addition, an increased individual variance across time was observed in medicated subjects. This drug-induced decrease and temporal instability in 5-HT levels may have contributed to some of the variability in the previous reports.

In the group of twenty-one unmedicated autistic individuals that we studied (Anderson et al., 1987), the distribution of blood 5-HT levels

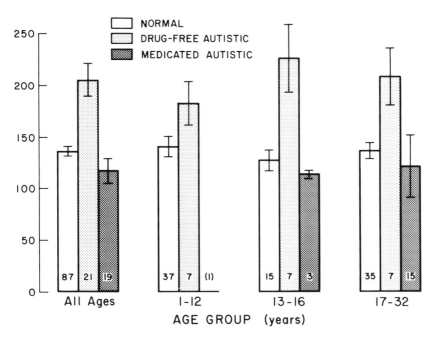

Figure 11.3. Mean concentrations (ng/ml) of whole blood serotonin (5-HT) in drug-free autistic, medicated autistic, and control individuals. The number of subjects is given within the bar; medications were anticonvulsants and neuroleptics, in some cases in combination.
Source: Anderson et al., 1990

was apparently Gaussian, suggesting that the group mean increase was not due to a subgroup of hyperserotonemic individuals. The possibility of a bimodal or multimodal distribution cannot be ruled out, however, given the size of the group examined. This question of modality is an open one, even though a group mean increase of platelet 5-HT has been very consistently observed in autism, because none of the groups studied have been large enough to address this important issue.

The factors that might be relevant to the platelet hyperserotonemia are presented in Figure 11.4. Studies of 5-HT metabolism and plasma 5-HT levels have attempted to determine whether changes external to the platelet could be causing the platelet elevation seen in autism. The issue of decreased catabolism of 5-HT has been examined by measure-

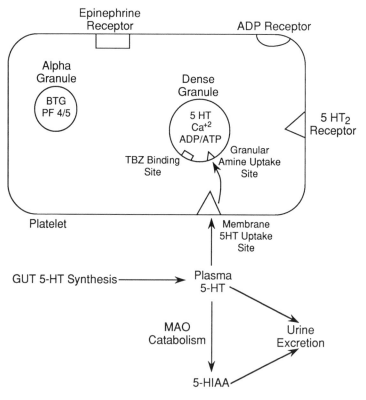

Figure 11.4. Peripheral serotonin (5-HT) metabolism and serotonin-related aspects of platelet physiology. Abbreviations: MAO, monoamine oxidase; TBZ, tetrabenazine; ADP/ATP, adenosine di-/triphosphate; BTG, -thromboglobulin; PF 4/5, platelet factors 4 and 5; 5-HT2, serotonin type 2 receptor.
Source: Anderson, 1992.

ments of platelet monoamine oxidase (MAO) activity, and by measuring monoamine substrates and metabolites. The studies of platelet MAO activity have consistently found no difference between autistic and normal subjects (Anderson, 1987). This approach is somewhat compromised, however, as platelets contain the B-form of MAO, while 5-HT is predominantly metabolized by MAO-A.

In a different approach, we attempted to assess in vivo MAO activity by determining urine concentration ratios for several substrate/metabolite pairs in autistic and normal subjects. Ratios of dopamine (DA)/homovanillic acid, NE/vanillylmandelic acid, NE/3-methoxy-4-hydroxyphenylglycol, and 5-HT/5-HIAA in the autistic group were either similar to (DA and NE) or slightly lower than (5-HT) normal values (Minderaa et al., 1987, 1989, 1992; Anderson et al., 1989). These results strongly suggest that MAO functioning is not decreased in autism.

The normal excretion rates that we observed for 5-HIAA in autistic subjects also strongly indicate that 5-HT synthesis is not increased in autism. Other findings related to this issue include our observations of normal whole blood levels of the 5-HT precursor tryptophan (TRP) (Anderson et al., 1987), and the presence of normal plasma levels of substance P in autistic subjects (G. M. Anderson, unpublished data).

While the data strongly suggest that 5-HT metabolism is unaltered in autism, they do not definitely indicate whether or not the circulating platelet is exposed to increased levels of 5-HT. This issue can be addressed most directly by determining plasma-free levels of 5-HT. We have developed a sensitive HPLC-fluorometric method that permits the analysis of 5-HT in platelet-poor plasma and plasma ultrafiltrate (Anderson et al., 1987). In addition to the clinical applications, the method has also allowed us to test a model developed for free 5-HT in blood (Anderson et el., 1987).

When the HPLC method was used by us and by Cooke and colleagues at the University of Chicago to determine platelet-poor plasma 5-HT levels in autistic subjects, the levels were similar to those seen in controls (Cooke et al., 1989; G. M. Anderson, unpublished data). In addition, we measured urinary excretion rates for 5-HT in autistic subjects and found the group mean to be slightly lower than that seen for normal subjects (72.8 ± 19.8 versus 104.0 ± 39.4 µg/g creatinine, $p = 0.04$) (Anderson et al., 1989). Jouvé and colleagues (1987) also reported that levels of urinary 5-HT are not increased in autistic children. These more direct measures of plasma 5-HT levels, as well as the evidence regarding 5-HT metabolism, indicate that the platelet is not exposed to increased concentrations of 5-HT.

We believe that the accumulated evidence warrants focusing research on the platelet. Aspects that bear close scrutiny are the uptake, storage, and release of 5-HT, as well as 5-HT-stimulated platelet responses. The specific questions to be addressed are grouped here into categories dealing with these four areas, as well as a fifth more general area of inquiry.

Plasma Membrane (5-HT) Uptake:
Is the maximum rate or affinity of platelet 5-HT uptake increased in autism?
Is the rate of 5-HT uptake at low, near physiologic, levels of 5-HT greater in autism?
Are there increased or more avid imipramine binding sites in autism?

Dense Granule (5-HT) Uptake and Storage:
Is the maximum capacity for platelet 5-HT storage greater in autism?
Is the platelet-dense granule 5-HT uptake rate or affinity greater in autism?
Is the density of the dense granule transporter or associated regulatory site (the tetrabenazine site) altered in autism?

Platelet 5-HT Release:
Is the stimulated release of platelet serotonin slower or reduced in autism?

5-HT_2 Mediated Responses:
Is platelet aggregation in response to 5-HT decreased in autism?
Is platelet shape change in response to 5-HT decreased in autism?

General Issues Regarding 5-HT and Platelets:
Is the mean platelet volume or lifespan increased in autism?
How do the various platelet function measures relate to the levels of 5-HT seen across subjects and groups?
Are 5-HT levels and the other measures normally distributed in the autistic group?
How do the measures relate to behavior in the autistic and retarded groups?
Is there some measure or group of measures that has a high degree of sensitivity and selectivity for autism or retardation?

It should be noted that although most of the questions are phrased with respect to autism, it will be of interest to contrast the findings in autistic individuals with those in the retarded group. The issue of whether hyperserotonemia exists in retardation has not been well studied.

We spent several years optimizing the methodology that can now be applied to answering these questions. This line of research has included work on characterizing the platelet-dense granule (Chatterjee et al.,

1990), development of an improved method for assessing the platelet release reaction (Anderson et al., 1992), studies on the regulation of membrane 5-HT uptake (Anderson and Horne, 1992), and improving the in-vitro assessment of platelet aggregation and shape change (Horne et al., 1991). By combining these methods, a very complete and careful assessment of 5-HT-related platelet physiology is possible. The clinical application of this battery has begun and will, it is hoped, provide answers to a number of the questions concerning the hyperserotonemia of autism.

The identification of the presumed platelet alteration that is responsible for the hyperserotonemia of autism would prove useful in several ways. It would be expected that assessment of the altered function would provide a marker having less overlap with the normal population than the multidetermined measure of blood 5-HT. Determination of the specific protein(s) involved in the altered platelet should lead directly to gene probes and chromosomal location. These, in turn, should prove useful for neonatal screening, subtyping, and more powerful genetic and family studies. Work of this sort might also allow early intervention and improved treatment. Finally, characterization of the physiologic alteration would provide a basis for focusing studies of brain neurochemistry and should also suggest modes of neuropharmacologic intervention. The confidence that one can have in the basic finding of hyperserotonemia in autism and the potential benefits to be derived from its explication make further research in this area of great interest.

NEUROPEPTIDES

Research over the past twenty years has revealed that peptides play critical roles in neurotransmission and neuromodulation (Emson, 1979; Snyder and Childers, 1979). There has been a special interest shown by autism researchers in the opioid peptides due to behavioral effects of agents that affect opioid peptidergic systems. It has been noted that some of the effects of opiates, such as decreased pain sensitivity, self-injurious behavior, and poor social relations, resemble symptoms of autism (Kalat, 1978; Panskeep, 1979).

The hypothesis that autism, and some forms of self-injurious behavior, may be a result of increased opioid peptide functioning has led to a large number of treatment studies using opioid antagonists. While initial open trial studies of naloxone, and the longer-acting naltrexone, were promising, small numbers of patients were examined. The few double-blind studies have not clearly demonstrated that the antagonists are of consistent therapeutic benefit (Campbell et al., 1990; Sandman, 1991). Most of the work has been performed in the last five years; at this point it appears that further careful study is warranted, both for the nonselective opioid antagonists and for other related agents, such as the adrenocorticotropin hormone (ACTH) analogue ORG 2766 (Buitelaar et al., 1990).

The neuropharmacology offers only slight support to the idea that the opioid systems are altered in autism. A parallel line of neurochemical research has attempted to assess the systems by measuring the levels of opioid, and opioid-related, peptides in the CSF, plasma, and urine. The compounds determined have included β-endorphin and ACTH (both derived from the precursor proopiomelanocortin) as well as met-enkephalin. A recent brief tabulation of the plasma and CSF studies appeared (Sandman, 1992). The studies, beginning with Coid et al. (1983) and including the later work of Herman et al. (1990) and Gillberg et al. (1990), have not revealed consistent differences between autistic and control groups. The disparate observations for β-endorphin emphasize the need for studies comparing carefully defined autistic, self-injurious, retarded, and control groups using specific assay procedures. Although the previous work can serve to guide the design of future studies, it, too, offers little in the way of support for the notion that opioid peptides are altered in autism.

Another line of peptide research has investigated patterns of urinary peptide excretion. Although several reports of marked differences in excretion patterns between autistic and control groups have appeared, the nonquantitative, subjective nature of the work has hindered replication and interpretation (Shattock et al., 1990). It is not clear whether further research in the area of peptide excretion is warranted.

FUTURE DIRECTIONS

A broad view of the previous neurochemical research on autism reveals a fairly disappointing picture. However, the future holds some promise for this approach for several reasons. The hyperserotonemia of autism offers a promising lead that should be pursued actively; further careful research on the opioid peptides also seems justified. Researchers also need to stand ready and able to apply relevant advances in the neurosciences to research on the neurochemistry of autism. The continuing advance of the field of developmental neurobiology will assuredly offer opportunities for increasingly informed and sophisticated neurochemical assessment.

The neurochemical research that is performed needs to be carried out in concert with the most complete and careful behavioral assessments. In this way the potential for delineating categorical subgroups and for defining behavioral dimensions that might be associated with neurochemical changes are maximized. Finally, there are very good reasons to suggest that postmortem brain research will be a fruitful area for investigation. Recent advances in other neuropsychiatric disorders, such as Parkinsonism, Huntington disease, and schizophrenia, demonstrate how useful direct neurochemical examination of brain tissue can be. Research in this area will require a significant recruitment effort as well as a commitment to establishing tissue handling procedures that assure that brain specimens are utilized to the greatest degree possible.

In conclusion, the next few years hold the promise for real advances in understanding the neurochemical changes that occur in autism. It is hoped that the promise is realized and that the knowledge gained leads to improved treatment and care of autistic individuals.

REFERENCES

Anderson, G. M. 1992. Serotonin in autism: Research strategies. In H. Naruse and E. M. Ornitz, eds. *Neurobiology of Infantile Autism.* 269–86. Tokyo: Excerpta Medica.

Anderson, G. M., Feibel, F. C., Cohen, D. J. 1987. Determination of Serotonin in whole blood, PRP, PPP and plasma ultrafiltrate. *Life Science.* 40:1063–70.

Anderson, G. M., Hall, L. M., Yang, J. X., and Cohen, D. J. 1992. Platelet dense granule release reaction monitored by HPLC-fluorometric determination of endogenous serotonin. *Analytical Biochemistry.* 206:64–67.

Anderson, G. M., and Horne, W. C. 1992. Activators of protein kinase C decrease serotonin transport in human platelets. *Biochimica Biophysica Acta.* 1137:331–37

Anderson, G. M., Home, W. C., Chatterjee, D., and Cohen, D. J. 1990. The hyperserotonemia of autism. *Annals of the New York Academy of Sciences* 600:333

Anderson, G. M., and Hoshino, Y. 1986. Neurochemical studies of autism. In D. J. Cohen and A. M. Donnellan, eds. *Handbook of Autism and Pervasive Developmental Disorders.* 166–91. New York: John Wiley & Sons.

Anderson, G. M., Minderaa, R. B., Choe, S. C., Volkmar, F. R., and Cohen, D. J. 1989. The issue of hyperserotonemia and platelet serotonin exposure: A preliminary study. *Journal of Autism and Developmental Disorders* 19:349–51.

Anderson, G. M., Stevenson, J. M., and Cohen, D. J. 1987. Steady-state model for plasma free and platelet serotonin in man. *Life Sciences* 41:1777–85.

Buitelaar, J. K., van Engeland, H., van Ree, J. M., de Wied, D. 1990. Behavioral effects of Org 2766, a synthetic analog of the adrenocorticotrophic hormone (4–9), in 14 outpatient autistic children. *Journal of Autism and Developmental Disorders* 20:467–78.

Buznikov, G. A. 1984. The action of neurotransmitters and related substances on early embryogenesis. *Pharmacology and Therapeutics* 25:23–59.

Campbell, M., Anderson, L. T., and Small, A. M. 1990. Pharmacotherapy in autism. *Brain Dysfunction* 3:299–307.

Campbell, M., Anderson, L. T., Small, A. M., Locascio, J. J., Lynch, N. S., and Choroco, M. C. 1990. Naltrexone in autistic children: A double-blind and placebo controlled study. *Psychopharmacol Bulletin* 26:130–135.

Chatterjee, D., Anderson, G. M., Chakraborty, M., and Cohen, D. J. 1990. Human platelet dense granules: Improved isolation and preliminary characterization of [³-H]-serotonin uptake and tetrabenazine-displaceable [³-H]-ketanserin binding. *Life Sciences* 46:1755–64.

Cohen, D. J., Caparulo, B. K., Shaywitz, B. A., and Bowers, M. B. 1977. Dopamine and serotonin metabolism in neuropsychiatrically disturbed children: CSF homovanillic acid and 5-hydroxyindoleacetic acid. *Archives of General Psychiatry* 34:545–50.

Cohen, D. J., Shaywitz, B. A., Johnson, W. T., and Bowers, M. B. 1974. Biogenic amines in autistic and atypical children: Cerebrospinal fluid measures of homovanillic acid and 5-hydroxyindoleacetic acid. *Archives of General Psychiatry* 31:845–53.

Cooke, E. H., Leventhal, B. L., and Freedman, D. X. 1988. Free serotonin in plasma: Autistic children and their first degree relatives. *Biological Psychiatry* 24:488–91.

Emson, P. 1979. Peptides as neurotransmitter candidates in the mammalian CNS. *Progress in Neurobiology* 13:61–116.

Fankhauser, M. P., Karumanchi, V. C., German, M. L., Yales, A., and Karumanchi, S. D. 1992. A double-blind, placebo-controlled study of the efficacy of transdermal clonidine in autism. *Journal of Clinical Psychiatry* 53:77–82.

Folstein, S. E., and Piven, J. 1991. Etiology of autism: Genetic influences. *Pediatrics* 87:767–73. (supplement)

Gillberg, C., and Svennerholm, L. 1987. CSF monoamines in autistic syndromes and other pervasive developmental disorders of early childhood. *British Journal of Psychiatry* 151:89–94.

Gillberg, C., Svennerholm, L., and Hamilton-Hellberg, C. 1983. Childhood psychosis and monoamine metabolites in spinal fluid. *Journal of Autism and Developmental Disorders* 13:383–96.

Gordon, C. T., Rapoport, J. L., Hamburger, S. D., State, R. C., Mannheim, G. B. 1992. Differential response of seven subjects with autistic disorder to clomipramine and desipramine. *American Journal of Psychiatry* 149:363–66.

Horne, W. C., Anderson, G. M., and Cohen, D. J. 1991. Reproducibility and temporal stability of ADP-induced platelet aggregation: Comparison of the anticoagulants sodium citrate and D-phenylalanyl-L-prolyl-L-arginyl-chloromethyl ketone. *American Journal of Hematology* 38:48–53.

Jouvé, J., Martineau, J., Mariotte, N., Bartkelemy, C., Muh, J. P., LeLord, G. 1986. Determination of urinary serotonin using liquid chromotography with electrochemical detection. *Journal of Chromotography* 378:437–43.

Kalat, J. W. 1978. Speculation on similarities between autism and opiate addiction. *Journal of Autism and Childhood Schizophrenia* 8:477–479.

Lauder, J. M., and Krebs, H. 1986. In W. T. Greenough and J. M. Juraska, eds. *Developmental Neuropsychobiology.* 119–74. Orlando, FL: Academic Press.

Markowitz, P .I. 1992. Effect of fluoxetine on self-injurious behavior in the developmentally disabled: A preliminary study. *Journal of Clinical Psychopharmacology* 12:27–31.

Mayford, M., Barzilai, A., Keller, F., Schacher, S., and Kandel, E. R. 1992. Modulation of an NCAM-related adhesion molecule with long-term synaptic plasticity in aplysia. *Science* 256:638–44.

McBride, A. P., Anderson, G. M., Hertzig, M. E., Sweeney, J. A., Kream, J., Cohen, D. J., and Mann, J. J. 1989. Serotonergic responsivity in male young adults with autistic disorder. *Archives of General Psychiatry* 46:213–21.

McBride, P. A., Anderson, G. M., and Mann, J. J. 1990. Serotonin in autism. In E. F. Coccaro and D. L. Murphy, eds. *Serotonin in Major Psychiatric Disorders.* 49–68. Washington, D.C.: American Psychiatric Press.

McDougle, C. J., Price, L. H., and Goodman, W. K. 1990. Fluvoxamine treatment of coincident autistic disorder and obsessive-compulsive disorder: A case report. *Journal of Autism and Developmental Disorder* 20:537–43.

McDougle, C. J., Price, L. H., Volkmar, F. R., Goodman, W. K., Ward-O'Brien, D., Nielson, J. R., Bergman, J. D., and Cohen, D. J. 1992. Clomipramine in autism: Preliminary evidence of efficacy. *Journal of American Academy of Child and Adolescent Psychiatry.* 31:746–50.

Minderaa, R. B., Anderson, G. M., Volkmar, F. R., Akkerhuis, G. W., Cohen, D. J. 1987. Urinary 5-HIAA and whole blood 5-HT and tryptophan in autism and normal subjects. *Biological Psychiatry* 22:933–40.

Minderaa, R. B., Anderson, G. M., Volkmar, F. R., Harcherik, D., Akkerhuis, G. W., and Cohen, D. J. 1989. Neurochemical study of dopamine functioning in autistic and normal subjects. *Journal of the American Academy of Child and Adolescent Psychiatry* 28:200–206.

Minderaa, R. B., Anderson, G. M., Volkmar, F. R., Akkerhuis, G. W., and Cohen, D. J. 1993. Noradrenergic and adrenergic functioning in autism. In submission.

Narayan, M., Srinath, S., Anderson, G. M., and Meundi, D. B. 1993. Cerebrospinal fluid levels of homovanillic acid and 5-Hydroxyindoleacetic acid in autism. *Biological Psychiatry.* 33:630–35.

Panksepp, J. 1979. A neurochemical theory of autism. *Trends in Neuroscience* 2:174–77.

Ross, D. L., Klykylo, W. M., and Anderson, G. M. 1985. Cerebrospinal fluid indoleamine and monoamine effects in fenfluramine treatment of autism. *Annals of Neurology* 18:394.

Sandman, C. A. 1991. The opiate hypothesis in autism and self-injury. *Journal of Child and Adolescent Psychopharmacology* 1:237–48.

Sandman, C. A. 1992. Various endogenous opioids and autistic behavior: A response to Gillberg. *Journal of Autism and Developmental Disorders* 22:132–33.

Synder, S. H., and Childers, S. 1979. Opiate receptors and endorphins. *Annual Review of Neuroscience* 2:35–64.

Todd, R. D. 1991. Fluoxetine in autism. *American Journal of Psychiatry* 148:8.

Whitaker-Azmitia, P. M., Lauder, J. M., Shemer, A., and Azmitia, E. C. 1987. Postnatal changes in serotonin₁ receptors following prenatal alterations in serotonin levels: Further evidence for functional fetal serotonin₁ receptors. *Developmental Brain Research* 33:285–89.

Whitaker-Azmitia, P. M., Murphy, R., and Azmitia, E. C. 1992. Stimulation of astroglial 5-HT₁ₐ receptors releases the serotonergic growth factor, protein S-100, and alters astroglial morphology. *Brain Research.* In press.

Winsberg, B. G., Sverd, J., Castells, S., Hurwic, M., and Perel, J. M. 1980. Estimation of monoamine and cyclic AMP turnover and amino acid concentration's of spinal fluid in autistic children. *Neuroleptics* 11:250–55.

Young, G. J., Cohen, D. J., Kavanaugh, M. E., Landis, H. D., Shaywitz, B. A., and Maas, J. W. 1981. Cerebrospinal fluid, plasma and urinary MHPG in children. *Life Sciences* 28:2837–45.

Young, G. J., Newcorn, J. H., and Leven, L. I. 1989. Pervasive developmental disorders. In H. I. Kaplan and B. J. Saddock, eds. *Comprehensive Textbook of Psychiatry.* 1772–87. Baltimore: Williams and Wilkins.

Yuwiler, A., Geller, A., and Ritvo, E. 1985. Biochemical studies of autism. In E. Lajtha, ed. *Handbook of Neurochemistry.* 671–91. New York: Plenum.

Yuwiler, A., Shih, J. C., Chen, C., Ritvo, E. R., Hanna, G., Ellison, G. W., and King, B. H. 1992. Hyperserotonemia and antiserotonin antibodies in autism and other disorders. *Journal of Autism and Developmental Disorders* 22:33–45.

Zhou, E. C., Auerbach, S., and Azmitia, E. C. 1987. Denervation of serotonergic fibers in the hippocampus induced a trophic factor which enhance the maturation of transplanted serotonergic neurons but not norepinephrine neurons. *Journal of Neuroscience Research* 17:235–46.

12

EPILOGUE

Margaret L. Bauman, M.D.
Thomas L. Kemper, M.D.

There have been considerable advances made in our understanding of autism since its initial description in 1943. Over the past decade, epidemiologic, clinical, and biologic research has provided insights into the underlying neurologic substrate for this disorder, as well as hypotheses as to how this substrate might lead to the characteristic features of autism. It has become generally accepted that the etiologies for autism are neurobiologic and there is evidence to suggest that the disorder may be of prenatal origin.

Autism is a behaviorally defined developmental disorder of brain function. There are currently no available identifying studies, and the diagnosis is based on a characteristic set of behaviors. These include atypical social interaction, disordered verbal and nonverbal communication, poor or limited imaginative play, a need for routine or sameness, and significantly restricted areas of interest and activity. The diagnosis can often be confusing, particularly in the toddler and preschool child. This is often due to the subtlety of early presenting abnormalities, difficulty differentiating autism from other causes of developmental delay in this age group, and significant variations in the severity of the clinical presentation.

The first chapter in this book discussed the history of autism and some of the diagnostic dilemmas encountered by the clinician. The broad spectrum of abnormalities in sensory perception, attention, language, cognitive abilities, and social functioning observed in this disorder were highlighted, and questions were raised about the appropriateness of the assessment tools that we traditionally use to evaluate individuals with autism. Further, it is clear that, although numerous theories attempt to clarify the nature of autism, no one theory has so far been able to adequately account for its uniquely characteristic features. Carefully planned and detailed longitudinal clinical studies in large populations of autistic individuals could contribute to a better understanding of the natural life history of the autism spectrum disorders, and thereby suggest more specific directions for neurobiologic research.

One of the major areas of interest at this time is the role of genetics as an etiologic factor in autism. It has been suggested that different genetic mechanisms could account for the mild cognitive and social abnormalities often seen in family members. Studies to date suggest that there is an increased liability for social, language, and cognitive deficits in both parents and siblings of affected individuals and that these may be milder in degree but conceptually similar to those seen in autism. In addition, it is possible that other factors such as sex, IQ, and prenatal factors may alter the basic genetic liability. While the exact mechanisms involved in autism remain unknown, genetic studies are likely to provide important information in the future about its cause.

The relationship between the behavioral and cognitive characteristics of autism and abnormal brain structure and neural processing have been explored with electrophysiologic techniques. Electroencephalographic abnormalities, involving all areas of the cerebral cortex, have historically provided the first indication of biologic involvement of the central nervous system in autism. Later, because of the frequent association of abnormal responses to sensory input in this disorder, including sound, auditory brainstem responses were studied. In general, the findings were inconsistent and lent little support for a pervasive dysfunction in the brainstem systems associated with auditory processing in most of the autistic individuals studied. However, a high percentage of autistic individuals were unexpectedly found to have a peripheral hearing loss, a finding that otherwise could have been overlooked in this population. More recently, research using event-related potentials have begun to focus on attentional control and modulation. Results have shown abnormalities in the frontal and parietal association cortex, impairment in orienting to novel stimuli and in the shifting of attentional focus in many autistic individuals. Future investigations will need to address variations in the modality-specific processing of information under differing circumstances and their relationship to brain localization and function.

With the advent of computerized tomography (CT) in the 1970s and, more recently, the availability of magnetic resonance imaging (MRI), the ability to study brain structure in vivo became possible. It has been disappointing that numerous reports of CT findings in autistic individuals resulted in inconsistent findings. Furthermore, it was suspected that the few positive observations that were noted might be related to central nervous system disorders other than autism. MRI studies in autism initially appeared to be equally unrevealing. However, quantitative analysis of brain structure has begun to suggest volumetric alterations in selected parts of the cerebral hemispheres and cerebellum. How these observations relate to underlying histoanatomic findings and whether there is any correlation with brain function remain to be determined.

Since volumetric measurement of brain structure may not necessarily be an accurate reflection of function, increasing interest has focused on studies of in vivo brain chemistry using positron emission tomography (PET) and magnetic resonance spectroscopy (MRS). Although there have been technical difficulties in the use of these tools, particularly with children and handicapped subjects requiring sedation, research to date appears promising. PET studies in autism have failed thus far to identify focal areas of abnormal brain metabolism under relatively non-demanding conditions. It has been suggested, however, that unlike acquired disorders associated with structural damage, subtle developmental abnormalities of brain function may require the added sensitivity of activation studies to localize areas of dysfunction. Pilot data from autistic subjects studied with MRS have shown alterations in high-energy phosphate and membrane phospholipid metabolism in the dorsal prefrontal cortex. These findings correlated with symptomatic severity and suggested an undersynthesis of brain membranes in affected systems. Thus, although MRS is in its infancy this technology, as well as PET, has the potential to significantly increase our understanding of normal and abnormal mechanisms of brain function.

Due largely to the fact that autism is a nonfatal disorder and that the brain abnormalities associated with it are subtle, relatively few neuroanatomic studies have been reported. Observations to date have shown abnormalities of the limbic system that are consistent with a curtailment of development. These findings may have implications for some of the deficits in processing information often associated with autism, particularly given the relationship of the limbic system structures to memory and to the sensory association cortices. Abnormalities have also been found in the cerebellum and cerebellar circuits, with preservation of neurons in the inferior olive. This latter observation has suggested that the onset of this disorder is of prenatal origin. Furthermore, large neurons have been found in the deep cerebellar nuclei and inferior olivary nucleus in the brains of autistic children, and small nerve cells have been noted in these same areas with cell loss in the cerebellar nuclei in the adult autistic brains. These findings have suggested the preservation of a primitive fetal circuit in autism. The functional relationship of these abnormalities to the clinical features of autism is unknown. However, there is growing evidence that the cerebellum may play a role in some types of memory and learning. Future research should attempt to correlate more closely clinical characteristics in well-studied cases, in both younger and older autistics, with the severity and distribution of microscopic abnormalities in the brain. In addition, it would be of great interest to study the neuropathology of disorders associated with autistic features such as tuberous sclerosis, phenylketonuria, and fragile X syndrome to determine the similarities and differences with classic autism.

Much of what we know about brain function in humans has been derived from research in animals. In this regard, lesion studies involving specific regions of the limbic system in neonatal monkeys have expanded our understanding of the development of certain types in learning, memory, emotion, and behavior. These and other observations have led to the conclusion that the representational memory and procedural memory circuits are both functionally and maturationally different. While the procedural memory system appears to develop very early in life, the representational system seems to mature more slowly. Clinical and experimental work indicate that these two subdivisions, while distinct from each other, interact in the adult to produce normal mnemonic functions. Although autistic individuals are not amnestic, they have significant difficulty processing certain types of information while, at the same time, retaining the unusual ability to recall large amounts of detailed rotely learned material. Based on our current knowledge, it could be hypothesized that this dichotomy in the handling of information in autism might relate, at least in part, to faulty development in the representational memory circuitry associated with the limbic system with relative sparing of the procedural memory pathways that involve the striatum and neocortex.

How a partial dysfunction of the limbic system may manifest itself, cognitively and behaviorally, during development is unknown. There is some preliminary evidence to suggest that variability in clinical expression in autism may be a function of which regions of the limbic system are more severely impaired. In addition, there is also the observation— in the monkey, at least—that varying phenotypic expression can result from identical surgically produced lesions, possibly in relationship to differences in normal brain development. Whether or not these factors, or still others as yet to be defined, explain the apparent heterogeneity of clinical expression in autism remains to be determined.

What contribution, if any, might be made by the cerebellum to higher cortical function in general and to the clinical presentation of autism in particular has become an area of increasing interest. Varying degrees of microscopic abnormality throughout the cerebellum have been reported in autism, and involvement of the cerebellar hemispheres and vermis have been observed with MRI in some cases. Anatomic studies in animals have found projections to the corticopontocerebellar circuit from behaviorally related areas of the temporal, frontal, and parietal cortexes and from the paralimbic regions. In turn, the cerebellum projects back to these regions via the thalamus. Thus, the cerebellum appears to have access to highly processed, behaviorally relevant information from the cerebral cortex, and is in a position to redirect this now-modified information back to the cerebral cortex. It is therefore possible that the cerebellar abnormalities observed in autism are not incidental findings; rather, they may reflect a disturbance in the pathways that include the cerebellum in the organization and modulation of emotion, language, and behavior.

Neurochemical changes may also contribute to the atypical processing of information in autism. Much of the major work has involved investigations of monoamines and neuropeptides and their metabolites in blood, urine, and spinal fluid. These studies, along with associated neuropharmacologic trials, have generally shown inconsistent results. Nonetheless, the neurochemical profile of the brain in autism remains an area of intense interest. Since it is now known that hormones such as oxytocin may have a significant impact on early brain development, neuroendocrinological studies of these relationships will also need to be considered.

We now have a wealth of descriptive information about the clinical and neurobiologic features of autism, without a clear framework with which to fully understand the implications of these observations. Given the developmental nature of the disorder, it is difficult to extrapolate from adult neurobiologic research. In contrast to a lesion in the adult brain, a prenatal insult may result in fundamentally altered neuronal circuitry with a substantially different outcome than would be predicted from the adult model.

How are we then to approach the puzzle of autism? An animal model would be invaluable. Lacking that, well-designed specific lesions in prenatal animals could yield valuable information. The identification of the etiology of autism would also increase our understanding of the nature of the prenatal insult and might suggest new avenues of investigation. Of major importance will be carefully designed neurochemical analysis of brain tissue from well-studied cases of different ages. The availability of new and improved technology, such as MRS and PET, may allow us to study both structure and function in the living subject in the future.

The topics included within this book represent some of the basic science research that has lead to our current understanding of autism. This research is beginning to offer further clues about and approaches to future investigations of the causes and neurobiologic mechanisms of this disorder. It is hoped that bringing these perspectives together under a single cover will stimulate autism research and lead to more useful and definitive diagnostic tools, and ultimately to more focused modes of intervention and treatment.

INDEX